A Guide to Compassionate Health care

A Guide to Compassionate Health care looks at how to maintain wellbeing in today's challenging health care environments, enabling practitioners to make a positive difference to the care environment whilst providing compassionate care to patients.

This practical guide focuses on strategies to maintain health and wellbeing as health care practitioners, in relation to stress management, resilience and positivity. Health and social care practitioners have been challenged over and above anything they have faced before due to the COVID pandemic. These situations have caused extreme trauma and stress to patients, their loved ones and those who have been struggling to care for them. The book highlights why resilience and good stress management are crucial, and how they can be achieved through a focus on wellbeing and positivity, referring to her RESPECT toolkit: Resilience, Emotional intelligence, Stress management, Positivity, Energy and motivation, Challenge and Team leadership.

This is essential reading for all those working in health care today who are passionate about compassionate care and want to ensure that they remain positive and well, particularly newly qualified staff.

Claire Chambers teaches on the Open University nursing and nursing associate programmes and is passionate about supporting students in practice and focusing on their excellent practice. She has previously led the community nursing and public health programmes at Oxford Brookes University and has practised as a health visitor and a nurse in a range of community and acute settings.

A Guide to Compassionate Health care

How to Develop Resilience and Wellbeing in Today's Stressful Environment

Claire Chambers

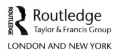
Routledge
Taylor & Francis Group

LONDON AND NEW YORK

Designed cover image: Getty Images

First published 2024
by Routledge
4 Park Square, Milton Park, Abingdon, Oxon OX14 4RN

and by Routledge
605 Third Avenue, New York, NY 10158

Routledge is an imprint of the Taylor & Francis Group, an informa business

British Library Cataloguing-in-Publication Data
A catalogue record for this book is available from the British Library

Library of Congress Cataloging-in-Publication Data
Names: Chambers, Claire, MSc., author.
Title: A guide to compassionate health care : how to develop resilience and wellbeing in today's stressful environment / Claire Chambers.
Description: Abingdon, Oxon ; New York, NY : Routledge, 2024. l Includes bibliographical references and index. l Summary: "A Guide to Compassionate Health care looks at how to maintain wellbeing in today's challenging health care environments, enabling practitioners to make a positive difference to the care environment whilst providing compassionate care to patients. This is essential reading for all those working in health care today who are passionate about compassionate care and want to ensure that they remain positive and well, particularly newly qualified staff"— Provided by publisher.
Identifiers: LCCN 2023050603 l ISBN 9781138093393 (hardback) l ISBN 9781138093409 (paperback) l ISBN 9781315106861 (ebook)
Subjects: LCSH: Medical personnel—Job stress. l Stress management. l Well-being. l Resilience (Personality trait)
Classification: LCC RC451.4.M44 C43 2024 l DDC 610.69/6—dc23/eng/20240215
LC record available at https://lccn.loc.gov/2023050603

ISBN: 978-1-138-09339-3 (hbk)
ISBN: 978-1-138-09340-9 (pbk)
ISBN: 978-1-315-10686-1 (ebk)

DOI: 10.4324/9781315106861

Typeset in Frutiger
by codeMantra

Contents

Figures

Tables

Case studies

Questionnaires

Foreword

Stressful. That's something of an understatement. Today's health professionals are facing unprecedented demands from every source. Those in their care are feeling the same intrapersonal, social, cultural, political and planetary stressors to which health professionals as fellow citizens are feeling too. We health professionals find ourselves in a fray each day. From an interaction with those in our care or our colleagues that did not go to plan and on through trying to take in truly sobering news about social conflict and planetary health, finding a real sense of relief feels impossible. We typically find ourselves considering our ability to bounce back, keep moving forward, and feel well as we try to support others in doing the same. Too often, resilience and wellbeing feel like buzzwords or unattainable goals as opposed to personal aims within our grasp.

Claire Chambers' book *A Guide to Compassionate Health care: How to Develop Resilience and Wellbeing in Today's Stressful Environment* is the fourth in a series she and her longtime colleague Elaine Ryder have offered to colleagues in the health professions over the past several years. Across six chapters, Chambers uses her trademark approachable and familiar style that I dare say many will find comforting at the outset. Reading her feels akin to chatting over a cup of tea. I'll take mine without milk, thanks. There's something of a conversation in how Chambers reaches through the page to talk to her readers. Her practical knowledge of health care in the United Kingdom resonates as Chambers supplies understandings of topics like "what is compassion?", building on that more conversational approach that she uses to teach to move into engaging the reader more closely. Chambers offers case studies, self-assessments, and aides mémoire among other activities and information displays to move from talking about why compassion and resilience matter to how to lead in compassionate practice for resilience and wellbeing for oneself and one's team.

I appreciate that Claire Chambers writes with others in mind. She deliberately and carefully offers selected information, tools and resources without presumption. Chambers doesn't convey that any of what she discusses is easy. Nor does she portray that she or indeed any of us can fully escape these times in which we live or magically make everything better. Rather, she conveys her goodwill, knowledge and experience in the manner of a comrade. Chambers shares authentically voiced case studies as easily as she does what she gleans from current and classic science. Through all her chapters, I hear Chambers return to learning how being positive is a strength and the power that positivity brings.

As I close in on four decades of nursing here in the United States, a sociocultural context with some marked similarities and many dramatic differences when compared to the United Kingdom, I am struck by the deliberate choice to be positive. That choice sometimes feels like a stretch for me. Can I smile today? Can I find the advantages in a gloomy situation? I took away several moments for thought and a variety of quick tips as I read Chambers' chapters in this fourth book. Time and again, she reminded me of something that my own clinical teammates at Pennsylvania Hospital, our nation's oldest, often comment upon. "You are so positive, Sarah, and always cheerful." Truthfully, I am not always positive and there are many moments each day when I cannot feel cheerful. No one of us is or can. But I use techniques much like those Chambers offers in the context of this book to beneficial effect. The "glass half full" vantage point that I've adopted over my years in nursing allows me to see ways forward that colleagues who are tired or distracted, who feel the weight of their distress more acutely, might struggle to see. I feel more able to share from my glass, if you will, because I see how full it is instead of focusing on how much I've lost.

Claire Chambers reminds me of popular neuroscience which reveals that smiles do really make us feel better. We health professionals know that negative emotions are easily shared. I'm not the first nurse to caution students and colleagues alike that anxiety is contagious. That caution is important in highly stressful situations. But Claire Chambers reminds me that we need to balance our admonishments about the contagion of anxiety, anger and even despair for those in our care and those with whom we work. Positivity, as a building block for resilience, is easily spread. Following her guidance and that from others whom we trust, let's all find a moment or two for ourselves each day even amid very real hardship and distress. Doing so won't wipe away all that surrounds us, but I think it will and can cushion the pain and exhaustion from which none of us are immune. A few seconds to several minutes might be all it takes to create just a little bit of positivity which can go on to strengthen a sense of resilience and helps us find a feeling of wellbeing for ourselves. Those feelings and abilities are a foundation on which we can build from day to day, even bridging the down days all of us will have as we move forward. Even more rewardingly, we can share what we've achieved with those around us as easily as a smile and as sustainably as switching up some of our tactics and habits.

Sarah H. Kagan
Philadelphia, Pennsylvania
October 2023

Preface

I have been writing about compassionate health care practice since 2007 because I passionately believe that certain values have to underpin the pursuit of excellence in compassionate care, and that this pursuit should lie at the heart of all health care practice. In the course of writing the first book on *Compassion and Caring in Nursing* in 2009, I confirmed that nurses are genuinely concerned about the care that is provided, and that when patients or clients feel they are not being cared for with compassion, we want to resolve these problems. The all too prevalent media reports of poor health care reflect on all our health care professions. It is therefore understandable that professional, conscientious and compassionate practitioners feel in some ways complicit, even though we were not ourselves responsible for these deficits in care. In the face of such publicity, we are likely to feel disillusioned, powerless, angry, and undervalued in our work. Once caught in this downward spiral we are less likely to feel empowered to become leaders of practice. Everyone involved in health care, whether we are in a professional, informal or formal caring role, has a duty to ensure that compassion, and the patient or client, stays central to all care and health care interventions. (Chambers and Ryder 2011)

Therefore, the second book, *Excellence in Compassionate Nursing Care: Leading the Change,* published in April 2012, focused on how nurses can challenge poor care, act as role models for excellence and take a leadership role in making a difference, whatever their position in their organisation. I started from the premise that compassion is based on kindness and deep awareness of the suffering of others, and a wish to help in some way. Patients, clients and practitioners themselves would view kindness as a key attribute of any practice; something that ensures patients and clients feel "cared about" as well as "cared for".

So, in attempting to single out the essential features of compassion in practice, I identified six main themes (Chambers and Ryder, 2009) that encompass what compassion would feel like from the patient or client perspective:

- empathy and sensitivity
- dignity and respect
- listening and responding
- diversity and cultural competence
- choice and priorities
- empowerment and advocacy.

Although clearly competence is paramount in health care, I do not believe that care is truly competent if it is not carried out with compassion. As Radcliffe says, compassion is "the thing that stops nursing being simply a list of acts aimed at wellbeing. Ask patients what makes the difference and they always say something that looks like compassion" (2010, p23). Yet in the incentive-driven, resource-constrained culture where we live and work, compassion and kindness may seem like a hindrance to achieving all-important targets. As Gilbert (2010) reminds us, modern life (and its organisations) tends to over-stimulate our incentive/resource seeking and threat/ self-protection systems to the detriment of our soothing/contentment systems. As practitioners who want to provide compassionate care, we are likely to feel stressed if the quality of the care that we provide is valued less highly than the more measurable aspects of our practice. According to Mooney (2009), when nurses are too busy they become less kind and compassionate. However, in my experience, the opposite is true: it is when individuals feel too busy to be compassionate that they burn out; compassion, in effect has a protective value. The King's Fund agree with this view:

> If finance and productivity are perceived as being the only things that matter it can have profound negative effects on the way staff feel about the value placed on their work as caregivers. This makes it more difficult to cope with the inevitable emotional and psychological demands of the job.
>
> (Firth-Cozens and Cornwell, 2009, p. 13)

Staff are the most valuable resource in any organisation, but particularly in those aspiring to care. So, if we are to develop compassionate approaches to practice we may have to shift from leadership based on targets, throughput and efficiency, to forms of leadership which value and model compassion, care and kindness. In these environments staff feel listened to, and wherever appropriate, are given choices They are also empowered and helped to develop cultural competence. Where strategic-level managers and leaders – whether in management, clinical specialist or education roles – all have that same vision, a consistent message still has to be conveyed vertically down to grass roots level. This extends from educationalists to mentors and to students, and from high level managers to team leaders and to practitioners working with patients or clients. We need to create systemic compassion, with firm foundations based on communication and collaboration, linking leadership and theory-practice, as well as joined-up thinking **and action.** These also need to become urgent priorities in all health care organisations. Practitioners need to act as role models for colleagues and students and I identified three kinds of potential obstacles to compassionate care (Chambers and Ryder, 2009).

- resourcing issues
- the culture of the organisation
- individual practitioner attitude.

Leadership at all levels will ensure that problems are identified and solved as quickly as possible (Chambers and Ryder, 2012). The focus has to be on the patient experience, on recognising, providing and valuing compassionate practice, and conveying its importance to all members of the multifaceted multiprofessional teams we work in. Everyone in the team contributes to the care experience, and acts of compassion do not rely totally on those with professional qualifications. Times of great change and challenge need great leadership and great leaders to maintain a climate of resilience and positivity.

Therefore, the third publication *Supporting Compassionate Health care Practice*, which was published in 2019, focused on how all health care professionals, not just nurses, can focus on excellent practice and energise others in these difficult financial times. The emphasis is on excellent health care, which by definition would need to be compassionate, and this is challenging to provide day after day. However, we as health care professionals decided on our career choice because we have the values, attitudes and attributes that help us to address the challenges of our daily roles. Attitudes and elements of care which clients and patients value are central to the care that we provide. In addition, health care practitioners need to have the following key attributes in order to create a culture of excellence (Chambers and Ryder, 2012):

Personal attributes
Quality attributes

Leadership attributes
Educational attributes
Team leading attributes

The benefits of a compassionate approach to patients and clients, ourselves, and our organisations are undeniable, and there is a growing body of evidence to demonstrate this. Therefore, I discussed these benefits after I discussed how we can address our own stress and build resilience and capitalise on our positivity and wellbeing. We are then able to develop strategies to combat stress and emotional burnout and find innovative ways to enhance patient and client care. We can then foster a culture of compassionate care, where insensitive practice is not tolerated, and excellence is the norm.

This book will build on *Supporting Compassionate Health care Practice* and is a practical guide on how to implement strategies to maintain our health and wellbeing as health care practitioners. This has never been more important than in these pandemic-challenged times, and I have focused some of the case studies and discussions around health care experiences during COVID. Many of these case studies have been written by my students in their reflections on practice, and they are genuinely moving and inspiring.

In all health care environments throughout the world, compassion is of paramount importance to patients and clients. There is no doubt that patients and clients, and their families and friends, value practitioners who are caring and compassionate, and that is why the books focus on case studies from the patient's or client's perspective. I have included case studies, exercises and questionnaires, as appropriate, to help focus on practical ways to enhance our own personal and professional lives and to help develop strategies for ourselves and others. I have then discussed ways in which we can make a positive difference in our working environment with colleagues and students.

I have used case studies and poems to make the discussion as accessible and user friendly as possible. The focus is on the integration of theory and practice throughout, and I have used articles and resources from a wide range of countries to give as much of an international perspective as possible. I have also included very recent articles, and others which are either seminal texts or major research studies, to give a strong historical perspective to add to the depth of the discussion. I want you to feel challenged, in terms of your own practice, and to recognise the dilemmas raised in the case studies. I hope that this style of writing will encourage you to review your current practice and take a lead in bringing about change within your own practice environment. I take the thinking further in this practice guide by developing specific exercises and questionnaires which focus on areas of my RESPECT toolkit to address stress in the health care environment. This RESPECT toolkit focuses on:

- **R**esilience
- **E**motional Intelligence
- **S**tress management
- **P**ositivity
- **E**nergy and motivation
- **C**hallenge
- **T**eam leadership.

I have included exercises and questionnaires to assess stress and enhance resilience, positivity and wellbeing against criteria and established thinking on each topic. You should then feel able to take the lead in developing strategies, for yourself and others in practice. I hope that these four books will create a combined approach to coping with the inevitable stresses within resource constrained health care practice today and enable you to take a lead in ensuring that compassion is central to all nursing practice.

Claire Chambers
September 2023

REFERENCES

Chambers C, Ryder E. (2009) *Compassion and Caring in Nursing*. Abingdon, Oxon: Radcliffe Publishing Ltd.

Chambers C, Ryder E. (2011) Excellence in Compassionate Nursing Care: Leading the Change. *Journal of Holistic Health care*, 8(3): 46–49.

Chambers C, Ryder E. (2012) *Excellence in Compassionate Nursing Care: Leading the Change*. London: Radcliffe Publishing Ltd.

Chambers C, Ryder E. (2019) *Supporting Compassionate Health care Practice: Understanding the Role of Resilience, Positivity and Wellbeing*. Abingdon, Oxon: Routledge.

Firth-Cozens J, Cornwell J. (2009) *The Point of Care: Enabling Compassionate Care in Acute Hospital Settings*. London: The King's Fund.

Gilbert P. (2010) *The Compassionate Mind*. London: Constable and Robinson Ltd.

Mooney H. (2009) Compassion is Early Casualty of Nurse 'Frustration and Burnout'. *Nursing Times*, 105(15): 2.

Radcliffe M. (2010) Compassion is No Harder to Measure than Rain. *Nursing Times*, 106(17): 2.

About the author

Claire Chambers MSc, PgDip (Prof) Ed, CPT, HV (Dip), RGN

I worked as a nurse in various hospital environments and then moved into health visiting. I was a health visitor, community practice teacher and lecturer practitioner before I moved into full-time education. During my teaching career I have worked with preregistration, post qualification and postgraduate students from many community and acute settings, but my prime interests have always been related to community practice, public health, patient and client-centred care, diversity, cultural competence and values-based practice.

Amongst other publications and conference presentations, I have co-authored three books with Elaine Ryder *Compassion and Caring in Nursing*, *Excellence in Compassionate Nursing Care: Leading the Change* and *Supporting Compassionate Health care Practice: Understanding the Role of Resilience, Positivity and Wellbeing* which reflect my belief in the centrality of compassion and excellent communication skills in nursing. I ensured that advanced communication skills and values-based care, focusing on positive attitudes to patients and clients, were central tenets of the Specialist Community Public Health Nursing and Community Specialist Practice programmes at Oxford Brookes University. I also facilitated sessions on compassion, emotional resilience and positivity within the acute hospital environment. I am now an associate lecturer at the Open University and was part of a team delivering the Mary Seacole programme which was developed by the NHS Leadership Academy, in collaboration with the Hay Group and the Open University. This programme was designed to help participants to develop leadership expertise in line with putting patients at the heart of health care systems. I now really enjoy supporting students and apprentices on the pre-registration nursing and nursing associate programmes as a practice tutor and academic assessor within the Open University, and enjoy teaching and supporting adult, mental health and children's nursing students. These students inspire me every day with their excellent, person-centred and compassionate practice and many of their reflections are included in this book.

This *Guide to Compassionate Health care: How to Develop Resilience and Wellbeing in Today's Stressful Environment* builds on the third book co-authored with Elaine Ryder *Supporting Compassionate Health care Practice: Understanding the Role of Resilience, Positivity and Wellbeing* which was published in 2019.

Acknowledgements

Firstly, I would like to thank Elaine Ryder, my co-author on the first three books, who was very much part of this book too. She joined me in my writing journey, and I would not have managed to carry on writing, alongside a very busy personal and professional life, if she had not been there. She works for Age UK Oxfordshire which gives an excellent service to those with dementia, and she has always been an excellent nurse, district nurse and nursing tutor. I am also lucky to call her my friend.

I would like to thank all those who have shown an interest in compassion being the central part of nursing. My patients, clients and students have always motivated me, and discussion with other health care professionals has also stimulated debate on this essential aspect of care. The sensitive understanding demonstrated by nurses and other health care practitioners in different areas of practice has helped me to think more deeply about taking a lead in compassion. I am very grateful to specific students for giving their permission to use their experiences and reflections as case studies in this book. Their contributions are not attributed to them by their full names, despite the fact that they have given their permission. They know who they are though, and how impressive I think their practice is. My colleagues, throughout my career in nursing, health visiting and education, have also been integral to my value system. They have discussed with me times when care of their loved ones, or themselves, has not been of a standard that any caring nurse would support. They have also provided me with key examples of excellent care. My students have always been exceptional and they inspire me every day.

During the writing of the books, I have found that each conference at which I speak has brought me into contact with others who feel as passionately as I do about compassion. This has stimulated my thinking about how practitioners, at all levels, can genuinely take a lead in influencing the quality of care in their practice areas.

I am also very grateful to Professor Sarah Kagan for her continuing invaluable support. Sarah has written the forewords for all the previous books and has been so encouraging about the work and my writing. She feels as strongly as I do about the importance of compassionate attitudes and values in nursing care.

Dr. Robin Youngson is particularly inspirational in his writing and speaking, and it has been very interesting to see how medical practice is embracing the centrality of compassion. He has also been supportive of my writing and he believes in the importance of more published material focusing on compassion and key values of practice.

I would like to thank all those at Cherry Blossom Manor Barchester care home in Bramley, Hampshire for the care they give to my mother who is a resident there. Their care is exceptional and the culture there exudes compassion at all times. All of those in the nursing and care team have a way of caring for residents in an individualised way. They genuinely like those in their care and find ways to engage with each resident, many of whom have dementia, using their knowledge of them and their preferences, and they use their sense of humour appropriately when this is helpful. The administration, domestic, catering and grounds staff also clearly enjoy what they do and contribute greatly to the experience there, and the care of the residents. I am so grateful to them all for the difference they make in my mother's life, and I hope they know how excellent they are. This is what care home, and dementia care, should look like, and this does not happen by accident. The leadership is very much part of making this happen, and all the staff clearly feel part of the team and enjoy working there. My mother means so much to me, thank you so much, all of you.

From a personal point of view, I would like to thank all those who have encouraged me in my writing. I would like to thank my parents Ken and Monica Hale who have made me the person I am. In particular, I would like to thank my wonderful nieces and nephew and their partners for their love and always being there: Dannii and Tom, Chris and Lizzy, Amy and John and Anna and now Gary too. Their children Jess, Ella, Louis, Rex, Ted, Isaac and Eli bring us so much joy and we love all of you to bits.

My special thanks goes to Alan, my ever supportive husband, who always encourages me in everything I do. He is always constructive in the help he gives me in so many different ways. He has been very much a part of this process, and he is very proud of my achievements. His unfailing support and love has helped me maintain my motivation throughout the writing of all the books. He is an exceptional person and is always positive and he means everything to me. Thank you so much sweetheart for all the joy and love you bring to our journey through life.

The importance of compassion and why positivity and resilience matters

- Introduction
- Discussion – main points and evidence with case studies, exercises, aide mémoires and questions

  - What is compassion?
  - Why do we need to focus on compassion, and manage our stress, and build on our positivity and resilience?
  - Are you an "aholic"?
  - The importance of self-compassion
  - The healing nature of compassionate practice
  - The importance of compassion for you, your patients, and the organisation you work for
  - Why do we need to be positive and resilient?
  - The challenges of happiness

- Recommendations for leadership as individual practitioners, and leaders and organisations

  - Focusing on compassionate care as individual practitioners
  - Focusing on compassionate care as leaders
  - Focusing on compassionate care as organisations

INTRODUCTION

I have written this book to build on the third book *Supporting Compassionate Health care Practice* (Chambers and Ryder, 2019) and this practical guide focuses on strategies to maintain our health and wellbeing as health care practitioners, in relation to stress management, resilience and positivity. Everyone working in health and social care has been challenged over and above anything they have faced before due to the COVID-19 pandemic, and many of you have had to cope with patient care experiences that you will remember for the rest of your lives. These situations have caused extreme trauma and stress to patients, their loved ones and those who have been struggling to care for them. I am sure that we are all truly grateful for all that you have done, and are still doing at the time of writing this, and hope that this book is helpful in trying to find practical ways to cope with your stress and resilience, and recapture positivity and wellbeing.

I have developed a model called RESPECT which is based on the importance of having respect for ourselves, our profession, our organisation and the patients in our care. RESPECT is a mnemonic which incorporates:

- Resilience
- Emotional intelligence
- Stress management
- Positivity
- Energy and motivation
- Challenge
- Team leadership which focuses on how practitioners can take a lead in implementing the RESPECT toolkit in their areas of practice. .

The chapters of this book will discuss these different elements, focusing on stress management, resilience and positivity. We need all the elements in our toolkit to be able to cope with the undoubted pressures of our professional roles, and to maintain our health and wellbeing. These tools will be central to all the discussions and in some cases they will be the focus of whole chapters.

Chapter 1 will focus on the importance of compassion in relation to positive and resilient approaches to care

Chapter 2 will focus on the challenges of compassionate care, and how these could be addressed

Chapter 3 will focus on stress management strategies

Chapter 4 will focus on strategies to increase our resilience

Chapter 5 will focus on reducing negativity and increasing positivity

Chapter 6 on our leadership in compassionate practice, stress management, resilience and positivity.

The chapters will incorporate case studies, to illustrate points in the discussion. They will include aide-mémoires, exercises and questions in the discussion to help us to develop our own strategies in relation to compassion, stress management, resilience, positivity and wellbeing. There will then be recommendations for individual and team leadership.

Chapter 1 will focus on why we need to focus on compassion, and why it is important to manage our stress and be as positive and resilient as possible. A compassionate approach is essential for patients, but it is also of paramount importance for us as practitioners, and to our organisations. The chapter will start by discussing what compassion means, its relevance in our health care roles, and the role of compassion in managing our stress, and keeping us positive and resilient. It will discuss the importance of self-compassion, and the healing aspects of compassionate practice for patients in our care. Following this there will be a discussion of the importance of compassion for ourselves, our patients, and the organisations we work for. It will then start to discuss the importance of a positive approach, and the challenges of happiness, which will also be the main focus of Chapter 5. Positivity is key to enhancing our resilience and it is one of our major tools in maintaining our wellbeing at work, and at home. The chapter will finish by focusing on leading on compassionate care, as individuals and as leaders.

DISCUSSION

Case Study 1.1

Tony's resilience in the face of extreme work pressures as a GP

Tony has been a GP for many years and despite all the changes and challenges in primary care he still enjoys his role. He makes an effort to build meaningful relationships with all his patients and they are very loyal to him and are largely very appreciative of his efforts. Even in a single consultation with a patient who is not known to him he tries to build a trusting, patient centred relationship, where the patient feels that he is generally interested in their health issues. Tony works in a very busy practice and in common with other practices nationwide it is proving difficult to recruit new partners to the practice. Therefore, the few partners that there are inevitably make the management decisions, and carry out a large proportion of the patient consultations. Other salaried and part time doctors take on the other patient consultations and the practice has now employed some nurse practitioners and a pharmacist who use their specialist expert knowledge to meet patient needs.

Tony, despite the challenges of his role, is perceived by patients as always compassionate, positive and caring. He needs to demonstrate resilience in the face of extreme workload pressures, but he sees this as being of paramount importance to keep these pressures away from the doctor/patient interface as much as possible. He receives a lot of positive feedback from his patients and colleagues, and he is aware that when colleagues become overwhelmed by the pressure of their roles, their stress is often very apparent to patients. Patients in that situation are then much more likely to feel more negative about their experience of patient care, and become more upset and angry, which further increases the load on the doctor.

The case study above clearly demonstrates how crucial a compassionate approach is in all patient care. Patients coming to see a doctor are largely unwell and concerned about their health. They do not want to be concerned about how hard their GP is finding their role. Being a health care practitioner is inevitably very stressful for all practitioners in the multidisciplinary team (MDT). The patient might be well known to the practitioner over many years, and it is hard to witness the emotions of patients and their loved ones, especially when they are acutely ill or when their lives are coming to an end. This is particularly the case when the person concerned is younger or a child, or close to you in age. Also, when they remind you of someone you love, or if the diagnosis has come out of the blue to someone who has been well up to that point. The fact that this is so stressful for the health care practitioner needs to be acknowledged, and steps need to be taken to ensure that compassion is also shown towards the person providing the care. That person also needs to harness their own resilience and positivity in order to be able to deal with the impact of this stress on their physical and emotional wellbeing.

We live in a time of deficit journalism where the media really likes to portray the problems and challenges that individuals, businesses or organisations face. Constant criticism, increased litigation and the need to cover our backs and meet ever increasing targets can make us feel under the microscope, undervalued and unappreciated. This in turn can make us feel stressed, anxious, unhappy and exhausted by our health care

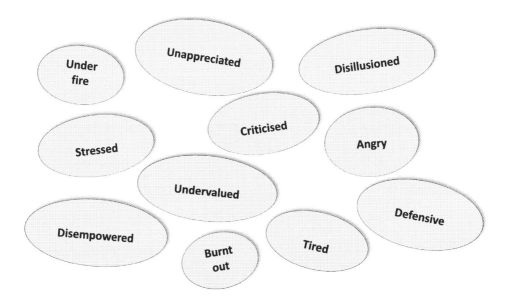

Figure 1.1 Practitioners in all roles can feel....

roles (see Figure 1.1). We need to be kind to ourselves, and our colleagues, as well as the patients in our care. We also need to develop strategies which help us to be less stressed and exhausted.

Questions to ask yourself

Your feelings about the work that you do

- Do you recognise any of the feelings above?
- Which feelings deplete your energy the most?
- Can you do anything to change these negative feelings?

What is compassion?

Compassion is crucial to how we carry out our health care roles, and yet it has become a challenging area to discuss. Some people feel that as compassion is so central we should not be discussing this at all. It can feel like an insult to caring health care practitioners to discuss the fact that compassion is sometimes challenging, or not as central to our care as it should be. Others feel that in these resource constrained times everyone is doing the best that they can and "you want us to be compassionate too?!" It seems like a step too far. Another perspective is that nurses need to be evidence-based in all that they do, and that focusing too much on compassion is perceived to be to the detriment of focusing on the highest quality clinical interventions that are needed in today's health care environment.

All of these arguments detract from what should be unique to health care practitioners, whatever role they have. Yes, we need to focus on the evidence-based science that underpins all that we do, but how we carry this out is more about the art of our practice, and this is needed too. The art and science of our roles should not be in conflict, we need both to carry out excellent care. Patients will forget exactly what we do, and even what we say in many cases, but they will never forget how we made them feel. We need to remember that we often meet patients at their worst times, and these times will be indelibly printed on their memories for the rest of their lives. We have the chance to make those memories better than they could be, or even worse than the circumstances dictate. It is a real privilege for us to be with them, and their loved ones, at times of illness and crisis, and although we might forget exactly what happened, or how we approached each patient, they might not. Yes, they want us to be as clinically effective as possible, but how we carry out care is of monumental importance to them. Therefore, it should be just as important to us. We cannot separate the art of what we do from the science (Carper, 1978), and we should not try to. So, to those who say that all this focus on compassion is less important than efficient, effective care, I would say why should we choose one over the other, why is it not possible to have both? I would say that evidence-based care should not be to the detriment of compassionate care, or vice versa, it is imperative to have both. I also think that continuing to examine what patients find so important about the way that we carry out our roles adds to our evidence base, it does not detract from it. It is part of who we are as health care practitioners, and this needs to be front stage in our discussions.

For those who argue that a compassionate approach is challenging when we are so short of time, we would agree wholeheartedly. To ignore this pressure on our roles would be to ignore the elephant in the room. However, if we have a big task to complete, we can do this if we approach it one step at a time. Baby steps make a huge impact on the patient's experience of our care. We can usually find ways to be kind as well as effective, by being both at the same time. We also need to acknowledge that at times the most time effective way to help a patient is to stop what we are doing, really listen, maximise our eye contact and take a couple of minutes to actively listen to their concerns. If not, their anxiety levels will increase, and the number of times they might press their call buttons, or make calls on health professional time, will also increase. So, on a purely practical level this is counterproductive. The "intentional rounding" approach where nursing staff proactively and regularly approach patients to assess what their needs are in relation to toileting, drinking, pain needs etc appears to demonstrate that patients are less likely to fall and also less likely to press their call bells. There is evidence to show that this maximises nursing time and encourages patients to feel that nurses are more responsive to their needs (Christiansen et al, 2018 and Mitchell et al, 2014). However, the authors of both these literature reviews highlight that more evidence is needed on intentional rounding and its impact on patients. There also needs to be more research focusing on how nursing staff perceive the benefits and potential disadvantages of this approach. On a human level, ignoring patients' needs, or not interacting with them in a sensitive manner, is actually "non care" (Chambers and Ryder, 2019) and this is distressing to both the patients and ourselves. Carrying out our roles in this way is not the reason we came into health care and the "ethical distress" (Mendes, 2017) that this causes to us is palpable. We end the day knowing that it should not be like this and that we have not been true to our ethical beliefs of what good care should be. This is what causes burnout and a distancing from patients, and stress. This is not good for us, and it is certainly not good for the patients in our care. We will discuss ethical distress in more detail in the next section of this chapter.

I believe that it is essential to carry on debating the nature of compassionate care, and what matters to our patients. I do not believe that being compassionate means that we are not evidence-based, we can be both. We also need to understand that resource constraints are a huge pressure on the care that we give, but also on our own self beliefs and wellbeing. We need to focus on what helps us to manage our stress most effectively and keeps us resilient. Positivity plays a major role in this, and if we remain positive this has a huge impact on our patients, our colleagues and ourselves.

So, what is compassion? Nussbaum (2001) takes Aristotle's perception of compassion even further. Both focus on the fact that it relates to a painful emotion caused by the misfortune of others. However, they also both focus on the fact that the misfortune needs to be **serious** enough to warrant that distress, and be **undeserved**, and we need to feel that this misfortune might also **befall us too**. Crisp (2008) highlights the fact that compassion is unusual in that the word is used to reflect the feeling and also the corresponding virtue, and that it is always seen as a positive feeling and virtue. He argues against this and says that Aristotle's term 'eleos' actually translates to pity and not compassion. He goes on to say that pity often involves contempt or condescension and does not necessarily cause us any real distress, or motivate us to act in ways to alleviate it. If our distress is only felt if we perceive the situation to be serious and undeserved, and if our main motivation focuses on the fact that it could also happen to us, then this involves more than a little self-interest, so is this always a positive emotion? Kyprianidou (2019) also discusses this and says that it is our perception of the size of the distress felt by others, as well as whether we think that someone is undeserving which makes the feeling very subjective. Added to this is whether we can only feel compassion if we feel vulnerable to that same misfortune, makes an interesting study on whether feeling compassion is largely about ourselves or others. However, working on the assumption that our motivation is positive, and that we do want to alleviate the suffering of others, then those of us who work in health care would want to convert feelings of compassion to actions to alleviate suffering when possible. We therefore need to understand that the patient's perception of what is serious is the only perspective of importance, and that whether this could befall us as well is not of any relevance to us in our compassion. We also need to move away from whether a misfortune is deserved or undeserved, because this is not up to us to assess, and judgmental views like this have no place in compassionate health care practice.

It can be difficult to articulate exactly what compassion is, but we know when it is not there (Chambers and Ryder, 2019). It is essential to focus on what compassion feels like, or what care does not feel like this, from the patient's perspective, because that is the perspective that really matters. Although there are many definitions of compassion, we like Gilbert's definition. "Compassion can be defined in many ways, but its essence is a basic kindness, with a deep awareness of the suffering of oneself and of other living things, coupled with a wish and an effort to relieve it" (Gilbert, 2010, p11). This awareness and understanding of another's distress and pain is essential to being in a position to relieve it. If we are unaware of that distress how can we help? If we have normalised that pain and distress, and distanced ourselves from it, then again we would find it difficult to do anything to alleviate it. We must have that desire to do all that we can to minimise distress and pain, in order to be effective. So, we have to use our assessment skills to identify pain and distress in its many manifestations, so that we can build on that and our relationship with the patient, in order to find strategies to help. So really compassion is about the ability to understand suffering, and the motivation to do as much as we can to help. Surely that is the essence of health care practice, wherever you work, and whatever your role. Doctors have been encouraged to think much more about their sensitivity and communication, and in some situations they can be more sensitive than their nursing colleagues. Compassion should be inbuilt in nurses, and a unique selling point of all who work in health care practice, because we are meeting people who are unwell, and perhaps having the worst time of their lives. Sensitivity is part of so many roles in social care, teaching, business etc, and it is an innate part of what makes us human as individuals. However, if people who work in health care cannot be role models for compassion, then this would leave a very large void in care that is provided, and we need to realise that compassion is therapeutic in its own right. When people appear to care about us, then we feel more able to cope with our life, and the challenges this brings.

Melissa, a student of mine wrote the following insightful reflection which demonstrates her empathetic, sensitive and compassionate practice, see below (Case Study 1.2).

Case Study 1.2

Melissa's adaptation of policy to ensure patient's distress was minimised

A patient came into the ward with congestive heart failure which made him so breathless that it affected his normal routine and caused him to be bedbound due to increased breathlessness. The patient was sitting upright in bed, but he had slid down the bed so his feet were touching the base board of the bed. This made him slouch more on the bed but the headrest on his bed was raised. His breathing was fast and heavy, despite the fact that he was sitting upright in bed with plenty of pillows to support his shoulders, back and head. He was looking exhausted, weak and tired and he could not keep his eyes open fully.

I was with another carer at the time, to support the patient with repositioning. I assessed the patient's ability to help himself to be more comfortable. He could not shuffle up the bed himself as this would have made his breathing worse, and the patient mouthed to me "I can't breathe" when the pillows were moved. He looked distressed, and his breathing was fast and short, and his face became red and he needed time to get his breath back.

The time spent observing his abilities and how they affected him was important as he was the person in distress, and not repositioning the patient could lead to other complications for his skin. I put myself in the patient's shoes and followed the pattern of his breathing and how different it was to mine. I could feel my whole chest moving, and I was becoming more tired in the few seconds I was with him. I thought about if I continued this for a whole day I would be exhausted. Not being able to breathe is not a nice feeling and I had experienced a little of this when I had a chest infection.

The training I had from the trust's manual handling training in "how to slide a patient with a slide sheet" was beneficial for this patient as there would be minimal physical activity for him, to ensure that his breathing was not compromised. However, using this approach would not be beneficial for his breathing as he would need to be laid flat to slide him safely and protect our backs.

So, I put the patient in the centre of this activity. I made sure that he was comfortable throughout the activity, with the help of my colleague. I knew the height position for his head that he could cope with, without getting too distressed in his breathing. We fully supported the patient with pillows in an upside-down V shape to support his head, shoulders and back at a height that the patient could tolerate. This allowed me to lower the head rest but still support him with his breathing. This adhered to the trust's training when I slid the patient up the bed with my colleague using the slide sheet and we continued to protect our backs. Each movement was carried out taking into account the patient's ability and giving him time to catch his breath.

Was the practice I carried out safe, and if so, where could I obtain the evidence to prove this? I researched practice on using a slide sheet for patients but the literature sources mostly stated that the patient would be lying flat, or using one pillow. However, from further reading I found that a patient could use pillows, especially if they were breathless or there was a restriction to their breathing. Despite obtaining the right information I needed to ensure that my practice was justifiable. I felt it was right for the patient at that time despite the fact that I did not have any evidence to back up my practice. By the end the patient was not distressed through the manual handling procedure and was more comfortable as he could stretch his feet out in bed.

Melissa has given permission for her reflection to be used in this book. She has used sensitivity and empathy to fully assess the patient, and their needs. She then adapted the moving and handling policy to ensure that she kept him as comfortable as possible, whilst protecting the health and wellbeing of herself, and her colleague. The fact that she breathed with the patient helped her to really appreciate his level of distress, and the extent to which his breathing was compromised. She then looked up the evidence for what she did afterwards. It would be really good for her to teach other students, and other members of staff about her strategies to adapt the policy to individual patient situations. Melissa's care encapsulates compassionate and evidence-based practice and the art combined with the science of nursing.

The first book in this series (Chambers and Ryder, 2009) identified six main themes in relation to compassion:

- Empathy and sensitivity
- Dignity and respect
- Listening and responding
- Diversity and cultural competence
- Choice and priorities
- Empowerment and advocacy

You might want to review your ability to be compassionate in your professional role by using the aide mémoire in Table 1.1 Once you have considered the statements in relation to the different areas of compassion identified above, you could use your findings to make plans to enhance your compassion in your work role.

Table 1.1 Compassion in your professional role – personal review

How compassionate are you in your professional role?					
How much does each statement apply to you?	Mark your score				
Read each statement and decide how strongly the statement applies to you. Score yourself 1–5 based on the following guide: 1 = none of the time 2 = a little of the time 3 = some of the time 4 = most of the time 5 = all of the time	Ring the number that shows how strongly the statement applies				
Compassion and taking a lead					
I am able to sense distress in others	1	2	3	4	5
I want to help alleviate this distress	1	2	3	4	5
I act when patient pain/distress is not well managed	1	2	3	4	5
I predict and resolve conflict in relation to patient care	1	2	3	4	5
Emotional intelligence					
I think that I understand myself and my feelings	1	2	3	4	5
I think that I am good at engaging with others	1	2	3	4	5
I feel that I can manage my own emotions	1	2	3	4	5
I feel that I can understand the feelings of others	1	2	3	4	5

(Continued)

Table 1.1 (Continued) Compassion in your professional role – personal review

Dignity

I focus strongly on maintaining the dignity of others	1	2	3	4	5
I make sure that patients have control over their care	1	2	3	4	5
I try not to appear too rushed and give time to people	1	2	3	4	5
I argue for appropriate time to meet my patients' needs	1	2	3	4	5

Respect

I always show respect to patients in my care	1	2	3	4	5
I am always non-judgmental towards patients	1	2	3	4	5
I always aim to be as person-centred as possible	1	2	3	4	5
I always question lack of sensitivity in others	1	2	3	4	5

Listening and Responding

I actively listen to patients when they talk to me	1	2	3	4	5
I do take in what patients are actually saying to me	1	2	3	4	5
I respond appropriately to patient concerns	1	2	3	4	5
I keep my focus on the patient and their needs	1	2	3	4	5

Diversity and cultural competence

I fight social exclusion and stereotyping	1	2	3	4	5
I aim for inclusive care and decision making	1	2	3	4	5
I value the importance of being culturally competent	1	2	3	4	5
I try to enhance my cultural knowledge and skills	1	2	3	4	5

Patient choice and priorities

I work in partnership with patients in my care	1	2	3	4	5
I ensure that patients are actively involved in decisions	1	2	3	4	5
I try to find out what my patients' priorities are	1	2	3	4	5
I make sure that care is based around patient priorities	1	2	3	4	5

Empowerment and advocacy

I encourage patient empowerment at all times	1	2	3	4	5
I argue strongly when patients are disempowered	1	2	3	4	5
I act as a patient's advocate when required	1	2	3	4	5
I encourage patients to be their own advocates	1	2	3	4	5

Compassion themes	Total score (out of 20)	Strengths	Needs attention	Developmental priority
Compassion and taking a lead				
Emotional intelligence				
Dignity				
Respect				
Listening and responding				

(Continued)

Table 1.1 (Continued) Compassion in your professional role – personal review

Diversity and cultural competence	
Patient choice and priorities	
Empowerment and advocacy	
Consider your results and identify one or two actions you can take immediately to enhance your compassionate approach	
Action 1:	
Action 2	

Questions to ask yourself

Your personal experiences of compassion in your workplace

- What does compassion mean to you?
- How do you incorporate compassion into your day-to-day role?
- What limits your ability to be compassionate?
- Do you feel guilty about limitations on your ability to practice compassionate care?
- Does this cause you distress because you are unable to fulfil your role in a way that you felt was important when you started your journey in health care?
- What areas in the questionnaire are you finding challenging?
- In what areas of compassion are you still able to excel?
- Are you able to teach, coach or lead others to be compassionate in these areas, if not could you consider doing so?
- What actions are you going to take having carried out this questionnaire?
- Could you use this questionnaire with your team?

Why do we need to focus on compassion, and manage our stress, and build on our positivity and resilience?

As effective and compassionate practitioners we should have a deep desire to alleviate suffering where possible, and to do this we need to focus on the person behind the patient and their manifestations of illness. We need to connect with patients and treat them holistically and build compassionate relationships. Many patients will not return to the healthiest versions of themselves, so we need to focus on caring and not merely curing. We need to **care about** people not just **care for** them. Caring for a patient is task orientated, whereas caring about someone involves "an attitude of concern and commitment on our attitude and commitment" (De Raeve, 2002, p 159). Being connected to patients makes us more effective, and this makes our job easier and potentially saves time. We need to appear to have a lot of time and focus our attention completely on the person we are talking to. This is because if we appear hurried we will fluster the patient and this will be distressing for them, but it will also require more of our time. If we use appropriate therapeutic touch and humour and appear cheerful, and be the best versions of ourselves, we are more likely to bring out positive communication in our patients and colleagues.

We chose to work in our health care roles because we want to care and if we are not able to do this we experience ethical distress (Mendes (2017) and feel diminished by this. This ethical distress creates conflict between the values that we feel are essential in health care, and our ability to carry out care in line with these values. Research carried out with newly qualified nurses found that they started with compassionate beliefs but these were crushed out of them after two years in the role. (Maben et al 2006). They became acculturalised by the covert rules and socialisation that were part of their practice environments. These norms were around hurried care being valued more than psychological care, and real work being seen to be about hard physical work rather than spending time talking to patients in their care. They saw it as important not to make waves or rock the boat, and to harden up and distance themselves from patients. This all increased their emotional labour and increased the stress of their roles.

We need to care and be compassionate to ourselves, as well as our colleagues and managers, and try to help create compassionate and healthy care environments. To do this we need to avoid the "error of the average" (Achor, 2011 and 2013). If we strive to just be normal and do things as everyone else does, we can only ever be average, and not the best versions of ourselves. We need to focus on happiness and positivity because we will perform at a higher level. So, if we change our thinking, and become more positive, we are more likely to see the positives in our lives. If we believe that we will be successful we will transmit positive messages to others, we can inspire them, so that they become more positive too. These virtuous circles (Campling, 2013/14) of ascending spirals will create more positivity, rather than vicious circles which take people down into ever increasing negativity. "Virtuous circles, or healthy cultures can take a long time to build, take a lot to sustain, and are easily destroyed" (Campling 2013/14 and Chambers and Ryder, 2019). Kindness creates more kindness, smiling at others makes others smile, and being happy creates more happiness.

Questions to ask yourself

The challenges of compassion

- Do you feel ethically compromised by not being able to be as compassionate as you would like to be at times?
- What sort of situations make you feel ethically compromised? For example, not being able to spend time with someone when they are dying. This could be because you have insufficient resources to meet all the needs in your placement at that time. It could also be because sitting with someone when they are dying is not valued by other members of staff?
- Do you feel pressured not to spend time with patients, and feel a need to "just get on with the work"?
- Can you spot virtuous and vicious circles in your practice area? Remember that negative circles are more difficult to resolve and can be more ingrained than more positive circles.
- Could you increase the opportunities for virtuous ascending spirals of kindness and positivity? If so, how would you do this?
- How could you influence your practice area, and teach and take the lead on compassion in practice?

Unfortunately, the opposite is also true in terms of unhappiness, and feelings of negativity are much easier to create and sustain.

Are you an "aholic"?

It is interesting to debate what draws people into working in a caring setting and being a member of a health care team. Are people who work in health care naturally caring, or do they develop these attributes by working in this environment? Conversely does the stress of working in a care setting have a negative impact on our ability to care for others? We would argue that caring for others is a privilege and an honour, and this opportunity gives us a great deal back and this is "sustaining not draining". We like the definitions of personality types that Clouston (2015) has adapted from the work of Schaef (2004 and 2006) and feel that these are represented strongly in the personalities of health care practitioners. The activities, which we really enjoy and find it difficult to stop, make us "aholics", and there are four different ways we can be addicted to certain aspects of our life. We can be addicted to caring, our work, being busy and rushing and this can have a negative impact on our health and wellbeing.

Firstly, we could be a **careaholic** and therefore overly involved with others and worrying about them all the time. Schaef (2006) says that we could over sympathise with how we think that they might feel, which might not be an accurate assessment of how they feel at all. Therefore, we might be communicating with them in a way that is not helpful for them, but also wasting our energy on concerns that might not be valid. We are ethnocentric in how we perceive life, and how we perceive the world and how we feel, and our only identity can be our perspective. So, we need to validate our perception of others' feelings before we make assumptions. In addition, if we are over caring we exhaust ourselves through being over committed and over belonging and carrying out too many activities which support our assumptions. Our view would be that if we are good communicators, we can check our understanding about how others feel and therefore reduce the risk of "suffocating" others with our caring. Also, that if we do not carry out the caring activities which we feel are in keeping with who we are, we can feel that we are letting ourselves, and others, down. This adds to our stress and the "ethical distress" of not being at one with our values (Mendes, 2017).

Secondly, we could be a **workaholic** and work, or thinking about work, to too great an extent (Schaef, 2006). This interferes with our ability to engage meaningfully with others and we become exhausted by doing too many work type activities. Our view would be that as Confucius says "choose a job that you love and you will never have to work a day in your life". If you are lucky enough to have a job like that it is not the burden that others might feel in their work role. Many people though are not that lucky, and their work does tire them, and they need to separate work from their life in order to recharge their batteries.

Thirdly, we could be **busyaholics** and always have to be doing something, and hate doing nothing. We can then become exhausted because we cannot focus on the important things in life, such as our relationships, feeling peaceful or being happy (Schaef, 2006). Personally, I find it very stressful having lots of things to do and knowing that I have empty time when I need to be waiting for something to happen. So, I multitask at times like this and use the time to sort out other things in my personal or professional life. So, if I am in a telephone queue or a traffic jam I might make a shopping list, or listen to music I like, reply to an email or plan my response to a work situation or continue doing a jigsaw on my iPad, whichever is most appropriate in the circumstances. I find that by making the most of my time in this way gives me more genuinely relaxing time and reduces the frustration of time that would otherwise be empty, but not relaxing time. However, everyone is different and how busy our lives are at any given point, and what fills our time, is also variable, so we need to work out what works for us.

Lastly, we could be **rushaholics** and constantly be worrying about what is next on our agenda. Potentially if we do this too much we are never in the moment and we become exhausted by never fully experiencing and enjoying the moment that we are in. It is possible that we can live in the past and we can find that we are never totally happy because we miss the things that we are no longer experiencing. So, if we are having a good evening out with friends but we let our mind go to what time we have to get up in the morning, how we are going to get home and what we need to do the next day, then we are not experiencing the happiness we should feel at the time. We then have a sense of bereavement the following morning, because we realise how enjoyable the evening was, and it is a shame that we did not take the time to enjoy it at the time.

So how much are we careaholics, workaholics, busyaholics and rushaholics? I think that I have all these traits but I like to reassure myself that at least I am balanced and not taking any of these traits too far. I have a particular fear of not having anything to do, so that if I watch a programme and someone is locked in a police cell I think of the stress of not even having a Sudoku or a book to read. Others might worry more about feelings of claustrophobia, or who is looking after their children or their pets, or whether what has happened has been reported in the press, or worry about what strategies might address what they are being accused of. We all worry about different things, but if we become overwhelmed by the needs of others, our work demands, or the need to rush or be busy all the time, this will be detrimental to our health and wellbeing. So, we need to think of strategies which work for us. If rushing around at certain times of the day gets a lot done and is very effective, then we need to make sure that we have times when we can focus on ourselves and relax with the people we love, or whose company we enjoy. So, we need to realise the importance of caring for ourselves, as well as others.

Aide Mémoire

Focusing on ourselves

Important self-help messages for ourselves (from ideas generated by Schaef (2004) in her book *Meditations for Women Who Do too Much*):

- The busier we are the more we lose our **humanness**, so we need to actively focus on reconnecting with our compassionate self.
- Sometimes our busyness helps us to feel less powerless. Maybe we need to admit that we sometimes feel powerless in order to recover our personal power. Admitting that we are **vulnerable** can help us to feel less so.
- It is not easy to find **happiness** within ourselves, but that is where it lives, not in what lies outside ourselves. Happiness is elusive, particularly if we look for it, but we can find it in ourselves, and in the moment we are in.
- We need to stop talking and start to **listen**, but busy people can talk too much and we can be afraid of silence, and being on our own.
- We can find it difficult to laugh, and we can feel like we need to suppress it. However, **laughter** is one of the gifts of being human and this is very therapeutic in its own right.
- Our constant busyness can stop us **feeling really alive** and this can kill us slowly.

- We can poison ourselves with our **negativity** and negative thoughts; we have the power to change this.
- We are very good at some things and sometimes we can play this down and make ourselves think that we are worthless and incompetent. **Celebrating our skills** is good and Schaef (2004) uses the example of Gingers Rogers, who did everything that Fred Astaire did, but backwards and in heels!
- We work hard to be accepted and to prove that we can do things, but working so hard at everything is **hard work** and exhausting.
- Sometimes we need to **ask for help**, this is not an admission of failure, but a sign of courage, strength, honesty and intelligence.
- Sometimes we miss out on the therapeutic and regenerative power of **sleep** when we are too busy to totally relax and renew ourselves after the previous day.
- Sometimes we give ourselves good advice, because we know ourselves well. If we cannot **act on our own advice** we should not beat ourselves up about that.
- Demanding too much of ourselves is bad for us and **self-battering** is arrogant and self-centred and does not help anyone.
- We do not have to do it all, we can **let go of some things** and not take responsibility for everything.

Questions to ask yourself

Your "aholic" tendencies

- What sort of "aholic" are you?
- Do you have many of these traits?
- Do you think that any of these traits are having a negative impact on you or anyone at home or work?
- Do you think that you need to change in any way in relation to these areas?
- What do you think that you need to do differently, and what is your timescale for this?

The importance of self-compassion

We need to accept that if we care about others, whether this is patients, colleagues, family or friends, this has to start with care of ourselves and we have to be compassionate to ourselves. Self-compassion is about "merciful and steadfast love" to ourselves (Neff, 2003). Being kind to ourselves is about not being too critical about ourselves, and our challenges and shortcomings. We need to be as warm and kind to ourselves, as we are to others. Seppala (2016) says that self-criticism is actually self-sabotage, because we can sabotage our ability to understand that we have done well in the circumstances, even if we know that we could have achieved more if the situation had been different. Inadequate staffing levels can really impact on the standards of care that we are able to provide, but if we have still managed to appear caring and nothing has been left undone we should be congratulating ourselves. We need to understand common humanity and realise that everyone suffers and fails at times, it is not unique to us. However, our standards can be too high in relation to what we think that we should be achieving, and therefore we do not accept anything other than perfection in ourselves. Mindfulness can help us to think about our difficult feelings in a balanced way so that we do not over identify with them. That allows us to practice self-forgiveness as well as self-compassion.

As health care practitioners we can expect too much of ourselves but we need to acknowledge the highly charged situations in which we work. If we experience a traumatic situation at work we can end up as secondary victims. So those health care practitioners who cared for the victims and the loved ones of the Manchester Ariana Grande concert bombing May 2017, or the Grenfell Tower fire or the London Bridge terrorist incident, both in June 2017, were deeply affected by what they witnessed. Catastrophic events worldwide can also be traumatising, such as the terrorist attacks in New York in September 2001, Paris in November 2015, Christchurch, New Zealand in March 2019 and in Sri Lanka in April 2019, the tsunami that hit Indonesia, Thailand and India in December 2004. There are many other extremely traumatic incidents which would have caused post traumatic symptoms in many people who witnessed these events. However, the impact of these, and other terrible situations would have also been felt by emergency personnel and health care workers who tried to save and care for those who were suddenly involved in life changing events. Many people put themselves at personal physical and psychological risk to help those who were dead and injured, and many witnessed situations that will affect them for the rest of their lives. So, not only are there many primary victims of incidents, there are also many secondary victims, some of whom are emergency and health care personnel. More still needs to be done to support secondary victims, particularly amongst the services who are more likely to be exposed to traumatic events. We need to be able to give and receive support when someone dies on our watch. Did that person remind you of someone else that you love, or was it a painful wakeup call of our own mortality? Do we know if our colleagues are hurting, or traumatised by a situation that they have been part of? If so, what help is there available? We need to create a culture of compassionate support, and challenge and take the lead if this is not in place.

We also need to be emotionally intelligent (Goleman, 1996) and be self-aware when we are traumatised by events, so that we recognise how this impacts on our wellbeing. We need to be aware of our relationships with others and how important these can be in the aftermath of traumatic events. This emotionally intelligent approach will allow us to manage ourselves and our relationships in a helpful way in order to minimise ongoing trauma to ourselves and those we interact with, at home and at work. We will be discussing secondary trauma, self-care and the importance of self-compassion in greater detail in Chapter 3.

Questions to ask yourself

Self-compassion

- Do you think that you are successful in being compassionate to yourself?
- Do you hold yourself to account in less caring ways than you would for the colleagues who you work with?
- What can you do to be more compassionate towards yourself?
- What can you do to become more compassionate towards others?
- Can you create more of a culture of caring and positivity in your team? If so, in what ways could you do this?
- Have you got a timescale for introducing more compassion towards yourself and others and encouraging a more positive team culture?

The healing nature of compassionate practice

Robin Youngson is an anaesthetist in New Zealand and he works in highly acute and specialised areas of practice. He is also an internationally accepted expert on compassion. He argues against mechanistic models of care and believes passionately in the importance of building therapeutic relationships with patients. He says that patients often have no way of assessing our clinical competence, but they can and do assess us on our ability to care. As he says "when you show kindness, compassion and an honest desire to help your patients, they will forgive you almost anything. I have learnt now to be the patients' friend and advocate". Amongst other advice that he would have given his younger self (Youngson, 2017) he says that it is important not to see the patient as a burden of demand, but as a resource of health and healing, because people can, and do, heal themselves. We need to help people to utilise their own healing powers, and their innate strengths and positivity to bring about the most positive outcomes. If we judge ourselves by their health outcomes, we will miss seeing the advantage of helping people achieve the most positive death experience, or the best outcome possible considering the challenges to their health. He says that all practitioners make mistakes, and we need to learn from them, we are only human. However, if we are positive and smile and actively build relationships with others the world becomes a much more positive and welcoming place to be, and our patients are more likely to thrive in our care.

Like Youngson, we believe that the "ethical distress" (Mendes, 2017) of compromising our ideals and values of what we came into our health care roles to do, leads to burn out amongst health care practitioners. There is a disconnection between our professional ideals and the prevalent culture of health care today. Maben et al's research (2006), which we have discussed already, carried out on newly qualified nurses demonstrated that their high ideals of compassionate, person-centred care were crushed within two years of qualification. So, we do not need to withdraw from our patients and distance ourselves from their care needs. Instead, we need to reclaim our original ideals, and our identity as healers (Youngson, 2019a), and see how we can maintain this in the challenging culture where we work.

As healers we need to recognise that this is why we were attracted to working in health care and that we want to be person-centric, rather than disease-centric, that we want to develop relationships with people in our care, and that we understand the need to sometimes stop "doing" and focus on the importance of "being with" our patients. We need to believe in the importance of holistic and compassionate care as being therapeutic in its own right. Emotional suffering has a negative impact on our health, and we need to try to alleviate this as much as possible. We need to try to capitalise on the person's own ability to heal themself and recognise that making a healing connection with others saves us time and brings us satisfaction, and pleasure at the same time. In order to do this, we need to care for ourselves so that we can continue to care for others, and take time to create a balance in our own lives, and also support our colleagues in developing their skills and knowledge and support them emotionally as needed (Youngson, 2019b). We need also to believe in our collective power and stand together to express the importance of our belief in compassionate care and in healing, and help others to see that the art of how we practice teams very well with the science of evidence-based practice. Carper's (1978) discussion of the art and science of nursing going hand in hand is still relevant today and as health care practitioners we need to embrace both in order to maximise our therapeutic impact.

Questions to ask yourself

The healing nature of compassionate practice

- Can you think of examples when compassion itself was therapeutic?
- Could you do more to teach others about the importance of compassion, and its healing properties?
- If so, what do you need to do to make compassion part of your therapeutic skills?

The importance of compassion for you, your patients and the organisation you work for

We need to understand the importance of retaining our compassion and positivity, because as we have said already, for many of us this was the reason we came into health care, and it is part of who we are. An American study of 1,600 pregnant women found that mothers who felt in control of their lives, and felt positive, had a positive impact on their babies' life outcomes (Nowicki et al, 2017). If both parents had an internal locus of control (Rotter's seminal work, 1954), and felt more in control of their own destiny, their children were more likely to eat and sleep better and have more control of their emotions. They were also more likely to achieve greater academic success, have fewer school related personal and social difficulties, and they were also more unlikely to be obese. The findings reinforce the need to ensure that mothers know how much impact their behaviour and their feelings could have on their children, now and in the future. So, positivity can change the lives of ourselves and others for the better.

From a personal perspective happiness and optimism have a real impact on our own health and wellbeing, as well as that of our patients. The following facts are rather surprising and I have cited these at various conferences:

Aide Mémoire

The impact of optimism on our health and wellbeing

- If we are pessimists we have a four times **higher death rate** from cardiac disease and a three times higher mortality rate from all causes of death whereas optimists have a lower risk of cardiovascular events and mortality from mortality for other reasons (Rozanski et al, 2019).
- Our long-term **survival rate** after a heart attack is greatly compromised, if we are pessimists rather than optimists (Youngson, 2012).
- In terms of l**ongevity** the effect of happiness is comparable to the difference between being a smoker and a non-smoker (Veenhoven, 2008).
- Stressed patients experience **delayed healing**, higher risk of wound infection and cancer recurrence, and immune responses are compromised (Gouin and Kiecolt Glaser, 2011, and Godbout and Glaser, 2006).

Aide Mémoire

Positive health outcomes of compassionate care

There is a great deal of research around these areas of health:

- When patients are on the receiving end of compassionate care they have **better surgical outcomes, better wound healing and are discharged quicker** (Youngson, 2012, Egbert et al, 1964).
- When we interact with compassion this has a positive impact on our patients' **autonomic nervous system** in terms of respiration and heart rate, and their stress levels are lower and their **sense of peace** is enhanced (Kemper and Shaltout, 2011, and Pereira et al, 2016).
- Patients who are treated with compassion in Emergency Departments are 30% **less likely to return to the ED** for the same problem (Redelmeier et al 1995).
- Patients with terminal lung cancer with early access to compassionate palliative care have **better quality of life, less depression, fewer interventions**, reduced cost of care, and survive on average 30% longer (Dahlin et al, 2010).
- Having a caring doctor cuts the five-year risk of a heart attack more than aspirin, and reduces overall **mortality** more than smoking cessation (Kelley et al, 2014).
- Patients with diabetes who rate their doctors as having high empathy have 42% **fewer emergency admissions** to hospital (Del Canale et al, 2012).
- Surgical trauma patients who rated their doctors as having high empathy were twenty times more likely to report **good outcomes** six weeks after discharge (Steinhausen et al 2014).
- Patient **adherence with treatment** is 62% higher when the physician has been treated with empathetic doctor-patient communication (Zolnierek and Dimatteo, 2009).
- Patients with the common cold who receive empathetic consultation have **less severe symptoms, recover earlier** and have greater changes in neutrophil counts (Rakel et al, 2011).
- The total **costs of health care in the whole system are 30% lower** when the primary care doctor provides above average patient-centred care (Bertakis and Azari, 2011).

Youngson (2012), having found the above papers, and accessed the research, sums up his findings and says there are ten top reasons why compassion is great medicine (Figure 1.2):

So, if compassion reduces health costs and improves patient survival, as well as their experience of care, it is a "no brainer" for us all.

It is also really important that we are treated with care and compassion, and that we treat others in this way as well.

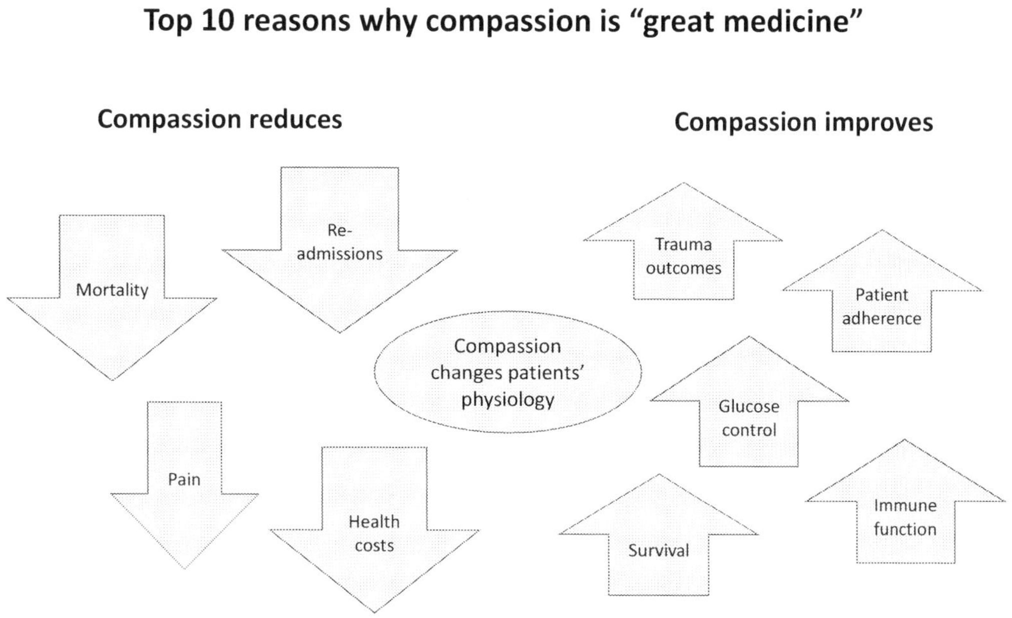

Top 10 reasons why compassion is "great medicine"

Compassion reduces

Compassion improves

Mortality

Re-admissions

Compassion changes patients' physiology

Trauma outcomes

Patient adherence

Glucose control

Pain

Health costs

Survival

Immune function

Figure 1.2 Why compassion is "great medicine"

Aide Mémoire

Organisational benefits of treating staff with compassion

- Staff who are well and happy have higher levels of **self-efficacy** and are more effective in their working roles.
- They have a higher **internal locus of control** and have more control over their lives
- They have healthier lifestyles.
- **Staff sickness** levels are lower.
- **Staff turnover** is lower.
- Being treated with compassion has a **positive impact on those we care for**, and those we work with.

(Cook and Chater, 2013)

So, if compassion is so good for us in terms of our health and wellbeing, and so positive for our patient in terms of their outcomes why is this not a major focus in health care today? After all, staff resourcing is also much improved in a compassionate environment, because staff absence through sickness and high staff turnover creates a much greater burden on those who are working. In addition, there are added risks because lower patient staff ratios are more likely to be responsible for adverse patient outcomes and higher incidents of poor care, missed care and mistakes. Health care costs are greatly reduced, and there are improved patient outcomes and lower burnout amongst health care staff. Bertakis and Azari (2011) found in their study that a more patient centred approach led to significantly fewer specialist visits, laboratory tests and hospitalisations over the year afterwards. So, it makes good therapeutic and economic sense to focus on helping health care staff to retain their compassion towards themselves, their patients and their colleagues. Trzeciak (2018) refers to the "compassionomics" of compassionate health care leading to reduced costs, alongside better outcomes for patients and lower burn out levels for staff. Kopp (2018) says that we just need to be intentionally compassionate, and we need to practice this. Goodrich and Cornwell (2011) agree with the health economics argument that enhancing care leads to less anxiety and pain, and also leads to better health and wellbeing and a faster recovery, which also gives better value for money and also makes sense economically too.

One study focused on measuring levels of empathy in students (Hojat et al, 2013). The researchers found that students who had watched video clips designed to enhance their empathetic understanding had higher levels of empathy after the activity. The same group was divided into two groups, one of which watched a lecture on empathy in patient care and their empathy levels were increased as a result. The other half of the group watched a movie on racism and their empathy levels were reduced as a result. The findings of the researchers were that empathy declines, but it can be enhanced, and in order for this to be the case and empathy levels to be sustained, the focus on empathy needs to be reinforced. So there needs to be a much greater focus in primary training for health care roles, but also in relation to ongoing training amongst health care practitioners. We need to understand what feels like empathy to patients, and why this is important, and how we can connect to people in a meaningful way. So how much time does it take to give a meaningful expression of compassion to a patient? The answer, from a study by Fogarty et al (1999) of healthy breast cancer survivors and a control group who were shown an "enhanced compassion" videotape, is around 40 seconds. Women who had been shown the video were significantly less anxious, and rated their physician as warmer and more compassionate. So, when we say that we do not have time to be compassionate this is clearly not the case. We can all afford 40 seconds, however busy we are. All we need to do is to stop and actively listen to each patient and give a strong message that we are supportive of them and that we want to help.

Case Study 1.3

Annie's adaptation of communication when a patient was distressed and did not speak English

Annie, a nursing student of mine was working in the emergency department when a French lady was admitted in a neck brace having fallen five feet from her bed in her cabin on a cruise. This lady spoke no English at all and she arrived before her husband and the interpreter. The patient was terrified and unable to move, she did not understand what was being carried out, and the student nurse could see her distress and tried to build a therapeutic connection. She held her hand, stroked her hair and put her face very close to the patient's and keeping her tone reassuring and low said "I am here, I know that you are frightened but I am here for you, you are not alone". The patient could not understand what was said but she understood the message and calmed down instantly. Annie also accompanied her to have a CT scan and X ray so that she had a familiar face with her. Later that day the patient was found not to have any serious injury and was going home. She went to find the student nurse and spoke to her in French and the interpreter said "What a lovely lady you are, you are so kind and I was not frightened any more, thank you, thank you, thank you". "Kindness is the language which the deaf can hear, and the blind can see" (Mark Twain). In this case it transcended linguistic barriers and made the patient feel much less frightened and she felt genuinely cared for.

Annie was well aware that it would not always be appropriate to touch someone in this way, and it would depend very much on the patient. She says:

> As nurses we touch our patients all the time with consent, we take observations, we give medications, we may change catheters and help with personal care and nearly all nursing interventions will require touch. We often take for granted the power touch can have when our patients are upset, confused or simply introducing ourselves. The impact of touch in a distressing situation can bring comfort, understanding and bring a sense of calmness. However, every situation is different, as our patients are different, and we have to be mindful of when this is appropriate and when it is not acceptable to that patient. Being able to read body language as well as nonverbal cues, as well as gaining consent as appropriate, can help touch to be a positive communication tool.

Therefore, being compassionate can clearly make a difference to ourselves, our colleagues and the patients in our care. It also can free up resources to allow care not to be adversely affected by high sickness levels and staff turnover. We are going to focus next on the power of positivity and resilience.

Questions to ask yourself

The importance of positivity

- Are you now more convinced of the importance of optimism and positivity in relation to your own health?
- Could you now start to convince others about the power of positivity and compassion in your practice environment?
- What actions could you take to spread the word about positivity and compassion?
- Are there any areas that you would like to focus on to increase compassion for patients in the practice area where you work?
- Could you find small pockets of time to increase your connection to patients in your care? Could you encourage others to do the same? If so, how?

Why do we need to be positive and resilient?

Maintaining positivity and personal and team resilience is not easy when the health care environment is so challenging. We can find that how we feel able to carry out our roles can have a real impact on our emotional response to challenges in our professional and personal lives. Davidson and Begley (2012) differentiate between the characteristics of our emotional responses:

- Emotional state refers to fleeting emotions at the time.
- Emotional mood refers to how we feel over a period of time.
- Emotional trait refers to feelings that characterise us over a period of years.
- Emotional style refers to how we consistently respond to life circumstances.

Therefore, it is easy to see how fleeting feelings can build up and influence us over a period of time, which can in turn start to characterise us over a period of time, or become part of our general personal emotional style. So, we need to be careful to try to make sure that our emotional responses are positive whenever they can be, so that our future responses tend to reflect positivity and resilience too.

Lyubomirsky et al (2005) say that we have genetically determined "set points" which provide a baseline or potential for our personal happiness. This is the point to which we return following setbacks and positive experiences. So, 50% of our happiness potential comprises our genetic disposition for happiness. On top of this, 10% of our happiness is influenced by our life circumstances and what happens in our life. However, that leaves 40% of our happiness potential being within our hands, and this is often influenced by intentional activities which we carry out which make us happy. So even if we are genetically predisposed to be less happy, and our life circumstances could be improved, we can make a real difference to how happy we are by making sure that we do things that are more likely to bring happiness to our lives. Happiness is more about the small things that go right every day, than in the big and rarer experiences like going on holiday or winning the lottery. So, if we can ensure that we keep our happiness quota up by thinking about what activities make us happy, we can then make sure that we expose ourselves to these experiences as frequently as possible, then we can have a strong influence on our ability to be happy.

We need to remember that nobody wakes up in the morning thinking that they want to be unhappy that day (Ricard, 2004). However, we know and work with people who appear to spend most of their time feeling this way, and they tend to have a negative impact on the dynamics of the group and individuals they meet each day. They therefore have the capacity to bring others down and make them feel less positive, and therefore they act as a **drain** on others. We also know that the opposite is true and some people always seem to brighten our mood and make us feel happier, and they **radiate** positivity. **So are you a drain or a radiator?**

Aide Mémoire

Maximizing our happiness potential

What can we do to make ourselves happier, which could help others to feel more positive too? We need to perhaps focus on the following:

- Make sure that we boost our energy getting **sufficient sleep**, organise our lives better and enhance our efficiency so we can spend more time on positive activities.
- We need to make time for **activities which make us happy**.
- Sometimes it can be a matter of lightening up, **seeing the funny side of life**, and **acting happy** even if we are not at that point. A "fake it until you make it" approach might be a starting point. If we smile and act happy others will respond to this and will respond in positive ways which will help us to feel more positive as well.
- We need to be as committed and **serious about our leisure** and play time as we are about our work and what needs to be done around our home. So, we need to find time for activities which make us laugh, and let us exploit the silly and fun side of our personalities.
- This means **making time for friends and family** and friendship.
- We need to **pursue our passions**, whether this is reading, writing, mastering new skills or making time for hobbies that we enjoy.
- We need to **use our money wisely** on things that bring us happiness or make our lives easier, or on people that we value and whose company we

---

enjoy. Too often we spend our hard-earned money on items that do not bring us, or anyone else, happiness.

- We need to focus in a mindful way on **being positive** and how we feel (Rubin, 2009).
- We need to spend as much time as possible **with people who increase our happiness** and make us feel better about ourselves. Do the people that we see regularly make us the best versions of ourselves, do they make us laugh, and make us feel cared for, and celebrate our achievements? Or are they jealous of our successes and achievements, and make us doubt ourselves and bring our confidence down? If they act in this way, they will drag us down and make us less happy. It can be difficult for us to **distance ourselves from negative people** in our lives, but we need to limit the time we spend with people like this, and offset these negative experiences by spending time with people who make us feel happier and better about ourselves. Toxic people can make us less likely to succeed and limit our aspirations, whereas successful and positive people will do the opposite.
- We should not be shrinking down to become lesser versions of ourselves, so that others do not resent us and feel threatened by our success. Our true friends will be inspired by our achievements and celebrate these with us. However, not everyone will like us. As Dita von Teese said "you can be the juiciest, ripest peach in the world, and there's still going to be people who hate peaches". So, we need to **stop being a people pleaser**, not everyone will like us, but those we most like and respect will do so.

Questions to ask yourself

Focusing on happiness

- What is your genetically determined set point for happiness? Is this above or below average? This counts for 50% of your happiness quotient.
- Taking into account life experiences which constitute 10% of our happiness quotient, what can you do to increase the intentional activities which could enhance your happiness, which constitutes 40% of your happiness potential?
- Are you a drain or a radiator? How can you radiate more positivity in your practice area?
- What are you going to do to increase happiness in your life?

The challenges of happiness

So, why do we struggle to be happy? Why is being happy so difficult for us? Sometimes it is because we confuse being happy with pleasure, and sometimes it is because we do not realise that we are actually feeling happy at that point. Pleasure is more reliant on particular objects or times, whereas happiness and positivity are more about states of mind. Wellbeing involves a sense of calmness, serenity and fulfilment, which is ongoing and not about fleeting emotions. However, we can miss out on our feelings of wellbeing because we fail to recognise them. Another challenge is that happiness uses itself as we experience it. On a cold winter's day when we are really cold we cannot help but focus on how cold we are and we fantasise about being by a fire and feeling cozy. However, when we do manage to get out of the cold we very soon forget about the feelings of cold and we stop appreciating the warmth, and in fact can start to feel too warm. So, our pleasure at feeling warm is very transitory and unappreciated. The same thing applies to eating chocolate. We might really want some chocolate and in fact really enjoy the first few squares. However, we could have satisfied our pleasure at eating the chocolate at that point and could stop eating it. Generally though, we carry on to finish the bar, then beat ourselves up for the next few hours about the fact that we ate it. The trick is to stop when we are finding the pleasure of eating the chocolate is diminishing.

Another problem highlighted earlier is that we are never totally happy because we miss things that we are no longer experiencing, but those experiences can be translated into happiness. So, if we are enjoying going to a concert or film or spending time with friends we can find it difficult to live in the moment. Therefore, we spend our time worrying about small details for the future rather than focusing on how much we are enjoying the evening. However, the following day we look back at the evening and think how much we enjoyed it, and wish that we were still there, and this can lead to feelings of discontent. Therefore, when we can, we need to realise that we are happy and content and enjoying life and that we are not having any difficulties. After all, when is the last time you celebrated NOT having a headache, or NOT having aches and pains anywhere?

Barriers to happiness are negative feelings such as arrogance, anger and jealousy so we need to realise when we are experiencing negative feelings and try to stop ourselves feeling this way because they are pointless emotions. Unless we can find ways to dissipate these they will stop us being happy and positive. We also need to stop looking outside of ourselves for others to "fix" our problems and realise that we are usually the agents for change in our lives, and we are more powerful than we realise. We will be focusing on happiness, wellbeing and positivity in greater detail in Chapter 5

Questions to ask yourself

Focusing on happiness in your life

- What brings you enjoyment or peace in life?
- Can you build in more time for activities that help you to feel calm or happy?
- What are the emotions that hinder happiness for you, and can you try to minimise these?
- Can you try to focus more on realising that you are feeling happy at the time that you are experiencing it?
- Can you be a stronger agent for change in your life?

RECOMMENDATIONS FOR LEADERSHIP AS INDIVIDUAL PRACTITIONERS, LEADERS AND ORGANISATIONS

This chapter has discussed what compassion is, and why it is important to our own positivity and wellbeing and also whether we are prone to particular tendencies and whether we are "aholics". It then discussed the importance of self-compassion, and the healing properties of compassion, before focusing on its importance for everyone in our work environment including ourselves. It finished by discussing the importance of positivity and resilience, and the challenges of happiness.

Each chapter concludes with pointers for leadership, for us as individuals, and then for us as leaders, in this case focusing on compassionate care.

Focusing on compassionate care as individual practitioners

I would like to conclude by discussing the following areas in terms of their key attributes and actions:

- Components and attributes of compassion
- Indicators of caring
- The BOND framework of compassionate care
- Caring conversations
- How can we develop our practice.

I feel that these attributes and actions are essential in demonstrating compassionate care in our health care practice:

Aide Mémoire

Components and attributes of compassion.

How do we recognise these and what aspects do we struggle with, what is missing and what characteristics do we need to work on? (Sheridan, 2016, p 179).

Key attributes:

- Motivation
- Sympathy
- Empathy
- Non-judgmental attitude
- Distress tolerance
- Unambiguous communication.

Actions:

- *Motivated* towards engaging with the suffering of others
- *Sensitive* and notice when others are distressed
- *Sympathetic* and moved by the distress of others and want to help
- *Non-judgmental* and accept people in all their different challenges
- *Empathetic* and identify with, and make sense of the feelings of others, and our emotional responses
- Have *distress tolerance* and cope with our own difficult feelings, as well of those of others
- Always focus on "the right message to the right people at the right time with the intended effect" (Ratzan, 2001) and on "clear **unambiguous two-way constructive exchanges**, without distortion of the message between what is given and what is received" (Ewles and Simnett, 2003).

Indicators of caring

We need to focus on what actually matters (Baughan and Smith, 2013 p 19).

Key attributes:

- Individualised holistic care
- Demonstrate compassion in action

- Communicate compassion
- Positive values
- Recognise emotions and actions in ourselves and others
- Listen
- Use professional knowledge
- Guide and monitor others
- Be aware of public concerns.

Actions:

- **Provide individualised, holistic care** *and respond to essential care needs, remembering that "small things matter".*
- Show **compassion in actions** with those who are in pain, distressed, anxious or in need.
- **Be approachable and comforting** and make the most of opportunities to be available for patient and family.
- **Communicate compassion** with warmth, transparency and kindness.
- Be aware of how language can transmit values and beliefs, and **communicate only positive values**.
- Recognise emotional and behavioural responses in ourselves and others.
- **Listen** to and reflect on stories from those being cared for and ensure that they also feel cared about so that we can become more knowledgeable about their perceptions of the caring process.
- **Use professional knowledge** (including theories and stories from experience) to ensure that practice is informed and compassionate.
- **Guide and monitor others** to whom we delegate care, helping them to demonstrate compassion and interest.
- **Be aware** of public concerns and keep up to date with government and professional reports and frameworks which promote quality care.

The BOND framework of compassionate care

We need to focus on the **BOND** principles of **B**eing and becoming, **O**vercoming obstacles, **N**oticing and **D**oing (Baughan and Smith 2013, p155):

Key attributes:

- **B**e and become compassionate
- **O**vercome obstacles
- **N**otice compassion actions and challenges
- **D**o (actions for compassion).

Actions:

- **B**e and become
    - Be a caring presence
    - Be empathetic
    - Become more emotionally intelligent

- ○ Be conscientious and ready to learn
- ○ Be adaptable, flexible and creative

- **O**vercome obstacles

  - ○ Foster resilience and capability
  - ○ Reframe the problem or issue
  - ○ Be non-discriminatory and non-judgmental
  - ○ Use preventative and restorative skills
  - ○ Work in effective partnerships

- **N**otice

  - ○ Systematic and holistic assessment
  - ○ The effects of cues and interactions
  - ○ Indicators of compassion fatigue
  - ○ The professional and ethical demands of caring

- **D**o

  - ○ Establish therapeutic relationships
  - ○ Understand and support informal carers
  - ○ Engage in critical analysis and evaluation of practice
  - ○ Influence the practice environment

Caring conversations

Dewar and Nolan (2013) built on this, again in the older person acute care setting, and focused on caring about caring and compassionate relationship centred care, and caring conversations.

Key attributes:

- Courage
- Connect emotionally
- Curiosity
- Collaborative
- Considerate
- Compromise
- Celebrate.

Actions:

- Be **courageous** and feel confident to ask questions and stand up and challenge established practice.
- *Connect* emotionally and share feelings about the emotions of others.
- Be **curious** and ask questions about others' feelings and experiences and think about new ways of communicating.
- Be **collaborative** and develop a shared responsibility for creating new ways forward.
- Be **considerate** about others' perspectives and use patient and loved one's views and ideas.
- **Compromise** and reach a consensus through discussions and reflections.
- **Celebrate** what works well and why.

How can we develop our practice?

Dewar and MacKay (2010) carried out a study to explore how to appreciate and develop compassionate care in an acute care setting caring for older people.

Key attributes:

- Care for your colleagues.
- Positive feedback.
- Talk about compassion.
- Confidence to speak out and be a patient advocate.
- Be more curious.

Actions:

- **Celebrate more openly what works well.**
- Engage at an emotional level to learn and **act upon the things that matter to people**.
- Develop ways in which **caring acts can move from the unconscious to the conscious** and encourage this across our whole practice area.
- **Care for and about other members of the team.**
- Be more conscious and deliberate about **giving positive feedback**, rather than thinking that compassionate care was just part of everyone's job.
- Value, legitimise and **articulate compassionate acts** so that members of the team are more aware of what is caring practice, and that it is very much valued.
- Feel **confident to speak out** about the way we do things round here, and be braver in challenging others and take a lead in standing up for important values and being clear about what these are.
- **Be curious and take another look** at what is done, for example really listening to patients with dementia when they do not appear to be making any sense and try to understand what they are saying.

I would like to present these perspectives from different authors in an individual compassionate care practice model, focusing on the key attitudes and actions which encompass compassionate care (Figure 1.3). Try to think about how you could apply these to your own area of practice.

Focusing on compassionate care as leaders

Whether we are in a formal management role or not, we all need to be leaders in relation to creating a culture where we are happy to work, and patients feel cared for. So how can we do this, whatever our role in the organisation? We need to be able to foster an attitude of compassion in our practice area as leaders. The health care environment is so complex and challenging that we need to have all members of staff taking a leadership role, whatever their position and status in the hierarchy. We need to move away from a "heroic" approach where strong determined individuals turn around organisational performance. Collective leadership has the greatest potential to create caring environments for patients in our care (West et al, 2014, The King's Fund, 2011). The heroic model is not effective because the challenge of leadership is too great for any one individual, however charismatic or knowledgeable they might be. In the heroic model there is only one leader, and in their absence leadership can be absent. In

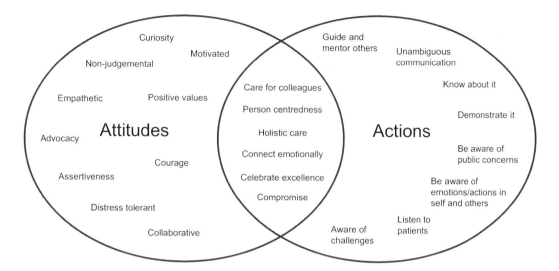

Figure 1.3 Individual compassionate care practice

addition, we can all make mistakes, and our mistakes could be devastating. The airline industry developed this approach first, in response to catastrophic events where plane crashes happened because of the captain being the only decision maker. Nowadays in health care multidisciplinary teams make decisions, not individuals. In operating theatres or in resuscitation situations the team leader asks if everyone is happy, and if anyone has any other suggestions. The Health care Leadership Model (NHS Leadership Academy, 2013) is an approach whereby leaders lead with care and inspire and engage others, and leadership ideas come from within the whole team. Therefore, even if you are not in a management role you can be a leader and suggest improvements in care, and your ideas are likely to be highly relevant and should be listened to. We learn by our relational connections with each other, and we lead by capitalising on these connections and relational approaches to leadership. In compassionate leadership we care for and about patients, but we also care for and about our colleagues, and if we want to lead with compassion, we need to demonstrate this in action.

Therefore again, we will focus on key attributes and actions, this time with our leadership role in mind, so that we can create more compassionate environments. In this case we will focus on:

- Staff wellbeing
- Appreciative inquiry
- Appreciative leadership
- Therapeutic communication
- Compassionate care culture
- A prescription for compassion
- Positive work strategies.

Aide Mémoire

Staff wellbeing

Maben et al (2012) discuss the importance of social support from line managers, colleagues and the organisation which encourages dedication to our work and is positively associated with wellbeing – The National Nursing Research Unit

(NNRU) says that staff wellbeing is the "antecedent rather than a consequence of patient care performance". So, if staff wellbeing at work is good, then they will perform better in their roles, not the other way round (Chambers and Ryder, 2019, p129). Seven wellbeing bundles are advised (see actions) and these are linked to good patient-reported experiences (National Nursing Research Unit (NNRU), 2013, p17).

Key attributes:

- Positivity.
- Focusing on staff wellbeing and a positive work climate.
- Being organised.
- Being supportive of others in the team.
- Focusing on strategies to address and prevent emotional exhaustion.
- Promoting staff satisfaction.

Actions:

- Promote good local teamwork and a positive team climate.
- Aim for a high level of perceived organisational support.
- Provide high levels of co-worker support.
- Aim for low emotional exhaustion.
- Create an environment where there is high job satisfaction.
- Ensure that there is high supervisor/mentor support.
- Create a good organisational climate.

Appreciative inquiry

It is important to focus on an "appreciative inquiry" approach (Cooperrider and Srivastva, 1987) within our teams. This focuses on what is going well and takes an asset approach which starts from the assumption that each person in the organisation has positive traits and motivations. Focusing on these and building more of the same helps us to appreciate ourselves and practice more self-compassion (New Paradigm, 2018 cited in Chambers and Ryder, 2019, p124)

Key attributes:

- Seeing everyone in the team as a potential asset.
- Focus on what is going well.
- Appreciating ourselves and our colleagues.
- Valuing our practice.

Actions:

- Discover – what works well in our team/organisation.
- Dream – what works well and what you like to see more.
- Design – what do we need to do to make the dream happen most of the time.

Appreciative leadership

Dewar and Cook (2014) took the idea of appreciative inquiry further and focused on appreciative leadership through creating a Community of Practice amongst a group of people who had the same ideals and passion and encouraging caring conversations. This helped to deepen knowledge and expertise by increasing interaction between colleagues. They also took part in action learning sets to explore issues in relation to caring conversations. Then they took part in work-based activities to help team members to develop their relational knowledge by understanding at a deeper level who people are, what matters to them and how they feel.

Key attributes:

- Focusing on your team's values and motivations.
- Encouraging discussions around care.
- Increasing relational knowledge.
- Focusing on what really matters to people in our care.

Actions:

- Promote more discussion between colleagues about their values and motivations in practice.
- Encourage caring conversations.
- Analyse practice in relation to how people relate to each other and relational knowledge.
- Work out who your patients are, how they feel, and

Therapeutic communication

Rungapadiachy (1999, p223–24) says that a therapeutic humanistic relationship-based communication is essential.

Key attributes:

- Warmth
- Acceptance
- Genuineness
- Empathy.

Actions:

- Demonstrate positive and affectionate feelings.
- Accept ourselves and others and try to feel accepted by others.
- Be authentic and express what we feel.
- See the situation from other person's point of view. This is "to sense the client's private world as if it were your own, but without losing the "as if" quality" (Kirschenbaum and Henderson, 1990, p226).

Compassionate care culture

A culture of compassionate care needs to be created and maintained (Baughan and Smith, 2013, p175).

Key attributes:

- Thinking like a leader.
- Being a supportive manager.
- Being a positive role model.
- Being a mentor and coach.
- Looking into the evidence.
- Working in partnership and collaboratively.

Actions:

- Be an effective leader and manager.
- Be a positive role model and help others to progress in practice.
- Be an effective mentor and plan learning in a systematic way.
- Ensure that there is preceptorship and clinical supervision in place.
- Ensure that there is a caring environment in which fundamental as well as advanced care needs are met.
- Help others to understand the legal, ethical and professional guidelines and requirements.
- Ensure that there is effective partnership with patients and service users.
- Work collaboratively with other professionals and agencies.

A Prescription for compassion

Youngson (2011, p7) promotes a prescription for compassion.

Key attributes:

- Compassionate care
- Positive reinforcement
- Focusing on others
- Positive challenge
- Compassionate values and behaviour
- Leading with compassion
- Ensuring diversity is valued
- Challenging discriminatory practice
- Working in partnership with patients and carers.

Actions:

- Declare "compassion" as a core value – and a patient right.
- Reward rather than punish compassionate caring.
- Hone communication and relationship skills.
- Provide space for staff to discuss difficult issues.
- Challenge models of professionalism and what is considered to be professional practice, this should be based more on empathy and compassion and loving kindness.

- Hard-wire new behaviours into the organisation – "hello, my name is…" "is there anything else I can do for you at the moment".
- Declare compassion as a management and leadership competence – role model compassion in the care of staff, challenge abuse, bullying and discriminate and celebrate diversity.
- Engage health consumers in the change.

Positive work strategies

Positive work strategies which could be helpful.

Key attributes:

- Awareness of our stress
- Awareness of balance in our lives
- Being resilient
- Being mindful
- Communicating well
- Focusing on wellbeing.

Actions:

- Stress management strategies and one to one support.
- An emphasis on work life balance.
- More education on resilience.
- Opportunities to practice mindfulness.
- Wellbeing and communication training for managers.

Having focused on key attributes and actions in relation to these areas of health care, it might be helpful to capture these as attitudes and actions in relation to compassionate care leadership (Figure 1.4).

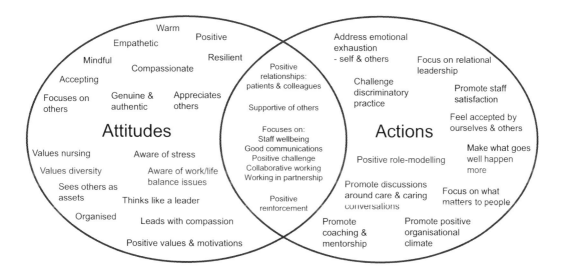

Figure 1.4 Compassionate care leadership

Having a strong focus on compassionate care helps us to remain positive. This in turn helps us to maintain a sense of resilience, for us and our teams, in a resource challenged care environment.

I have developed a toolkit for compassionate and positive practice based on the acronym RESPECT (Chambers and Ryder, 2019) (Figure 1.5):

- **R**esilience – bending but not breaking
- **E**motional intelligence – self and relationship awareness and self and relationship management
- **S**tress management – awareness and strategies
- **P**ositivity – optimistic attitudes to trigger positive emotions
- **E**nergy and motivation - turn challenges into opportunities
- **C**hallenge – "tipping point" to challenge the culture
- **T**eam leadership –practitioners need to take a lead in implementing the **RESPECT** toolkit in their areas of practice so that they are compassionate but conflict aware and challenge where necessary.

I have then incorporated my thoughts on the traits of compassionate individuals and leaders into the RESPECT model (Figure 1.6). We can then focus on what we need to do to take practice forward, as individuals and leaders.

Human interaction is paramount to nursing practice, and how we function in a socialised society. We can change how the brain works if we are compassionate, and can change each other physiologically if we are compassionate so there is a strong neurophysiological connection between compassionate interactions and how the body responds to this behaviour (Egan (2019] citing Kerr founder and CEO of NeuroTech Institute based in Australia). In addition:

- If we are warm and respectful, we make the person feel valued and heard.
- We also get a synchronisation of brains and neurophysiological things happen. If you hold someone's hand then therapeutic touch sets off other chemicals.

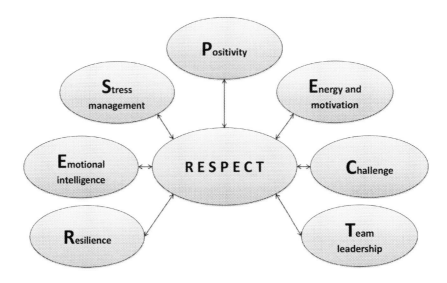

Figure 1.5 RESPECT toolkit for compassionate and positive practice (Chambers and Ryder, 2019)

	Resilience	Emotional Intelligence	Stress	Positivity	Energy & Motivation	Challenge	Team Lead
As Individuals we need to be:	Curious Person-centred Compromising	Non-judgmental Empathetic Emotionally connected Unambiguous communicators Aware of emotions/actions in self and others Actively listening to patients	Distress tolerant	Positively valuing Celebrating excellence	Motivated Courageous Holistically caring Knowledgeable about compassion Able to show compassion	An advocate Assertive Aware of public concerns Aware of challenges	Collaborative Caring of colleagues A guide and mentor for others
As Leaders we need to be:	Supportive of others Resilient Mindful	Warm Empathetic Genuine Compassionate Building positive relationship (patients/colleagues) A good communicator Authentic	Stress aware Aware of work/life balance Emotional exhaustion Aware of, prevent and address emotional exhaustion	Appreciative & accepting of others Positive Positively valuing & motivated Able to see others as assets Valuing nursing A positive role model Focusing on what is going well and what matters to people Positive reinforcers Give positive messages	Valuing of diversity Organised Focusing on staff wellbeing Promoting staff satisfaction Focusing on others Feeling accepted by others & ourselves	Positive challengers Working in partnership Collaboratively working Challenging of discriminatory practice	Leading with compassion Thinking like a leader Coachers Mentors Promoting discussion around care & caring conversations Promoting a positive organisational climate Finding out about relational leadership and what promotes this

Figure 1.6 Compassionate care for individuals and leaders – the RESPECT approach

- When we show compassion our mood lifts and our capacity for giving and for picking up nuanced information increases so we make better decisions.
- The person receiving compassion has increased immune responses and also better decision making.
- Self-compassion allows us to be able to accept the good and bad in ourselves, which makes us more able to do the same for others and be more tolerant.
- People who have no self-compassion and are hard on themselves are often hard on others too.
- A compassionate organisational approach needs to be modelled from the top down and the level of potential compassion an organisation has is determined by its values, beliefs and structures.

I hope I have managed to convince you of the importance of compassion and how this has a really positive impact on ourselves, our colleagues, and those in our care. In order to do this we need to show compassion to ourselves, build on our positivity and resilience and combat the challenges of happiness. Then we can become the best version of ourselves at home and in our personal relationships, and in our health care roles with colleagues and patients. Moreover, we can become leaders in our practice environments and take the lead in ensuring that others also become the best version of themselves, whether we are in a management role or not. This would be true whether we are a health care assistant, student, newly qualified or experienced practitioner or a ward manager. I hope that I have given you the tools to do just this, and I wish you every success in making any changes that you feel are necessary to make this happen.

Focusing on compassionate care as organisations

In order for us to maximise our potential as individual practitioners and leaders we need to have the support of our organisation. Organisational support will be discussed more in future chapters but all the issues raised in this chapter need structures in place to promote excellent practice, challenge poor practice and escalate concerns appropriately. Teams need support to ensure that compassionate care is the norm and there needs to be strong leadership and management from the top to ensure that this is the case.

The next chapters focus on the challenges of compassionate care, strategies to cope with stress and promote resilience, positivity and wellbeing. Strong leadership is needed in order to support practitioners and teams. Each chapter will end by discussing leadership as individuals, leaders and organisations and the last chapter will focus on this exclusively.

REFERENCES

Achor S. (2011) *The Happiness Advantage: The Seven Principles of Positive Psychology that Fuel Success and Performance at Work*. London: Virgin Books.

Achor S. (2013*) Before Happiness*. London: Virgin Books.

Baughan J, Smith A. (2013 2nd ed.) *Compassion, Caring and Communication: Skills for Nursing Practice*. London: Routledge.

Bertakis K.D, Azari R. (2011) Patient-Centered Care is Associated with Decreased Health Care Utilization. *Journal of the American Board of Family Medicine*, 24(3): 229–39.

Campling P. (2013/14) Intelligent Kindness: Reforming the Culture of Health care in the Wake of the Francis Report. *Journal of Holistic Health care*, 10(3): 5–9.

Carper B. (1978) Fundamental Patterns of Knowing in Nursing. *Advances in Nursing Science*, 1(1): 13–24.

Chambers C, Ryder E. (2009) *Compassion and Caring in Nursing*. Abingdon: Routledge.

Chambers C, Ryder E. (2019) *Supporting Compassionate Health care Practice: Understanding the Role of Resilience, Positivity and Wellbeing*. Abingdon: Routledge.

Christiansen A, Coventry L, Graham R, Jacob E. Twigg D, Whitehead L. (2018) Intentional Rounding in Acute Adult Health care Settings: A Systematic Mixed-Method Review. *Journal of Clinical Nursing*, 27(9–10): 1759–92.

Clouston T. (2015*) Challenging Stress, Burnout and Rust Out*. London: Jessica Kingsley Publishers.

Cook E, Chater A. (2013) Are Happier People, Healthier People? The Relationship Between Perceived Happiness, Personal Control, BMI and Health Preventive Behaviours. *International Journal of Health Promotion and Education*, 48(2): 58–64.

Cooperrider D, Srivastva S. (1987) *Appreciative Inquiry in Organizational Life*. In: Pasmore W, Woodman R. (eds.) *Research in Organisational Change and Development* Vol 1. Greenwich: JAI Press; CT 3–27.

Crisp R. (2008) Compassion and Beyond. *Ethic Theory and Moral Practice*, 11(3): 233–46.

Dahlin C.M, Kelley J.M, Jackson V.A, Temel J.S. (2010) Early Palliative Care for Lung Cancer: Improving Quality of Life and Increasing Survival. *International Journal of Palliative Nursing*, 16(9): 420–23.

Davidson R, Begley S. (2012) *The Emotional Life of your Brain: How its Unique Patterns Affect the Way You Think, Feel, and Live, and How You Can Change Them*. London: Hodder & Stoughton Ltd.

De Raeve L. (2002) Trust and Trustworthiness in Nurse-Patient Relationship. *Nursing Philosophy*, 3(2): 152–62.

Del Canale S, Louis D.Z, Maio V, Wang X, Rossi G, Hojat M, Gonnella J.S. (2012) The Relationship Between Physician Empathy and Disease Complications: An Empirical Study of Primary Care Physicians and their Diabetic Patients in Parma, Italy. *Academic Medicine: Journal of the Association of American Medical Colleges*, 87(9): 1243–49.

Dewar B, MacKay R. (2010) Appreciating and Developing Compassionate Care in an Acute Hospital Setting Caring for Older People. *International Journal of Older People Nursing*, 5(4): 299–308.

Dewar B, Nolan M. (2013) Caring About Caring: Developing a Model to Implement Compassionate Relationship Centred Care in an Older People Care Setting. *International Journal of Nursing Studies*, 50(9): 1247–58.

Dewar B, Cook F. (2014) Developing Compassion Through a Relationship Centred Appreciative Leadership Programme. *Nurse Education Today*, 34(9): 1258–64.

Egan N. (2019) Experts Share Evidence on How to Care and Lead with Empathy, Compassion. *Australian Ageing Agenda*. https://www.australianageingagenda.com.au/clinical/social-wellbeing/experts-share-evidence-on-how-to-care-and-lead-with-empathy-compassion/#.XUzT3Zp83vg.email (Accessed 12/9/23).

Egbert L.D, Battit G.E, Welch C.E, Bartlett M.K. (1964) Reduction of Postoperative Pain by Encouragement and Instruction of Patients. A Study of Doctor-Patient Rapport. *The New England Journal of Medicine*, 270: 825–27.

Ewles L, Simnett I. (2003) *Promoting Health: A Practical Guide*. 5th ed. London: Bailliere Tindall.

Fogarty L, Curbow B, Wingard J, McDonnell K, Somerfield M. (1999) Can 40 Seconds of Compassion Reduce Patient Anxiety? *Journal of Clinical Oncology*, 17(1): 371–79.

Gilbert P. (2010) *The Compassionate Mind*. London, Constable and Robinson.

Godbout J, Glaser R. (2006) Stress-Induced Immune Dysregulation: Implications for Wound Healing, Infectious Disease and Cancer. *Journal of Neuroimmune Pharmacology*, 1(4): 421–27.

Goleman D. (1996) *Emotional Intelligence: Why it Can Matter More Than IQ*. London: Bloomsbury.

Goodrich J, Cornwell J. (2011) Seeing the Person in the Patient: The King's Fund Point of Care Programme. *Journal of Holistic Health care*, 8(3): 10–12.

Gouin J, Keicolt-Glaser J. (2011) The Impact of Psychological Stress on Wound Healing: Methods and Mechanisms. *Immunology and Allergy Clinics of North America*, 31(1): 81–93.

Hojat M, Axelrod D, Spandorfer J, Mangione S. (2013) Enhancing and Sustaining Empathy in Medical Students. *Medical Teacher*, 35(12): 996–1001.

Kelley J.M, Kraft-Todd G, Schapira L, Kossowsky J, Riess H. (2014) The Influence of the Patient-Clinician Relationship on Health care Outcomes: A Systematic Review and Meta-Analysis of Randomised Controlled Trials. *PLOS ONE*, 9(4): e101191.

Kemper K.J, Shaltout H.A (2011) Non-Verbal Communication of Compassion: Measuring Psychophysiologic Effects. *BMC Complementary and Alternative Medicine*, 11: 132.

Kirschenbaum H, Henderson V. (1990) *The Carl Rogers Readers*. London: Constable & Robinson.

Kopp J. (2018) *Compassionomics 101: How Kindness Can Make a Big Difference in Health Care*. https://www.phillyvoice.com/compassionate-care-kindness-difference-healthcare-cooper-jefferson-temple-doctors-empathy (Accessed 12/9/23).

Kyprianidou E. (2019) (ed. and Introduction). *The Art of Compassion*. Athens: Nissos Publications.

Lyubomirsky S, Sheldon K, Schkade D. (2005) Pursuing Happiness: The Architecture of Sustainable Change. *Review of General Psychology*, 9(2): 111–31.

Maben J, Latter S, Macleod Clark J. (2006) The Theory-Practice Gap: Impact of Professional-Bureaucratic Work Conflict on Newly-Qualified Nurses. *Journal of Advanced Nursing*, 55(4): 465–77.

Maben J, Peccei R, Adams M, Robert G, Richardson A, Murrells T, Morrow E. (2012) *Exploring the Relationship Between Patients Experiences of Care and the Influence of Staff Motivation, Affect and Wellbeing*. London: NIHR Service Delivery and Organisation Programme.

Mendes A. (2017) How to Address Compassion Fatigue in the Community Nurse. *British Journal of Community Nursing*, 22(9): 458–59.

Mitchell M.D, Lavenberg J, Trotta R, Umscheid C. (2014) Hourly Rounding to Improve Nursing Responsiveness: A Systematic Review. *Journal of Nursing Administration*, 44(9): 462–72.

National Nursing Research Unit (NNRU). (2013) Does NHS Staff Wellbeing Affect Patients' Experiences of Care? *Nursing Times*, 109(27): 16–17.

Neff K. (2003) The Development and Validation of a Scale to Measure Self-Compassion. *Self and Identity*, 2(3): 223–50.

New Paradigm. (2018) *Appreciative Inquiry* http://www.new-paradigm.co.uk/Appreciative.htm (Accessed 12/9/23).

NHS Leadership Academy. (2013) *Health care Leadership Model*. https://www.leadership-academy.nhs.uk/wp-content/uploads/2014/10/NHSLeadership-LeadershipModel-colour.pdf (Accessed 12/9/23).

Nowicki S, Iles-Caven Y, Gregory S, Ellis G, Golding J. (2017) The Impact of Prenatal Parental Locus of Control on Children's Psychological Outcomes in Infancy and Early Childhood: A Prospective 5 Year Study. *Frontiers in Psychology*, 8: 546.

Nussbaum M. (2001) *Upheavals of Thought: The Intelligence of Emotions*. Cambridge: Cambridge University Press.

Pereira L, Figueiredo-Braga M, Carvalho I.P. (2016) Preoperative Anxiety in Ambulatory Surgery: The Impact of an Empathic Patient–Centered Approach on Psychological and Clinical Outcomes. *Patient Education and Counseling*, 99(5): 733–38.

Rakel D, Barrett B, Zhang Z, Hoeft T, Chewning B, Marchand L, Scheder J. (2011) Perception of Empathy in the Therapeutic Encounter: Effects on the Common Cold. *Patient Education and Counseling*, 85(3): 390–97.

Ratzan S. (2001) Health Literacy: Communication for the Public Good. *Health Promotion International*, 16(2): 207–14.

Redelmeier D.A, Molin J.P, Tibshirani R.J. (1995) A Randomised Trial of Compassionate Care for the Homeless in an Emergency Department. *Lancet*, 345(8958): 1131–34.

Ricard M. (2004) *The Habits of Happiness*. TED Talk: https://www.ted.com/talks/matthieu_ricard_the_habits_of_happiness (Accessed 12/9/23).

Rotter J.B. (1954) *Social Learning and Clinical Psychology*. Englewood Cliffs, New Jersey: Prentice Hall.

Rozanski A, Bavishi C, Kubzansky L, Cohen R. (2019) Association of Optimism with Cardiovascular Events and All-Cause Mortality: A Systematic Review and Meta-Analysis. *JAMA Network Open*, 2(9): e1912200.

Rubin G. (2009) *The Happiness Project*. London: Harper Collins Publisher.

Rungapadiachy D.M. (1999) *Interpersonal Communication and Psychology for Health Care Professionals*. Oxford: Butterworth-Heinemann.

Schaef A.W. (2004) *Meditations for Women Who Do Too Much*. New York: HarperCollins.

Schaef A.W. (2006) *Meditations for Women Who Do Too Much*. Revised Edition. New York: HarperCollins.

Seppala E. (2016) *The Happiness Track: How to Apply the Science of Happiness to Accelerate Your Success*. New York: Harper Collins.

Sheridan C. (2016) *The Mindful Nurse: Using the Power of Mindfulness and Compassion to Help You Thrive in Your Work*. USA: Rivertime Press.

Steinhausen S, Ommen O, Thum S, Lefering R, Koehler T, Neugebauer E, Pfaff H. (2014) Physician Empathy and Subjective Evaluation of Medical Treatment Outcome in Trauma Surgery Patients. *Patient Education and Counseling*, 95(1): 53–60.

The King's Fund. (2011) *The Future of Leadership and Management in the NHS: No More Heroes*. London: The King's Fund.

Trzeciak S. (2018) *Can 40 Seconds of Compassion Make a Difference in Health Care?* https://knowledge.wharton.upenn.edu/podcast/knowledge-at-wharton-podcast/the-compassion-crisis-one-doctors-crusade-for-caring/ (Accessed 12/9/23).

Twain M. https://www.azquotes.com/author/14883-Mark_Twain/tag/kindness (Accessed 12/9/23).

Veenhoven R. (2008) Healthy Happiness: Effects of Happiness on Physical Health and the Consequences for Preventive Health. *Journal of Happiness Studies*, 9(3): 449–69.

Von Teese D. https://www.goodreads.com/author/quotes/106288 (Accessed 12/9/23).

West M, Eckert R, Steward K, Pasmore B. (2014) *Developing Collective Leadership for Health Care*. London: The King's Fund.

Youngson R. (2011) Compassion in Health care. *Journal of Holistic Health care*, 8(3): 6–9.

Youngson R. (2012) *Time to Care: How to Love Your Patients and Your Job*. New Zealand: Rebel Heart Publishers.

Youngson R. (2017) *Five Things I Wish I Had Known as a Young Doctor*. https://tiapana.co.nz/five-things-i-wish-i-had-known-as-a-young-doctor/ (Accessed 12/9/23).

Youngson R. (2019a) *Reclaiming Our Identity as Healers?* https://neuroscienceofhealing.com/reclaiming-our-identity-as-healers/ (Accessed 12/9/23).

Youngson R. (2019b) *A (draft) Healers' Creed*, https://tiapana.co.nz/a-draft-healers-creed/ (Accessed 12/9/23).

Zolnierek K.B, Dimatteo M.R. (2009) Physician Communication and Patient Adherence to Treatment: *A Meta-Analysis. Medical Care*, 47(8): 826–34.

Why is compassionate care challenging and how can I overcome these challenges?

- Introduction
- Discussion – main points and evidence with case studies, exercises, aide mémoires and questions

  - What are the potential challenges to compassionate care?
  - Effective use of resources and the impact of compassion on organisations
  - What can we do to create a more compassionate culture in our care environments?
  - How can we focus on our individual attitude in relation to compassionate care in our team?
  - Am I suffering from burnout and how can I recognise this in myself and others?
  - What can I do if I do not feel compassionate towards someone, or colleagues are not demonstrating compassion?

- Recommendations for leadership as individual practitioners, leaders and organisations

  - Focusing on compassionate care as individual practitioners and leaders
  - Focusing on compassionate care as organisations

INTRODUCTION

This chapter will initially focus on the challenges of compassion in relation to resourcing, culture and individual practice. Next, it discusses compassion burnout and how we can identify this in ourselves and others. It will then focus on what we can do if we do not feel compassionate towards others, and what can we do about colleagues who are not showing compassion. Finally, it will discuss strategies to move forward as individuals and leaders. The culture of every organisation, and every team, is crucial to compassionate care, and the chapter will focus on organisational strategies to prevent, ameliorate and address burnout and increase compassionate care. Strategies for us as individuals and leaders, and for the organisations where we work, will be revisited at the end of each chapter throughout the whole book. Compassion burnout and strategies to mitigate against this will also be discussed in detail in Chapter 3.

DISCUSSION

Case study 2.1

Justin's intuitive and sensitive approach to ensuring that the qualified nurse was able to talk to a patient and his wife separately

Justin was in his second year community placement with a district nursing team and this was a totally different experience to his other hospital-based placements. He was enjoying his time in the team and it was very busy. He could not understand why his hospital-based colleagues seemed to think that nothing happened in the community. They appeared to think that care needs in the community were relatively minor and that community nurses just sat drinking tea all day. This was not his experience at all, and he loved the busyness of each day. He also enjoyed the diversity of patient care. Some patients were only seen once and it was so important to realise that it was a privilege to be welcomed into their homes, and that you were a guest. You might be the only person that they saw that day so it was important to make the most of the time you had to create a meaningful encounter where the patient felt valued and cared for. However, in other cases there was the opportunity to develop ongoing relationships with patients and their families, and have more continuity of care. He had felt from the start that he should do all that he could to learn from practitioners and patients, and to learn new skills, and that his community experiences would help him in his hospital-based care too. However, he soon found that he really wanted to work in district nursing when he was qualified.

At the review meeting with Liz his practice assessor and his practice tutor he explained why he found district nursing work so interesting and enjoyable. To his surprise his practice assessor said how unusual it was to have a student like him in the team. She explained that students were more likely to watch care being carried out, and not take much of an active part in what was taking place. Whereas just that morning she had been so impressed with how he had supported her in a distressing situation with a couple she was visiting.

Sanjeev had not needed care for very long, but it was clear that he was nearing the end of his life. His pain had escalated and Liz needed to discuss this with him. His wife Bel was very distressed as well. As Liz started to talk to Sanjeev, Justin asked Bel how she was managing, and asked about their children. Bel took him into another room to show him pictures of their grandchildren, and Justin could see how proud she was of how they were doing in school and in their dancing and judo. She also talked about their children, and how close Sanjeev and her were to them. Justin could hear Liz talking quietly to Sanjeev and when she came into the room Justin pointed to the photos and explained who they were. As Liz started to speak to Bel, and ask how she was, Justin went back into the room with Sanjeev and said what lovely grandchildren he had. Sanjeev said how sad he would be to leave them and his eyes filled up with tears. Justin held his arm and they talked about his life. He heard Liz and Bel come back into the room and Liz reassured them that she would be discussing increasing his analgesia with his GP. They left the house and both Sanjeev and Bel appeared to be reassured that Liz had taken his escalating pain so seriously.

Liz said that she had never had a student who had taken such a proactive role in helping her to have time alone with both a patient and his loved one, and that Justin had seamlessly swapped from talking to Bel to talking to Sanjeev. This had taken a great deal of advanced communication skills and empathy, but also intuitive knowing of what Liz needed from him, in order to facilitate the sensitive discussions with them both.

Justin felt reassured about his level of communication skills and his ability to be supportive of colleagues in a situation which was new to him. He had felt uncertain of Liz's expectations of him, and of his role in the visit. However, he knew that he wanted to help and to make sure that they both had the opportunity to discuss their individual concerns with Liz. He had felt quite challenged by being there and felt as if he could be intruding on their very personal distressing situation, so he was very pleased to hear that his presence there had been so helpful.

What are the potential challenges to compassionate care?

We have discussed already the fact that compassionate care can be challenging in health care but it is useful to try to identify the different challenges that can be factors in providing compassionate care. A previous book (Chambers and Ryder, 2012) identified three potential barriers (Figure 2.1):

- Resourcing
- Culture of the organisation
- Individual attitude.

The case study above clearly demonstrates how a student's presence in the interaction enabled care to be carried out in a way that was helpful to another member of the team, as well as to Bel and Sangeev. Justin was a clear asset to the team because his instinctive wish to make a very challenging situation easier enabled him to see that spending time with Bel, so that Liz could talk to Sangeev alone, allowed Liz to have a different kind of discussion with Sanjeev. This was also then possible in her interaction with Bel because Justin was talking to Sanjeev at that point. Many students would not have had the confidence to take the initiative in the way that Justin did, but the fact that he did this enabled Liz to maximise her time and clear excellent practice, for the benefit of the couple. Firstly, in terms of resourcing, time is always short in health care practice, and this is very true of community nursing and district nursing practice. Because of Justin's actions Liz's time was used to best effect for all involved. Secondly, the culture of the team was one that encouraged students to take the initiative and act as one of the team, and Justin worked with Liz to ensure that compassionate care was central to this visit. Finally, Justin's individual attitude to care meant that he could see the distress that the couple were experiencing, and he was able to work out what might be most helpful to Liz so that her expertise and compassionate approach were used to best effect. Justin is now working as a qualified nurse in this district nursing team. He is very much enjoying his role and is a real asset to the team. This is just one example of how the challenges health care practitioners face in carrying out best practice can be overcome in relation to the three challenges we have highlighted (Figure 2.1), and these will each be discussed separately.

Effective use of resources and the impact of compassion on organisations

It is clear that resource constraints are a genuine problem in health care today. However, in many situations there is no greater staffing in the practice areas where care is good than in care environments where patients do not feel cared for. So, what is it that makes the difference between the different care environments? The boxes below identify the potential challenges that arise in relation to resourcing, and some strategies that might be helpful for us to address these challenges.

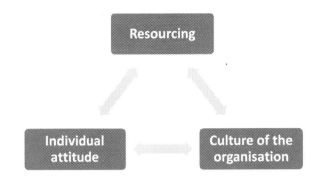

Figure 2.1 Potential barriers to compassion

Aide Mémoire

The impact and challenges of resource issues on provision of care

- Resource constraints
- Inadequate staffing levels
- Limited time to build relationships
- Fragmentation of care provided by different individuals
- Lack of continuity of care
- Lack of opportunity to build relationships with patients
- Too much focus on outcomes and targets
- Increased technology
- Nurses feeling "too busy to care".
- Too much focus on what can be cured, to the detriment of those who need care (Chambers and Ryder, 2009).

Therefore, as health care practitioners we need to:

- Challenge inadequate resources when they impact on care or ourselves.
- Understand that we could always benefit from greater resources.
- Maximise the use of available resources.
- Focus on the quality of care that we provide, and not just the quantity of tasks that we carry out.
- Focus on what patients and clients actually value.
- Consider lean thinking principles, where appropriate, to focus on constant quality improvement measures to eliminate waste.
- Focus on person-centred care.
- Ensure that there is continuity of care whenever possible.
- Maximise the specific skills of different members of the multidisciplinary team.
- Understand that time and professional expertise are key resources.
- Make the most of technological time to communicate positively.
- Minimise interruptions where possible to ensure that tasks are completed as fast as possible, which frees up time and minimises mistakes, which are distressing and time consuming.

- Improve the quality of care with systematic approaches that make the most of the time and resources available.
- Keep administrative tasks containable.
- Reduce the emphasis on targets, outcomes and task to time ratios.
- Do not use the nursing "minute" by saying that we will be back in a "minute".
- Ensure that all practitioners take a leadership role, however junior their position, because their ideas could really take practice forward.
- Increase opportunities for students and more junior members of the team to share their thoughts.
- Keep our motivation alive.

Focusing on what patients actually value is important. It could be that from their perspective little things that do not take much time to carry out could have a great impact on their experience of care. For example, while nursing staff are washing their hands, or preparing to carry out care, some words of comfort, or just talking to a patient, could make the difference between someone feeling cared about, rather than just being treated as just one more patient.

Lean thinking is a controversial issue. This involves focusing on reducing what would not be missed. Maybe much of the care that is provided would not be missed by patients, and would not result in any increase in risk or health needs either. Womack and Jones (2003) say that lean thinking combines adapting to change with continual improvement and elimination of waste. We need to think about the least wasteful way to provide what our patients and clients want. A great deal of time and resources can be spent on things that the client or patient does not even know about, does not value and would not miss. However, lean thinking is not necessarily an approach which is helpful in health care at all because it comes from the world of manufacturing and production line type practices, rather than from a person-centred care environment.

Having a focus on targets, and tick box driven approaches, can create additional stress for practitioners, and have a major impact on the morale and motivation of those who work in care environments (Mehri, 2006) and students can witness this in their placements. Kelly (2013) makes a really valuable point when he says:

> lean's relentless pursuit of the more obvious "added value" components of care can risk eliminating the hidden "added value" of high level interpersonal person-centred care. For example, lean thinkers might say that time is being "wasted" on the subtle nuances and everyday interactions that benefit patients (p 17).

So again, it is really important to ascertain what genuinely matters to patients and clients, rather than merely making incorrect assumptions about what matters to them. However, it could be said that lean thinking and person-centred care are so much at odds with each other that no health care service should be even thinking that lean principles apply to patient or client care. Winch and Henderson (2009) say that applying lean strategies in health care settings creates a tension between health care provision and protection of the patient. Kitwood (1997) also says that that even thinking about human services in the same way as manufacturing services is a travesty. Although I would fundamentally agree with these points, I would suggest that if lean principles were applied in a way that genuinely focused on what patients value this approach could maximise overstretched resources so that they could be used to best effect.

Continuity of care is really important when someone is feeling vulnerable, and this should be prioritised whenever possible. However, making effective use of different members of the team is also important to make the best use of the resources which are available. Focusing on continually improving care also keeps people's motivation alive and this is really important for staff morale. We need to understand that time and professional expertise are key resources and that we need to use these appropriately. However, if we make the best use of technological time, or time when we are carrying out tasks, to communicate with patients, they will feel much more positive about the care experience and more nurtured as a result. Many nurses use the nursing "minute" in a way that can cause distress. If a nurse says that they are coming back in a "minute" and do not return for an hour, or not at all, it makes patients feel vulnerable and unsafe. Health care practitioners also need to use the resources that they do have to best effect by using strategies like productive wards to make best use of their time. The Productive Ward initiative in the UK (www.institute.nhs.uk) has tried to empower staff to improve the quality of care in their environments by systematic approaches that make the most of the time that they have available, and the resources that they have at their disposal. This approach ensures that interruptions are kept to a minimum and tasks like drug rounds and writing patient notes can be carried out as quickly as possible. This also minimises the risks of mistakes and frees up staff more quickly to carry out more patient care. Keeping administrative tasks containable is important, as is reducing the emphasis on targets, outcomes and task to time ratios. It is important that all practitioners take a leadership role, however junior their position, because their ideas could really take practice forward. So, we need to increase opportunities for students and more junior members of the team to share their thoughts, so that they feel valued and important members of the ward team, and that their ideas will be taken seriously. When this is the case and they are listened to, this can create the impetus for other members of the team to see that small changes can result in patients feeling much happier with their care.

Patients feeling much happier with their care makes a real difference in terms of making the best use of limited resources. Redelmeier et al (1995) found that homeless adults often left the Emergency Department in Toronto feeling dissatisfied with their care and were more likely to return more often. In this study these homeless patients averaged seven visits a year, with a third making another two visits within two days of each other. When compassionate contact with trained volunteers was offered there was a reduction of a third return visit in comparison with the control group. The compassionate care involved giving them food and drink and time to talk about their challenges and experiences at other hospitals. This resulted in not only a higher quality of care but less resources used in return visits.

Having too few nurses and lower patient-staff ratios is associated with more negative interactions with patients, even if the numbers of staff are increased with larger numbers of health care assistants. Having more unqualified carers only helps if there are enough qualified nurses to supervise them. If there are insufficient qualified nurses to deliver care and supervise colleagues then this sets staff up to fail and for patients to receive sub-standard care (Bridges et al, 2019).

We also need to move away from, and challenge, stereotypical, dehumanising and judgemental terminology. For example, when we define someone in terms of their health issues, we depersonalise them. So, Ken Smith is not merely "a diabetic" but a man with a life and hopes and dreams. He is not just a task either or "the leg ulcer dressing in bed 4" and describing him as such reduces him to just one item on a "to do" list. We also need to challenge the use of the term "compliance" and "non-compliance" which are common terms in health care today. We do not want our patients to merely comply with our wishes and our professional opinions. We are aiming for relationships with our patients to be based on genuine understanding, partnership and concordance, not on blind and uncompromising obedience. Using the term compliance is bad enough, but non-compliance has very judgemental undertones.

Case Study 2.2

Elaine's focus on empowerment and concordance

Elaine had just come back to her second year placement on the medical ward after a couple of days off and at handover she heard that Bill was "non-compliant" in relation to restricting his fluids. Bill had developed some concerning symptoms which pointed to the fact that his kidneys were struggling to cope and the medical team had recommended that he restrict his fluid intake. He had become more breathless and his legs were oedematous. Restricting his fluids would reduce his symptoms and decrease the load on his kidneys and other vital organs. Elaine questioned why Bill was not following this advice and nobody seemed to know why.

An hour later Elaine approached Bill. She had assessed the needs of her other patients and everyone seemed to be stable and many had visitors at their bedside. Bill did appear to be more breathless than he had been a few days ago. She asked him how he was feeling and he said that he was not feeling well and he was finding it more difficult to breathe. She started to discuss the possible reasons for this and how his kidneys were struggling, and he looked interested in what she had to say. He said that he hated feeling this way and his grandson was going to be visiting at the weekend and he did not want to worry him. Having found out that he wanted to feel better, and not worry those he loved, she started to explain the part that fluids played in how he felt. He suddenly seemed to realise that something that had been said by the registrar about fluid intake could be relevant here. She agreed that this was why he had been advised to reduce his fluids. Bill said that it did not mean much to him in terms of amounts so she used his water jug to explain how all fluids needed to be taken into account, including soup, tea, coffee, milk in his cereal, yoghurt and ice cream. Starting with a full jug which was the amount of fluids he should have per day she explained that each time he had food or fluids he should remove the same amount from his jug so that he knew how much he had left for the day.

Bill looked as if he was taking on board how best to do this so Elaine asked him which fluids were particularly important for him each day. Together, they wrote a list of what he liked to drink and he decided not to have soup because this was less important to him, and that he would reduce his salt intake too. When he had decided what he would like to drink in the 24-hour period he changed his food choices for the following day and they worked out what he had already had to drink that day. Elaine explained that it would be good for the housekeeping staff to know what he was planning and he was happy for her to discuss this with them. Elaine approached the member of the housekeeping team who covered Bill's bay and they discussed his specific needs with her together.

Bill thanked Elaine for taking the time to explain why lower fluids were important and how he could manage this in his day-to-day life and by the time her shift finished she could see that he was following through on his plan. At handover she explained to the rest of the team what Bill was planning to do and she explained that he had had no idea of what restricting his fluids meant, why this was important and how he could go about this. So, he was not being "non-compliant" because he had never agreed to reduce his fluids or understood the importance of this for his health and symptoms. Bill had also not understood what he needed to do to make this possible. Mike, the charge nurse encouraged her to explain the importance of not labelling patients as non-compliant and she explained to other students who were at the handover that non-compliance is not a positive term and that a concordant understanding could only be based on a patient's understanding and agreement. She could see how other members of the team were starting to see that their assumptions were incorrect, and Mike used this opportunity as charge nurse to encourage ward staff not to use the term compliance in the future, and to try to find out the reasons why patients were not able to make positive health changes in their lives.

This case study from one of my students clearly demonstrates how judgemental terminology, like non-compliance, could prevent health care practitioners from having health enhancing conversations and this can detract from partnership orientated relationships between staff and patients. I feel that compliance is a term that should never be used in health care, though it is so often used. There are situations where patients are in prison or being detained under the Mental Health Act (CQC, 2018) where they have no choice but to comply. However, in other situations they can, and do, make their own life choices, and they have a right to do so. Using persuasive discussion and focusing on what motivates them has the greatest chance of success. Motivational interviewing is based on expressing empathy through reflective listening and avoiding argument and direct confrontation. It helps to help the patient to understand the discrepancy between their goals, values, motivations and intentions and their current behaviour. Therefore, this approach helps to adjust their thinking and behaviour, rather than opposing their actions and behaviour. This in turn increases their self-efficacy and optimism. Motivational interviewing is effective in behaviour change and works on the principles that a person's ambivalence to change is normal and that all of us vary in our readiness to change (Miller and Rollnick, 2002 and 2012). The theoretical underpinnings of motivational interviewing can help us to understand how to use motivational interviewing to increase healthy behaviour and focus on a person's own motivations and to help stimulate their desire to change. This is a very effective use of resourcing and health practitioner's time, so it is helpful to base our discussions on the stage of change they are at and using change talk strategies, and the principles of RULE, PACE and OARS (Haque and D'Souza, 2019 and Hall et al, 2012) can be really effective. (Table 2.1). Elaine, in her case study, was focusing on Bill's motivations and trying to help him channel these to help him to reduce his fluid intake. The more that a person defends their poor health choices, the less likely they are to make changes in the future, and the more disempowered and dispirited they become. Elaine's discursive, empathetic and non-judgemental approach was a really good use of time and Bill would have been able to return home more quickly and maybe have fewer hospital admissions in the future.

I have created the following aide mémoire to help to maximise our resources and our ability to provide compassionate care and have created a visual representation (Figure 2.2) of attitudes and actions which help us to achieve this.

Table 2.1 Motivational interviewing approaches

Stages of Change and Intention to Change (change talk)	RULE
• Precontemplation – not ready • Contemplation – getting ready • Preparation – ready • Maintenance – sticking to it • Relapse – learning (Prochaska and DiClemente, 1986) Change talk: • Disadvantages of the status quo • Advantages of change • Optimism for change • Intention to change (Hall et al, 2012)	• **R**esist the righting reflex – resist making suggestions • **U**nderstand the person's motivations to encourage discussions on their motivations • **L**isten – patient-centred and empathetic • **E**mpower – to be in control over their actions and feel a desire to change and take steps towards that change
PACE	OARS
• **P**artnership/collaboration • **A**cceptance, absolute worth, affirmation– non-judgemental • **C**ompassion and empathy towards the person's struggles and experiences – never punitive • **E**vocative – strong feelings and emotions High empathy = High positive outcomes	• **O**pen ended questions • **A**ffirmation of positive traits • **R**eflective • **S**ummaries – of experiences to encourage more exploration of their behaviour

Aide Mémoire

Maximising resources

- See time and professional expertise as key resources and focus on how to use these as wisely as possible.
- Make the best use of time and use time with patients to focus on communication.
- Focus on what patients want and reduce what would not be missed.
- Be caring and non-judgemental and avoid judgemental and dehumanising terminology for example non-compliance or the "diabetic in bed 1". Terminology like this can alienate patients who then feel devalued and unsupported. They are then less likely to make positive life changes which maximise their health potential. Using motivational interviewing strategies can be highly effective in maximising time and the impact of health conversations.
- Communicate effectively but in shorter times (Brief, Ordinary, Effective (Wigens, 2006) and Solution Focused Brief Therapy (Berg, 2003) (*see next section on culture*).
- Use bottom-up resources to change management in relation to the best use of resources. So, encourage ideas and leadership from more junior members of the team.
- Use emotional intelligence to improve team dynamics and keep others positive, because this tends to create a more caring environment which has

a positive impact on staff and patients. Happy staff are more likely to increase positive feelings in patients which in turn can shorten hospital stays and maximise healing. (See *Chapter 5 for more on emotional intelligence).*

- Reduce interpersonal conflict because this takes time away from the patient and increases staff absence and turnover, reduces motivation and leaves staff feeling disempowered. This is a poor use of time and resources. Also happy staff have more chance of experiencing happy patients (See *Chapter 4 for more on conflict management).*

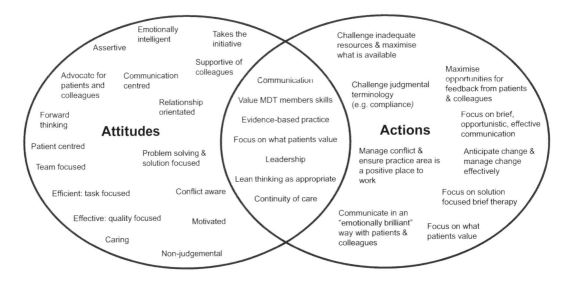

Figure 2.2 Maximising resourcing for compassionate care

Questions to ask yourself

Focusing on resources

- Could your practice area make better use of resources, and could there be greater continuity of care?
- What improvements could you suggest to ensure that resources are used to best effect to maximise compassionate care?
- Can you think of ways to increase the emphasis on quality of care rather than focusing on quantitative measures to assess performance indicators?
- What would patients in your practice area identify as their priorities for nursing care? Can you think of ways to focus on these areas more strongly?
- Can you think of ways in which judgemental or stereotypical terminology could be challenged in your placement area?
- How could you encourage patients to make effective changes in their lives through a motivational interviewing approach?
- How can you positively challenge members of your team to take a motivational interviewing approach?
- Think about creating an action plan to move forward in relation to maximising resources and compassionate care in your placement area.

This section focused on the first challenge to compassionate care, namely inadequate resourcing, and challenged how we could make the best use of the resources that we do have, such as our time. The next challenge is the culture of practice environments, and how this could be used to best effect to increase compassionate care.

What can we do to create a more compassionate culture in our care environments?

We know that wards, units or services with the same resources can feel very different in relation to how compassionate the environment feels. As a tutor visiting different care environments, I find that it is possible to sense how a ward or hospital feels within a few seconds of being there. Various senses can be involved in this assessment. What do I hear people saying, what visual cues can I see, is there any noticeable smell of food, urine, mustiness? Does a member of staff look up from what they are doing, do they appear welcoming? In one hospital I visit all members of staff will approach someone who looks lost and ask if they can help. I had given an elderly neighbour a lift to visit a friend, when I was visiting a student, and a phlebotomist asked if she was lost and then said that she was going that way and that she would take her to the ward she needed. This member of staff was undoubtedly busy but she took a caring approach and helped my neighbour to find the ward that she needed. I have seen this happen many times and staff seem to take responsibility for helping visitors to their hospital, rather than just continuing on their way. In other care environments this would not happen, and staff are no less busy. At this hospital it seems like everyone, including catering and portering staff and professional health care staff, have a pride in where they work and want to help. The culture of a care environment, and how it feels, makes a massive difference to how caring somewhere feels. This can come from senior management at the top or could be just absorbed from seeing how others behave. Either way, it is very effective in helping people feel good about the environment. Again, the following boxes highlight the challenges a negative culture can have, and the strategies that can be helpful in addressing these.

Aide Mémoire

The impact and challenges of culture on provision of care

- Stereotyping people and acceptance of non-inclusive and judgemental attitudes.
- Cultural norms and values misunderstood.
- Culture of the environment does not support sensitive approaches.
- Lack of leadership focusing on compassion.
- Inappropriately high focus on outcomes and task-centred approaches.

Therefore as health care practitioners we need to:

- Take a lead in promoting a positive culture.
- Challenge poor practice in a supportive and developmental manner.
- Promote a positive team environment and good team dynamics.
- Encourage feedback from patients and others.
- Work in partnership with our patients and colleagues.
- Focus on enhancing our provision and recognise that we are in a competitive and commissioned environment.
- Make change a personal mission.

Where there is a culture of judgement, and people are stigmatised and criticised, this impacts on the team morale and patient care. If there is a happy team of staff patients are also more likely to feel valued and accepted and their health outcomes are better, as discussed before. Empathetic and sensitive practice has to be encouraged from the top. There needs to be strong leadership and staff will then feel that poor standards are unacceptable, and that they can challenge care that is sub optimal. There needs to be a focus on understanding the norms and values of a diverse range of patients and on quality of care, rather than more quantifiable outcomes and targets. Many services are assessed in terms of patient feedback, whether the service is commissioned or not, and many care decisions are played out on the front pages of newspapers and on social media. We need to understand that if we are not part of the solution, then we are potentially part of the problem and need to initiate and promote change whenever it is needed.

Crawford et al (2014) talk about different ways in which the culture can be "warmed up" and suggests the BOE model for health care communication (Crawford et al 2006). BOE stands for **brief, ordinary and effective and it focuses on building therapeutic communication** in an environment where time is limited. This model of communication combines non-verbal communication such as eye contact, touching and smiling, with respectful and valuing comments, the appropriate use of questioning and clarifying, and confirming points. This can be carried out even in very complex situations, and in fact is even more important in these situations. Crawford et al (2006) also say that **creating more "hominess"** in the clinical environment, whereby more comforts of the home environment are introduced, can be helpful. With the emphasis on infection control this might create challenges in many health care environments, and sometimes the perceived evidence base can discourage these practices, and yet the evidence is not sufficient to support excluding these homely touches from a clinical environment. Initiatives such as the **Schwartz Centre rounds** (Schwartz 1995), could also have a positive impact because they allow practitioners to discuss the emotional impact of challenging patient and client situations with each other. This can have a normalising effect and creates a more compassionate culture within any care environment. Sometimes a care environment could benefit from some of these approaches, but the person making the suggestions might not have the influence to make these possible. In that case they could introduce these thoughts into discussions at team meetings, because it is likely that a higher level intervention would be required to create this degree of organisational change. Compassion burnout and the importance of a positive culture will be discussed in detail in Chapter 3.

Cole-King and Gilbert (2011) have defined key attributes necessary for engaging with, and understanding suffering: These are:

- Motivation – being committed to being caring and supportive to others
- Sensitivity – noticing when others need help
- Sympathy – being moved by another's distress
- Distress tolerance – ability to be with others in their distress without being overwhelmed by it
- Empathy – understanding another's needs even when the person themselves might be unaware of them
- Non-judgement – accepting and validating another's distress and pain, rather than judging them for it.

Again, many practitioners could benefit from thinking about their practice in this way. Education and CPD (Continuing Practice Development) activities focusing on these points might be helpful, as would planned clinical supervision opportunities focusing on these areas of practice. Knight (2011) makes the point when discussing her area of clinical practice as a General Practitioner (GP) that you would not expect a highly tuned and expensive car to carry on operating without regular servicing and repair. In the same way all health care practitioners should be required to service and repair their own practice. However, the emphasis of CPD activities tends to be on specific health care interventions or new systems or management imperatives, rather than on topping up the oil and retuning the engines on the highly experienced and unique aspects of our care provision, namely our humanity and compassion. As Burgess (2015) says "medical treatment should be the servant of genuine human caring, never its master" (p 25). Knight (2011) goes on to say that we have to recognise the fact that we are vulnerable, and that we are not cars or robots and we do need compassion in our lives. We need to demand, prioritise and focus on compassion driven education and discussions, and we need to find ways to be compassionate to ourselves. As Knight (2011) says "to compassionately care for our patients, we need also to compassionately care for ourselves" (p 53), as already discussed in Chapter 1. The next three chapters take this further by focusing on our stress management, resilience, wellbeing and positivity, followed by a discussion of how we can lead on positivity in Chapter 6.

Pamela Wible is a doctor who is a family physician and runs a clinic in Oregon on the west coast of America. She talks about how burnt out she was with the treadmill approach to medicine. She wanted to set up an "ideal clinic", which is one perceived to be that way by patients. Having done just this she is very happy in her work and much happier in herself. She makes the extremely good point that:

> If doctors are victims, patients learn to be victims. If doctors are discouraged, patients learn to be discouraged. If we want happy, healthy patients, why not start by filling our clinics with happy, healthy doctors?
>
> (Wible, 2012, p. 127)

Wible (2012) talks about the difference between professional distance and professional boundaries. This is often discussed in relation to empathy and compassion. Some people feel that in order to provide effective care, and protect ourselves from burnout, that we need to maintain a professional distance. However, if we can live the experience of our patients with empathy and sensitivity, we can walk beside them at their times of need, without becoming completely incapacitated by it. We will go home happy that we have done a good job that day, rather than being unhappy with all that we have not done to alleviate someone's distress. Wible (2012) gives her patients her personal phone number and does not feel that they abuse this. In return she gains happiness in her work. She does not believe in keeping a professional distance, but she does believe in maintaining professional boundaries, and she does not believe that she ever compromises this in her person-centred approach to her family medicine role. In my own way as a tutor I would agree with Wible. I also give my mobile phone number to my students and invite them to text me if they need anything or want to arrange review meetings with practice assessors. I find that they are very respectful of my time and rarely contact me at weekends, and if they do it is because they are working with their assessor and are trying to arrange a meeting. They do not expect me to respond then and are very grateful when I do. They know that I work long hours and am very accessible in the week so they value my weekend time and holidays. Like Wible, I find that increasing my availability does not cause people to abuse this, in fact quite the opposite tends to be true. We can maybe learn from this in relation to differentiating between professional distance and professional boundaries. Also, by really knowing the difference between showing compassion to ourselves and not becoming overwhelmed by people's terrible situations, whilst at the same time allowing ourselves to respond to the privilege we have in having the opportunity to walk alongside people at their darkest times.

NHS England Fifteen Steps Challenge (2017) focuses on the patients' or carers' perspective of care seen through their eyes and, as one family member says, "I can tell what kind of care my daughter is going to get within 15 steps of walking on to any new ward". This is a point that I made earlier, and I would agree with this. The 15 step challenge is a service/quality improvement approach that focuses on "walkarounds" using a "15 steps challenge" team that includes patients; carers; staff; and board members. The team members consider their first impressions of the ward/service from the perspective of a service user, recording how it appears, looks, sounds, smells, etc. Then outcomes can inform improvement actions at a ward/service and organisational level, linking into other relevant initiatives as appropriate. It might be worth considering taking this approach within your practice area and think about what visitors might feel in response to coming into your care environment. You could even ask students to contribute to this assessment because they are often a fresh pair of eyes, and they might come up with some insightful views.

Case Study 2.3

Peter's fears on coming into hospital and how nursing and ward staff alleviated his concerns

Peter had never been in hospital in his life, and he was now 80 and did not want to change this impressive record. However, he had had to agree with his daughter that he was not well, and he had had some investigations and was now waiting to go to theatre.

However, he had been pleasantly surprised to arrive at the ward and they seemed to know who he was and were clearly expecting him. The ward clerk explained how the bed worked and a member of the housekeeping team asked him to choose food for the following day, and she was smiley and knew that he would be having surgery and advised him about the sort of food to choose when he had just had an operation. The student nurse and her staff nurse colleague prepared him for theatre and both were friendly and understood his worries. So really nothing was as he had feared from reading his daily papers, and he started to feel more positive about his hospital stay.

Peter is not unusual in reading negative news items about NHS care and this makes people rightly apprehensive when they need to access any NHS health care. It makes such a difference when health care staff seem positive and want to get to know patients as people. This makes them more able to feel relaxed and confident about the care that they receive. They are then more likely to appear more positive, and this positive mirroring can make nursing staff feel more positive about their role and their care. A patient who is challenging and negative runs the risk of making nursing staff reflect back their negativity. Positive emotions are contagious, as are negative ones, and this results in an upward or downward spiral which impacts on staff, the patient, other patients and the whole team. The following aide mémoire identifies some strategies to encourage a positive culture in our practice areas. It is followed by a focus on attitudes and actions which help to build and maintain a positive and compassionate culture (Figure 2.3).

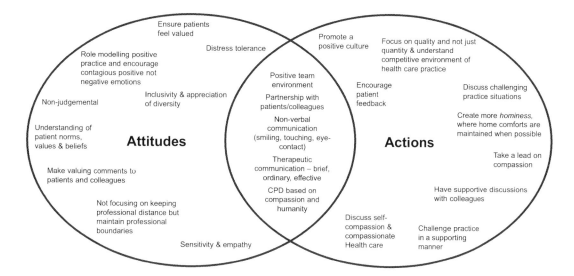

Figure 2.3 Building and maintaining a compassionate culture

Aide Mémoire

Promoting a positive health care culture

- Discuss challenging patient situations and ensure that there is time to debrief from distressing and worrying experiences.
- Be positive, non-judgemental, appreciative and valuing to patients and colleagues.
- Understand that we have an impact on the culture of our practice and this has an effect on others' beliefs and values.
- Avoid being a negative role model because negative mirroring encourages negative spirals of stress and demotivation in patients and colleagues.
- Instead be a positive role model so that positive mirroring of body language and leadership creates upward spirals of motivation.
- Realise that emotions are contagious, so stay as positive as possible and make others feel valued, respected and empowered by giving positive feedback.

Questions to ask yourself

Creating a compassionate health care culture

- Could you take a greater lead on building and encouraging a more compassionate culture within your practice area?
- What improvements could you suggest to ensure that patients feel cared for, cared about and valued in your practice area?
- Can you think of ways to increase the emphasis on quality of care and what patients actually value, rather than focusing on quantitative measures to assess performance indicators?
- Could you take a lead on encouraging self-compassion and encouraging a positive team culture and having more supportive discussions with your colleagues?

- Can you think of ways in which inclusivity, and an appreciation of diversity, and acceptance of different norms and beliefs, could be encouraged in your work area to a greater extent?
- Think about how contagious feelings and emotions actually are. How could you create upward positive spirals and discourage negative downward spirals within your team discussions?
- How can you challenge practice in a supportive and positive manner?

Think about creating an action plan to move forward in relation to building and maintaining a positive culture in your practice area.

The challenge of resourcing in relation to the ability to provide compassionate care has now been discussed, as has how a compassionate and caring culture can enable all members of the team to focus on positivity and excellent compassionate nursing care. The next discussion is on how individuals can focus on their own health care practice and become role models for compassionate care.

How can we focus on our individual attitude in relation to compassionate care in our team?

The discussion has now covered two areas of challenge in relation to compassionate care. First, the ever-present challenge of insufficient resourcing which is a challenge for any aspect of health care delivery. Secondly, the culture which prevails in any practice environment, which has the ability to act as a positive or negative influence on all practitioners who work in that care environment. The next section focuses on the importance of our own individual attitude in relation to compassionate practice. If poor practice is not tolerated and good practice strived for, then each individual health care practitioner is more likely to adhere to that culture. Unfortunately, the opposite is also true, and caring practitioners can become demotivated and disengaged by a negative care culture. In which case they are more likely to reduce their own practice in line with that of others. So, we are now going to focus on the importance of the motivations, standards of care and attitudes that an individual practitioner has, and how this can drive up the care throughout the whole team. An example of this is in the case study below where Annie, one of my students, challenged the approach of a much more senior colleague in the multidisciplinary team. Annie has given her permission for her reflection on this incident to be used here. At the time of the incident Annie was a highly experienced health care assistant but was only in the first week of her practice in the first year of her nursing programme. She was in her base unit of Surgical Outpatients and was with a consultant seeing patients. She could see how a patient was shocked by the response to a question she asked of the consultant and raised this with him after the patient left. From the perspective of later being in the second stage of her programme she rightly questioned her practice in terms of patient advocacy, because she was unable to question this whilst the patient was still in the room. However, it is important to recognise the fact that she was only in the first week of her programme, yet she managed to question the approach that the consultant took. She discussed this using her excellent communication skills in such a way that her medical colleague understood the seriousness of her concern but also asked her to give him feedback after every consultation. Annie is now a qualified nurse and her standards of care remain impressively high.

Case Study 2.4

Annie's reflection on being an advocate for a patient in discussion with a senior medical colleague

As I look back on how I have developed from a new student nurse to a second year student I look back on a reflection I had written in the first few days of my first placement, in my core base. I am surprised how far I have come and so I have decided to reflect on this case study.

During my first few days as a student nurse I was able to sit in on a surgical cancer clinic. A lady, who I shall refer to as Elise for the purpose of this reflection within the code of practice set down by the Nursing and Midwifery Council (2018) "Respect people's right to privacy and confidentiality". Elise was attending a surgical oncology appointment at a local outpatient department. She had had some lesions removed and skin grafts carried out and had presented with another lesion. While talking to the consultant about the planned surgical removal she asked if the growth would be sent off to see if it would develop into cancer. I was somewhat shocked by this question as the patient had had cancerous growths before, and clearly had had previous surgery, so I wondered why she would question the fact that the growth was malignant. The consultant replied that the lesion was cancerous. He proceeded to fill out the consent form for surgery, but I noted the shocked look on the patients face and she became tearful and the colour drained from her face. However, she remained composed, although clearly shocked by the comment. As was her husband whose eyes were darting from me to the consultant and then to his wife.

My instincts were screaming at me to offer comfort and support however I was unsure whether this was an appropriate course of action for a student nurse. So, I remained seated, which made me very uncomfortable, and I felt uncaring which I found very alien to me as a nurse.

When the patient left I felt I needed to raise my concerns to the consultant. I drew on my communication skills and built on my respect for this consultant's extensive experience and asked whether he was aware of the patient's reaction. I explained that I had felt that the patient had not realised that she had had skin cancer in the past, despite her previous treatment and surgery. Up until this consultation maybe the word cancer had not been used and maybe there had been a breakdown in communication. As health care professionals we often forget and use terms that our patients do not fully understand, and they do not always bring their lack of understanding to our attention. The consultant was interested in how I had come to this conclusion and asked me to explain further. I explained my reasoning with him and he seemed interested in what I had to say. He then agreed with my observation and said that this could have happened, although this was rare, and then proceeded to ask me for feedback after each consultation. At the end of the clinic I was given some very encouraging feedback and was told that I had very good observational and communication skills and that I had shown intelligence and I would make a very good nurse.

At the beginning of the day I felt totally out of my depth sitting in a multidisciplinary team meeting with some very experienced and knowledgeable clinicians and I was only a first year student nurse, However, I was given the opportunity to speak to a highly trained member of staff and question what I had felt had been missed, without upsetting or putting the consultant's clinical judgement into question. I gained some valuable feedback that I would use as I went forward in my training.

I was left feeling this was a really good experience for myself as a student nurse as I was able to draw on my communication skills, show that I am respectful to other professionals, but I am also able to question their practice in an effective manner. I was listened to and then asked to give feedback which was a real confidence builder.

I do not think I would do anything differently again except to explore how I could offer comfort and support to a service user within my capacity as a student. I need to explore my professional boundaries more in these situations. As I read this account I realised that I could have spoken out for my patient rather than allow her to leave the clinic without highlighting her reaction to the consultant at the time, as I had done in this case. The NMC Code (2018) states that we need to "recognise when people are anxious and distressed and respond compassionately and politely" If I was in this situation again I would feel more confident to speak up and bring to the attention of the consultant the patients visible confusion so that any misunderstanding could be addressed then. I look back now and I feel that I really let this patient down. When she left the clinic she may have felt confused and frightened and had I spoken out at the time the consultant could have had a more in-depth conversation and addressed her confusion. The NMC Code (2018) also states that "checking peoples" understanding from time to time keeps misunderstandings or mistakes to a minimum.

"The Code contains the professional standards that registered nurses, midwives and nursing associates must uphold". We are advocates for our patients, we must remember that sometimes we may be the only voice who speaks up for an individual in our care. We need to act within their best interest and work to 'keep and uphold the standards and values set out in the NMC Code (2018).

This case study demonstrates how someone in quite a junior role can drive the practice of very senior colleagues if this is carried out in a constructive and positive manner. Annie knows how impressed I was with her practice, and with her permission I have used this scenario, and her practice, as an example with other students. The fact that she has continued to learn from her new perspective as a more senior student is very much to her credit. It is true that she would have been a more effective advocate for her patient now and would have been able to "reflect in action", and not just "on action" after the patient left the room now that she is more experienced. However, she did question a senior medical colleague's practice in a manner that encouraged him to ask for her feedback after every consultation, and this is very impressive. If Annie could do this at such an early point in her nursing career, then we can all learn from this and take a greater lead in ensuring that our patients receive the care they need and deserve.

Molly Case's highly moving and insightful poem "Nursing the nation" was originally published in "Underneath the roses where I remembered everything" (Case, 2015). The full text of the poem is below and Molly has very kindly agreed that we can publish this here in its entirety. If you would like to hear Molly speaking the poem in her extremely powerful and sensitive manner, please access this YouTube clip. (https://www.youtube.com/watch?v=XOCda6OiYpg). Molly's book "How to treat people: A nurse at work" (I always aim to be as person-centred as possible) also gives many examples of her sensitive and compassionate practice. Molly read her poem at the

RCN Conference in 2013 whilst she was still a student nurse, and she makes a very effective point about the negativity with which the media often sees health care practice. She clearly explains how stressful and distressing her role can be, but also how rewarding nursing is. She also answers the critics who say that we are not doing enough, and says that we will do more, but that her care and compassion shines out in every verse of her excellent poem.

Nursing the Nation by Molly Case

> A woman comes in,
> too young to bear this;
> she's got a disease that will make her miss –
> her daughter's wedding day,
> her first grandchild being born,
> How would that feel, to have that all torn
> away from you?
>
> I can't answer that question,
> it's not my place to say,
> but I can tell you what we did for her,
> how we helped her get through the day.
> A cup of tea there and one for all her family,
> as they came, throughout the night,
> what a sight; there were loads of them.
> To help her fight the awful pain of it,
> paying last visits, we wouldn't let them miss it –
> farewell from a brother,
> last kisses with their mother –
> holiest love, love like no other.
>
> Maybe there's bad ones,
> no doubt that there are,
> but for this list I'm writing
> we don't want the same tar-brush,
> crushing our careers before they've even started;
> how could you say this
> about people being so big-hearted?
> Who would have thought we'd be having to defend?
> We don't do this for our families,
> we don't do this for our friends,
> but for strangers.
> Because this is our vocation
> and we're sick and tired
> of being told we don't do enough for this nation.
> So listen to us, hear us goddam roar;
> you say we're not doing enough?
> Then we promise we'll do more.
> This time, next time,
> there's nothing we can't handle,
> even if you bring us down,
> show us scandal, scandal, scandal.

You remember that man covered in burns head to toe?
I don't think you do
'cause you were on that TV show:
lipgloss-kissed women on daytime TV,
come into our world, see things that we see.

One lady, passing, had no relatives to stay.
We sang her to sleep, let angels take her away.
Were you there that day when we held her hand?
Told her nothing would harm her,
that there was a higher plan.
Saw her face as she remembered a faith she'd once held,
watched her breath in the room as she finally exhaled.

Why don't you meet us? Come, shake our hands.
Try to fit in between having tea with your fans.
Your hands are so soft and mine are cracked.
Why don't you let us on air?
Let us air the facts.

We've washed and shrouded people
that we've never known,
pinned flowers to the sheet
and told them they're still not alone.
Shown families to the faith room
and watched them mourn their dead,
then got back to work, bathed patients, made beds.

Hindus, Muslims, Jews and Sikhs,
Buddhists and Christians and just people off the street,
we've cared for them all and we love what we do,
we don't want a medal, we just want to show you.
So listen to us, hear us goddam roar;
you say we're not doing enough?
Then we promise we'll do more.

These highly positive examples of excellent practice, demonstrated in both Annie's case study and Molly's poem, should inspire us to be the best health care practitioners that we can be. Watson (2018 and 2020) also writes about examples of nursing practice which focus on compassion and kindness, and they are also very accessible books to read if you are interested in looking into this further. So, the discussion now focuses on the potential challenges to a positive compassionate attitude for individual practitioners, before going on to discuss what strategies can be used to address these.

As health care practitioners working in stressful situations, often with inadequate resources, we can take on board the stress of the people we are caring for and feel emotionally pressured by this. We can worry about not being able to provide the service that we want to, and this can translate into inappropriate attitudes, such as blaming the people in our care, using inappropriate humour and distancing ourselves from those in our care. We could also perhaps respond with less empathy and less sensitivity than we might do normally. We can then justify this by focusing on tasks to be carried out and the science of what we need to do, rather than the art of nursing in terms of how these actions could be carried out with greater sensitivity and compassion. I have summed up these points in the box below.

Aide Mémoire

The challenges for individual practitioners in relation to compassionate care

- Stress and anxiety
- Emotional overload
- Distancing ourselves
- Insensitive care
- Judgemental attitudes
- Poor use of humour
- Moral distress of not being able to give as good a service as we would want
- Lack of empathy.
- Lack of focus on the art of nursing (and not just the science)

However, I feel that practising in a purely task centred way demeans us as individuals and as health care practitioners. In order for us to be as effective as possible in relation to compassionate care we need to focus strongly on our emotional intelligence. This involves self-awareness and self-management and relationship awareness and relationship management. So, we need to understand our own emotions, and those of others (Goleman et al, 2002) in order to effectively manage our emotions and our interactions with patients and colleagues. When emotions and stress levels rise we need to maximise our emotional intelligence and demonstrate "emotional brilliance" (Goleman, 1996). When our ability to cope is most threatened we particularly need to ensure that we are relating to others at the peak of our emotional intelligence. We need to be as personally effective as possible and Thompson (2009) says that we need to be self-aware and manage our time, information and our stress as well as possible. We also need to be assertive and be effective advocates for our patients and think in creative yet realistic ways. We need to ensure that we state our opinions and views in a way that is acceptable to patients and colleagues, so that we are not perceived as using bullying or harassing strategies. We also need to ensure that we make best use of supervision and continuous professional development (CPD) opportunities to maximise our personal effectiveness.

We have many types of intelligences at our disposal and Furnham (2008) sums these up:

- Intelligence quotient (IQ) which involves processing information, a good memory and the ability to learn.
- Technical/Operational quotient (TQ) which involves our ability to manage ideas and projects, understand relevant technology and generally get things done.
- Motivational quotient (MQ) knowing where we want to achieve, lead and succeed.
- Experience quotient (XQ) which relates to the quality and quantity of our experience.
- People quotient (PQ) which relates to our self-awareness and self-management including knowing our motives, emotions, actions and the impact of these on others.

- Learning quotient (LQ) which involves our ability to think, manage and solve problems in different ways (Furnham, 2008, pp9–10).

I would also add another intelligence (Chambers and Ryder, 2012, p112):

- Cultural intelligence (CQ) which involves the ability to adapt to new cultural contexts and acquire new ways to deal with new situations (Gudykunst and Hammer 1983, cited in Berry et al, 2011).

The importance of cultural competence will be discussed in greater detail in Chapter 5. We need to ensure that we use all the resources at our disposal from a personal point of view in order to relate to others as effectively and compassionately as possible when so much is being expected from us in our professional roles and our relationships with others.

The questions below are designed to help you to identify where your positive strategies already lie, or where they could be enhanced further.

Questions to ask yourself

Enhancing your personal effectiveness as a compassionate practitioner.

- Do you need to revisit your communication skills and express more empathy and be more sensitive to the needs of patients and colleagues?
- Could you do more to support colleagues who are finding it difficult to cope? If so, what could you do differently?
- Do you always challenge insensitive care and judgemental attitudes? If not, what stops you and could you be more assertive and a better advocate for those in your care?
- Have you thought about asking others for feedback on your compassionate care behaviour and standards in practice?
- Do you ever pass on your stress to patients or colleagues? When does this happen and could you change how you behave under pressure?
- Could you focus on an individual patient and think about how to build a supportive relationship, however brief your time with them? How do you make this happen and could you teach this to others? If so, how could you do this?
- Do you ever compare yourself to others who appear to practice less well to justify when you know you could have related better to others in a recent situation? Can you take steps to change this?
- Can you identify times of positive communication strategies and compassionate communication with colleagues as well as patients? What can you learn from this?
- Thinking about your emotional intelligence, what sort of situations need you to be "emotionally brilliant". What would this look like and how could you help others to emulate this?
- Could you be more personally effective in relation to your:
  - Self-awareness
  - Time management
  - How you deal with information
  - Assertiveness
  - Putting pressure on others and being "too strong" with them

- ○ Being a better advocate for others
- ○ Being more creative and problem solving
- ○ Being more realistic in terms of work pressures
- ○ Accessing more CPD opportunities
- ○ Taking part in supervision

- • Could you put your different intelligences to better use?

    - ○ Using your intelligence quotient
    - ○ Being more emotionally intelligent
    - ○ Being more technologically or operationally intelligent
    - ○ Using your motivational quotient more
    - ○ Putting all your experience to better use
    - ○ Being more intelligent in relation to people
    - ○ Becoming more learning intelligent
    - ○ Being more aware of cultural issues and change

I have summed up the attitudes and actions that I believe are necessary to maximise our strategies in relation to compassionate care as individual practitioners (Figure 2.4).

The challenges of compassionate practice have now been discussed, in relation to resources, the culture of our workplace and our own personal attitude. This can be summed up in the diagram below (Figure 2.5) and we need to focus on positive principles and actions in relation to these areas of challenge, as discussed in this chapter. If we follow these principles and actions through, we can genuinely take a lead in promoting excellence in our practice environments (Chambers and Ryder, 2012).

Am I suffering from burnout and how can I recognise this in myself and others?

The challenges of resourcing, culture of our practice environment and our own attitude to compassionate practice have already been discussed, as well as the importance of taking a lead on this in our practice areas. However, there are concerns

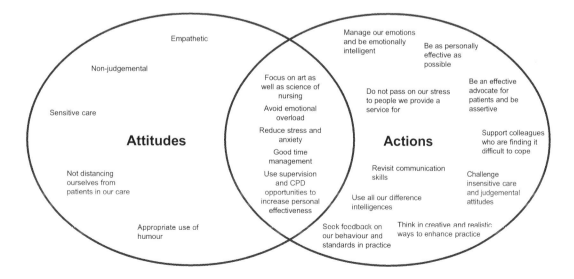

Figure 2.4 Enhancing our compassionate care attitude as individual practitioners

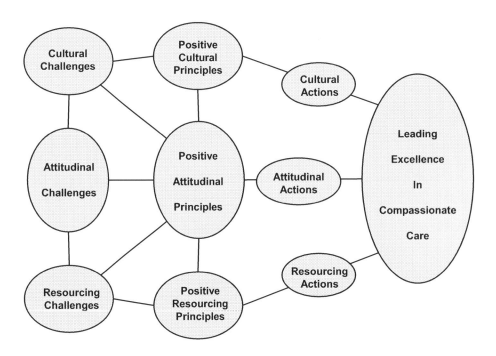

Figure 2.5 Key contributors to leading excellence in compassion

about the extent to which we, or our colleagues, could be suffering from compassion burnout. There is no doubt that caring for others at home and at work can potentially increase our stress levels, and we will now discuss the symptoms of compassion fatigue and burnout and how this can be manifested in our health care practice.

I want to make several points in relation to sympathetic distress and how this differs from compassion fatigue:

- Sympathy can be painful because we can become secondary victims in relation to another person's distress.
- Over time we can become sad, angry and fearful and can become distressed ourselves.
- We can then want to isolate ourselves and avoid contact with others.
- We can then become unable to connect with our patients and clients and can become overwhelmed.
- Compassion, on the other hand, means that we do not overidentify with the pain of others. We feel positive caring emotions and are motivated to help.
- Compassion builds resilience and strength and an increased capacity to care and we do not then become worn out and burnt out.

Symptoms of compassion fatigue can be similar to signs of stress (Lombardo and Eyre, 2011).

Work related and physical symptoms:

- Avoidance or dread of working with particular patients/clients
- Less empathy towards patients/clients
- Frequent sick time
- Lack of joyfulness
- Headaches and muscle tension

- Digestive problems
- Sleep disturbances and fatigue
- Cardiac symptoms.

Emotional symptoms:

- Mood swings
- Restlessness
- Irritability and oversensitivity
- Anxiety
- Depression
- Excessive use of substances
- Anger and resentment
- Intrusive thoughts
- Sleep problems
- Loss of objectivity
- Memory issues
- Poor concentration, focus and judgement.

Slatten et al (2011) make the point that many practitioners feel compassion satisfaction when dealing with people in need, which acts as a cushion and enables us not to suffer from compassion fatigue. However, compassion fatigue occurs when dealing with the traumatic experiences of patients and this can develop fast. Burnout develops over a longer period of time and occurs when people are working in organisational environments which are unhelpful and stressful. Skovholt and Trotter-Mathison (2016) say that burnout is a profound weariness which can incorporate feelings of "fatigue, frustration, disengagement, stress, depletion, helplessness, hopelessness, emotional drain, emotional exhaustion and cynicism" (p 103). Slatten et al (2011) state that management strategies would therefore vary between both situations. With compassion fatigue, managers would focus on changing where the practitioner is working, clinical supervision, mentoring and CPD opportunities and trying to create a compassionate organisational culture. When burnout is prevalent managers need to focus more on endemic and chronic organisational problems.

Skovholt and Trotter-Mathison (2016) differentiate between *meaning burnout* and *caring burnout*. Meaning burnout occurs when the real meaning of the work that you do, and what attracted you to your professional role at the start disappears, and without this meaning the purpose for the work has gone. Another form of meaning burnout occurs when we think that the work we do is no longer beneficial to the people we work with. Caring burnout focuses particularly on the relationships and attachments we have with patients in our care. When we detach from specific patients, and form new relationships with others, this can deplete us, and if this deficit is too great we can find it difficult to summon up the energy to form new relationships. So, too fast a turnover of patients in our care and a lack of continuity of care can have an impact on our ability to care.

In my previous writing (Chambers and Ryder, 2012) I have identified unhelpful attitudes and behaviours that practitioners can demonstrate:

- Stress and anxiety
- Being judgemental
- Insensitive care

- Emotional overload
- Distancing ourselves from the patient in our care
- Poor sense of humour
- Personal moral or emotional distress
- Lack of empathy
- Overemphasis on the science of our practice and insufficient emphasis on the art of our practice (Chambers and Ryder, 2012, p144).

Skovholt and Trotter-Mathison (2016) in their book on the resilient practitioner identify five areas that cause haemorrhaging of the caring self. These are:

- Burnout – the extinguished flame which is the motivational force in what we do and we can become unable to attach to new patients because we are too cumulatively depleted by previous attachments.
- Compassion fatigue – the overinvestment in the traumatic circumstances of people we are caring for.
- Vicarious trauma – the cumulative effect of hearing about traumatic circumstances of others.
- Ambiguous endings – not achieving closure and not knowing the results of what we do in our care of others, and how they are now.
- Professional uncertainty – not knowing exactly what is the best course of action.

Skovholt and Trotter-Mathison (2016) say that there are three dimensions of engagement or burnout. If we are fully engaged we are energetic, involved and have a sense of self-efficacy. Whereas when we are burned out we are exhausted, cynical and ineffective. This leads to other problems and makes us unable to view issues in a more positive light.

So, how can we recognise what creates and prevents burnout in our lives? Skovholt and Trotter-Mathison (2016) identify the following seven areas (p 106) in Table 2.2.

It is important for us to be able to focus on what prevents burnout in our lives, and to try to avoid roles which create potential burnout for us. I have designed the following questionnaire (Questionnaire 2.1) to identify where we are in relation to compassion fatigue. We could also use this to help others to assess their own levels of compassion fatigue and burnout.

Table 2.2 Burnout creation and prevention

Burnout Creation	Burnout Prevention
Work overload	Sustainable workload
Lack of control	Feelings of choice and control
Insufficient reward	Recognition and reward
Breakdown of community	A sense of community
Unfairness	Fairness, respect and justice
Significant value conflicts	Meaningful, valued work
Lack of fit (incongruence) between the person and the role	High job–person fit

QUESTIONNAIRE 2.1 Assessment of compassion fatigue and strategies

Assessment of your current feelings in relation to your personal and professional life

Please read each statement and circle the term that best fits your response and please use the spaces provided to comment in response to the prompts.

I feel stressed by the demands of my role at the moment

Very strongly agree	Strongly agree	Agree	Neither agree nor disagree	Disagree	Strongly disagree	Very strongly disagree

Please comment further if you would like to:

I feel positive about my professional role

Very strongly agree	Strongly agree	Agree	Neither agree nor disagree	Disagree	Strongly disagree	Very strongly disagree

Please comment further if you would like to:

I do not feel as if I can make a real difference in my work situation

Very strongly agree	Strongly agree	Agree	Neither agree nor disagree	Disagree	Strongly disagree	Very strongly disagree

Please comment further if you would like:

My stress at work is primarily due to caring for patients

Very strongly agree	Strongly agree	Agree	Neither agree nor disagree	Disagree	Strongly disagree	Very strongly disagree

Please comment further if you would like to:

My colleagues add significantly to my stress at work

Very strongly agree	Strongly agree	Agree	Neither agree nor disagree	Disagree	Strongly disagree	Very strongly disagree

Please comment further if you would like to:

My employer/manager causes me additional stress

Very strongly agree	Strongly agree	Agree	Neither agree nor disagree	Disagree	Strongly disagree	Very strongly disagree

Please comment if you would like to:

I feel that my work/life balance is generally good.

Very strongly agree	Strongly agree	Agree	Neither agree nor disagree	Disagree	Strongly disagree	Very strongly disagree

Please comment further if you would like to:

My home life helps with the stress I experience at work

Very strongly agree	Strongly agree	Agree	Neither agree nor disagree	Disagree	Strongly disagree	Very strongly disagree

Please comment further if you would like to:

I feel able to be compassionate towards my patients

Very strongly agree	Strongly agree	Agree	Neither agree nor disagree	Disagree	Strongly disagree	Very strongly disagree

Please comment further if you would like to:

I feel able to be compassionate towards my colleagues

Very strongly agree	Strongly agree	Agree	Neither agree nor disagree	Disagree	Strongly disagree	Very strongly disagree

Please comment further if you would like to:

I feel valued within my working environment

Very strongly agree	Strongly agree	Agree	Neither agree nor disagree	Disagree	Strongly disagree	Very strongly disagree

Please comment further if you would like to:

I feel as if I have good coping strategies to combat stress at work

Very strongly agree	Strongly agree	Agree	Neither agree nor disagree	Disagree	Strongly disagree	Very strongly disagree

Please comment further if you would like to:

I feel that I have strategies to make a positive difference at work

Very strongly agree	Strongly agree	Agree	Neither agree nor disagree	Disagree	Strongly disagree	Very strongly disagree

Please comment further if you would like to:

I feel that I have strategies to make a positive difference to my health and wellbeing

Very strongly agree	Strongly agree	Agree	Neither agree nor disagree	Disagree	Strongly disagree	Very strongly disagree

Please comment further if you would like to:

Overall, I feel satisfied with my working environment.

Very strongly agree	Strongly agree	Agree	Neither agree nor disagree	Disagree	Strongly disagree	Very strongly disagree

Please comment further if you would like to:

Any further comments:

It can be very difficult to offer support to colleagues when they are struggling emotionally. A very courageous article written by Steve Robson (Robson, 2018), a senior doctor in Australia, about his near-miss suicide ideation and follow-through 30 years ago was very emotional to read. A medical colleague of his when he was a junior doctor interrupted his plan to commit suicide but they never spoke about his suicidal feelings and he never knew that that colleague was aware of his extreme distress. When he posted an account of this situation in order to try to reduce the stigma for doctors who are mentally unwell and to encourage honest conversations, the colleague who had intervened that night responded to his article. They apologised for not having the skills as a 23 year-old to encourage that discussion and for giving the impression that their presence that night was accidental. They were very concerned for his wellbeing and had gone to visit purposely. It is really important to encourage colleagues, and take the same advice ourselves, to speak out and get help when we are feeling overwhelmed

Beyond Blue is a website (https://www.beyondblue.org.au) which offers help to Australians who are anxious, depressed or suicidal. There is also a doctor's health part to this website (https://www.beyondblue.org.au/general/search-results?keywords=doctors&page=1). It would be good if more resources like this were available to help people in caring roles to assess their mental health, stress levels and potential burnout.

Duffy (2018) talks about the importance of recognising the "brokenness and woundedness" of physicians, nurses and everyone in health care. Less than half of physicians would choose a career in medicine if they led their lives over again, and 73% of physicians would not recommend medicine as a career to their children and 53% of doctors report some degree of burnout. These statistics come from America, but this is a worldwide problem and the importance of being able to care with compassion and empathy is seen as being crucial in caring for patients, but also in helping health care practitioners to feel less burdened by their roles.

In the NHS staff survey of 2017 although 38% of staff reported feeling unwell due to work related stress in the last 12 months, a rise of 1% since the previous year, 81% of staff said that they were satisfied with the quality of care that they give to patients, and 90% felt that their organisation took positive action on health and wellbeing. Staff were going over and above to deliver high quality care in resource constrained environments and 57% of staff reported being at work in the last 3 months despite feeling unwell. (NHS Staff Survey, 2017)

It is of paramount importance that we recognise when our colleagues are suffering from compassion fatigue, burnout or mental health issues. We have a responsibility for the wellbeing of our colleagues, as well as for the wellbeing of the patients in our care. If we encourage others to be honest and express their feelings or stress levels then we can be supportive. If we do not encourage this openness and create opportunities for discussion of emotional issues, then it is not surprising that people we know will keep their inner distress hidden from us. We need to be the ones to make ourselves available to others who we know, so that they can discuss their stress, distress and mental health concerns. Also as we have said in the past if we show compassion patients can be less challenging, and need less analgesia. This can make our professional lives better and patient outcomes are enhanced so they can be discharged from our care earlier (Youngson, 2012), freeing up bed space and time which could be used for other patients.

Sometimes people feel that it is more professional to be more detached, and this can hide insecurity. Patients have no way of knowing whether we are clinically competent most of the time and the most important part of our interactions with them is showing that we care. They assess us on our compassion, kindness and our desire to help them and if this is found wanting then they do not trust our competence as readily either. Admitting that we do not have all the answers, but that we will find out if we do not know, gives confidence too, but that is easier when we are very experienced than when we are new in a post.

Chapter 3 will be discussing stress management and compassion burnout, and resilience in Chapter 4, but we need to recognise the importance of salutogenic approaches to safeguard our mental health, and that of our colleagues. Salutogenesis is a medical approach which focuses on health and wellbeing and the relationship between, health, stress, resilience and coping. Lindstrom and Eriksson (2010) refer to the salutogenic umbrella which helps us to cope with life's challenges. In order to activate the umbrella we need to focus on:

- Being grateful for the good aspects of our lives.
- Self-efficacy to be as effective as we can be.
- Hardiness which refers to how much we feel in *control* of our lives, our *commitment* and having a strong sense of purpose and *challenge* where we see the challenges we face as being issues we want to overcome, rather than stressors in their own right (Kobasa, 1979). This gives us a strong defence against stress.
- Empathy which is about genuinely understanding the impact of situations on others.
- Sense of humour – which mitigates against stressful situations for many health care practitioners.

We need to assess ourselves in relation to these attributes and see where we stand in relation to all these areas. Then we can think of how to develop these further, at home and at work.

What can I do if I do not feel compassionate towards someone or colleagues are not demonstrating compassion?

We need to recognise that we are all human and that some people's life circumstances can immediately trigger our empathy and compassion. However, sometimes people do not present the best versions of themselves when they come into our areas of practice. They can be angry, exhibit signs of substance abuse or be verbally or physically aggressive. Whilst we should not be expected to be subjected to the aggressive behaviour of others, we should have the advanced communication skills to diffuse their challenging behaviour. We also understand that there are possible reasons for how they are behaving. They could be suffering from dementia, have acute mental health issues, or be frightened. They could also be suffering from flashbacks about other times they were cared for in your department, or have other physical causes for their aggression such as a head injury or a brain tumour.

All this behaviour is challenging for us as practitioners, but I always find it helpful to think about what might have gone before their aggressive behaviour on that day. Many people lead lives that we would not want to live, and are experiencing low self-esteem, a lack of compassion and love in their lives and judgement wherever they go. This can lead to them being defensive and aggressive in how they behave towards us. It is helpful to believe that most people are not bad people, they might just be behaving badly today. As health care practitioners we are trying to help people with their challenging lives and their health issues, and that means being as non-judgemental as possible. It is at times like this that we need our communication skills to be at their best, and for our emotional intelligence to be at its most "brilliant". It can be helpful to think about what sort of people or behaviour we find hardest to cope with.

Also, it can be helpful to discuss strategies with our colleagues, particularly with those who manage to stay most calm when faced with the bad behaviour of others. Can they see the fear and past experiences behind the challenging behaviour, and how do they manage their thinking and responses so that they can make up for the deficits in the behaviour of others?

Feelings are contagious. If we are positive, smiley and caring of others we are more likely to be met with colleagues and patients who are also more likely to act this way. In the same way if we bustle about and are not engaged with patients, they are more likely to be grumpy and offhand with us. It is so easy to pass on our stress to those in our care, and it is of paramount importance that we do not do this, because they have enough challenges of their own, and they should not be taking on our pressures as well. So, we need to nurture virtuous rather than vicious circles (Campling 2013/2014) where positive communication is prioritised and we are kind to others (Chambers and Ryder, 2019). As Caroline Flack posted on her Instagram page in December 2019 before her tragic death from suicide on February 15th 2020 "in a world where you can be anything, be kind". Unkindness can stimulate more unkindness, and negativity breeds more negativity whereas the opposite is also true, and kindness creates more kindness and positivity breeds more positivity. So, we need to take a lead on creating and maintaining a culture of kindness and compassion and encourage this in our colleagues. However, if patients are being treated in an uncompassionate manner, and we are not being listened to when we speak to those who provide care in this uncaring way, we have a duty of care and need to escalate our concerns to more senior members of staff. I hope though that a lack of sensitivity is caused more by hurried unthinking practice, rather than deliberately purposeful unkind care. If this is the case, then we can challenge this in a constructive and supportive manner through one-to-one discussion and clinical supervision sessions. We also need to revisit our communication skills and enhance these as necessary. We can then seek feedback on our own behaviour and standards in practice, from our health care colleagues, but even more importantly from the patients in our care.

RECOMMENDATIONS FOR LEADERSHIP AS INDIVIDUAL PRACTITIONERS, LEADERS AND ORGANISATIONS

This chapter has discussed the potential challenges to compassionate care in terms of resourcing, the culture of the practice area, and our own individual attitude. It would be useful to look at each section and create a personal resume of attitude and actions strategies to address each of these challenges. There is then a discussion of compassion burn out, and how to recognise this in ourselves and others and address the thorny issues of what we can do if we do not feel compassionate towards someone, or we can sense this in others through their attitude and behaviour.

Focusing on compassionate care as individual practitioners and leaders

This chapter has expressly focused on our own individual attitude in relation to compassion, and so covered key issues in relation to this important area of practice. Strategies in the area of our individual attitude are summed up in Figure 2.4 earlier in this chapter. Chambers and Ryder (2012) discusses the importance of being a leader in compassionate care. We clearly need to question poor practice and escalate concerns if necessary because this is highlighted as essential in the NMC Code (NMC, 2018). However, we also need to take a lead and maximise the opportunities for patients in our practice areas to receive evidence-based individualised and compassionate nursing care. We need to ensure that we lead with compassion, as well as lead on, compassion. So, we need to role-model sensitive and empathetic nursing care, as well as relate to our colleagues throughout the multidisciplinary team (MDT) in a compassionate manner, and foster processes which actively support us and our colleagues. As Seagar says:

> without compassionate leadership it will be hard for compassionate practice to survive, let alone flourish. Therefore, creating a culture of empathic support and supervision for health care staff is more likely to be effective than one-off teaching sessions or courses; although obviously to do both would be ideal.
>
> (Seagar, 2011, p 5)

I have identified five key attributes which help us to lead on excellence and compassionate care (Chambers and Ryder, 2012, p 157) and these are (Figure 2.6):

- Personal attributes
- Quality attributes
- Leadership attributes
- Educational attributes
- Team leading attributes.

So how can we focus on our important role as leaders of excellence in compassionate care? First, by concentrating on our personal attributes such as:

- Emotional intelligence and emotional brilliance
- Positive approach to practice
- High levels of motivation
- Assertiveness
- Understanding what compassion means to patients, clients and colleagues and conveying this to all in our team
- Finding new ways to demonstrate compassion to patients, clients and colleagues.

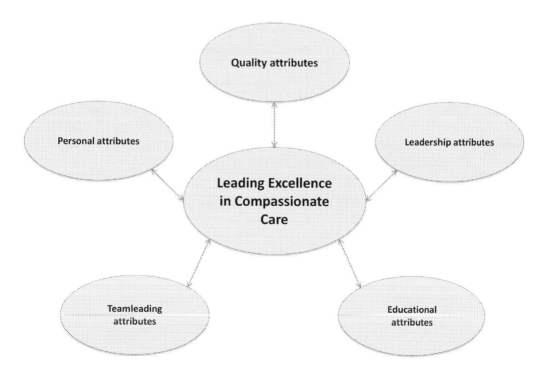

Figure 2.6 Leading excellence in compassionate care: personal and professional attributes

Second, by concentrating on our quality attributes such as:

- Mobilising and maximising resources
- Focusing on enhancing person-centred care
- Challenging inappropriate resourcing
- Challenging inappropriate standards of care
- Challenging inappropriate cultural norms
- Challenging inappropriate attitudes in others.

Third, by concentrating on our leadership attributes such as:

- An internal locus of control
- A sense of self-efficacy
- Strategic and visionary leadership – make your vision a reality
- Development and support of future leaders
- Maximising leadership opportunities at all levels
- Making change a personal mission.

Fourth, by concentrating on our educational attributes such as:

- Compassionate role modelling
- Ensuring students and colleagues focus on excellence in practice
- Positive mentoring
- Teaching others about excellence and compassion
- Influencing the practice curriculum of students in your practice area
- Maximising education and training opportunities.

Last, by concentrating on our team-leading attributes such as:

- Developing positive team relationships
- Developing positive team dynamics
- Focusing on positive team communication
- Maximising team skills
- Enhancing team learning
- Encouraging team intelligences.

(Chambers and Ryder 2012 and Chambers, 2013)

Why do we need to take such a strong lead on compassion? The King's Fund report (2011) *No More Heroes* says that the heroic model of leadership, where individuals almost singlehandedly lead the organisation towards success, has been replaced by the post-heroic model of leadership. This model involves collaborative and shared leadership working formally and informally across professional boundaries. Turnbull James (2011, cited in the King's Fund report 2011, p. 19–20) says:

> However, enticing in a pressurised environment, the fantasy that getting the right leader in place will be enough to change the system, this is untenable. The health care context requires people who do not identify with being a leader to engage in leadership. Leadership must be exercised across shifts 24/7 and reach to every individual: good practice can be destroyed by one person who fails to see themselves as able to exercise leadership, as required to promote organisational change, or leaves something undone or unsaid because someone else is supposed to be in charge. The NHS needs people to think of themselves as leaders not

because they are personally exceptional, senior or inspirational to others, but because they can see what needs doing and can work with others to do it.

Focusing on compassionate care as organisations

The organisations where we work also need to focus on fostering an environment where resources are available to ensure care can be maximised. They need to escalate concerns when this is not evident. However, this is not a perfect world and resources are stretched beyond the point where care can always be carried out to the standard that we would want. The COVID-19 pandemic is a very obvious example of this, which will be discussed more in the next chapter. However, managers and leaders within the organisation also need to help develop positive cultures and have escalation strategies in place if there are concerns. Patient Advocacy and Liaison Services (PALS) can be very helpful in listening to patients and their loved ones, and in taking their concerns forward. Performance management strategies need to be in place to ensure that individuals with poor attitudes are challenged appropriately, and measures put in place to address concerns. Strategies need to be in place to identify and manage individual and team burnout. Positive and compassionate cultures, where patients and staff feel valued, need to be encouraged. Clinical supervision, mentoring and CPD opportunities also need to be in place to encourage high standards, stress management and resilience strategies.

I hope that you have found this chapter helpful in identifying potential challenges to compassionate practice and in identifying compassion burnout in yourself and others. I also hope that you can develop strategies to overcome these challenges, and take a lead in compassionate care, in your area of practice. Chapter 3 will focus on stress management and strategies to prevent and alleviate stress in your professional roles, before moving on to discuss resilience in Chapter 4.

REFERENCES

Berg K. (2003) *Solution Focused Therapy: An Interview with Insoo Kim Berg.* http://psychotherapy.net/interview/Insoo_Kim_Berg (Accessed 12/9/23).

Berry J, Poortinga Y, Breugelmans S, Chasiotis A, Sam D. (2011) *Cross-Cultural Psychology: Research and Applications.* Cambridge: Cambridge University Press.

Bridges J, Griffiths P, Oliver E, Pickering R. (2019) Hospital Nurse Staffing and Staff-Patient Interactions: An Observational Study, *BMJ Quality and Safety*, 28(9): 706–13.

Burgess J. (2015) Improving Dementia Care with the Eden Alternative. *Nursing Times*, 111(12): 24–25.

Campling P. (2013/2014) Intelligent Kindness: Reforming the Culture of Health care in the Wake of the Francis Report. *Journal of Holistic Health care*, 10(3): 5–9.

Care Quality Commission (CQC). (2018) *Mental Health Act*, London.

Case M. (2015) *Underneath the Roses Where I Remembered Everything.* Portishead: Burning Eye Books.

Case M. (2019) *How to Treat People: A Nurse at Work.* London: Penguin Random House UK.

Chambers C, Ryder E. (2009) *Compassion and Caring in Nursing.* Abingdon: Radcliffe Publishing Ltd.

Chambers C, Ryder E. (2012) *Excellence in Compassionate Nursing Care.* London: Radcliffe Publishing Ltd.

Chambers C, Ryder E. (2019) *Supporting Compassionate Health care Practice.* Abingdon: Routledge.

Cole-King A, Gilbert P. (2011) Compassionate Care: The Theory and the Reality. *Journal of Holistic Health care*, 8(3): 29–37.

Crawford P, Brown B, Bonham P. (2006) *Communication in Clinical Settings.* Cheltenham: Nelson Thornes.

Crawford P, Brown B, Kvangarsnes M, Gilbert P. (2014) The Design of Compassionate Care. *Journal of Clinical Nursing*, 23(23–24): 3589–99.

Duffy B. (2018) *Ending Physician Burnout: It's Time for Physicians to Take Back Control of Their Environment and How They Deliver Care* https://www.linkedin.com/pulse/ending-physician-burnout-its-time-physicians-take-back-duffy-md/ (Accessed 12/9/23).

Furnham A. (2008) *Management Intelligence: Sense and Nonsense for the Successful Manager*. Basingstoke, Hampshire: Palgrave Macmillan.

Goleman D. (1996) *Emotional Intelligence: Why it Can Matter More Than IQ*. London: Bloomsbury Publishing.

Goleman D, Boyatzis R, McKee A. (2002) *The New Leaders: Transforming the Art of Leadership into the Science of Results*. London: Sphere Books.

Gudykunst W, Hammer M. (1983) Basic Training Design: Approaches in Intercultural Training. In Landis D, Brislin R (eds). *Handbook of Intercultural Training*, London: Pergamon Press.

Hall K, Gibbie T, Lubman D. (2012) Motivational Interviewing Techniques: Facilitating Behaviour Change in the General Practice Setting. *Australian Family Physician*, 41(9): 660–67.

Haque S.F, D'Souza A. (2019) Motivational Interviewing: The RULES, PACE and OARS. *Current Psychiatry*, 18(1): 27–28.

Kelly J. (2013) The Effect of Lean Systems on Person-Centred Care. *Nursing Times*, 109(13): 16–17.

Kitwood T. (1997) *Dementia Reconsidered: The Person Comes First*. Buckingham: Open University.

Knight R. (2011) The Doctor, the Patient and Compassion. *Journal of Holistic Health care*, 8(3): 50–53.

Kobasa S. (1979) Stressful Life Events, Personality, and Health: An Enquiry into Hardiness. *Journal of Personality and Social Psychology*, 37(1): 1–11.

Lindström B, Eriksson M. (2010) *The Hitchikers Guide to Salutogenesis,* Helsinki: Folkhalsn Research Centre.

Lombardo B, Eyre C. (2011) Compassion Fatigue: A Nurse's Primer. *Online Journal of Issues in Nursing*, 16(1): 3.

Mehri D. (2006) The Darker Side of Lean: An Insider's Perspective on the Realities of the Toyota Production System. *Academy of Management Perspectives*, 20(2): 21–43.

Miller W.R, Rollnick S. (2002) *Motivational Interviewing: Preparing People for Change*. New York: Guilford Press.

Miller W.R, Rollnick S. (2012) Meeting in the Middle: Motivational Interviewing and Self-Determination Theory. *International Journal of Behavioral Nutrition and Physical Activity*, 9(25).

NHS England (2017) *The Fifteen Steps Challenge*, London: NHS England.

NHS Institute (2009) *The Productive Ward: Releasing Time to Care*, https://webarchive.nationalarchives.gov.uk/ukgwa/20150401102711/http://www.institute.nhs.uk/quality_and_value/productivity_series/productive_ward.html (Accessed 12/9/23).

NHS Staff Surveys, (2017) *Results Archive for 2017 Survey* https://www.nhsstaffsurveys.com/results/results-archive/ (Accessed 12/9/23).

Nursing and Midwifery Council (2018) *The Code*. London: NMC

Prochaska J, DiClemente C. (1986) Towards a Comprehensive Model of Change. Cited in: Miller WR, Heather N. (eds.) *Treating Addictive Behaviours: Processes of Change*. New York: Pergamon Press.

Redelmeier D, Molin J-P, Tibshirani R. (1995) A Randomised Trial of Compassionate Care for the Homeless in an Emergency Department. *The Lancet*, 345(8958): 1131–34.

Robson S. (2018) *Learn From Me: Speak Out, Get Help, Get Treatment*. https://insightplus.mja.com.au/2018/41/learn-from-me-speak-out-seek-help-get-treatment/ (Accessed 15/9/23).

Schwartz K. (1995) A Patient's Story. *The Boston Globe Magazine* 16 July 1995. Available at https://www.theschwartzcenter.org/members/media/patients_story.pdf (Accessed 12/9/23).

Seager M. (2011) Compassionate Health Reform Must be Strategic. *Journal of Holistic Health care*, 8(3): 5.

Skovholt T, Trotter-Mathison M. (2016) *The Resilient Practitioner*. Abingdon: Routledge.

Slatten L, Carson D, Carson P. (2011) Compassion Fatigue and Burnout: What Managers Should Know. *Health Care Management*, 30(4): 325–33.

The King's Fund. (2011) *The Future of Leadership and Management in the NHS. No More Heroes*. London: The King's Fund.

Thompson N. *(2009) People Skills 3rd Edition*. Basingstoke: Palgrave Macmillan.

Turnbull James K. (2011) Leadership in Context: Lessons from New Leadership Theory and Current Leadership Development Practice. Cited in The King's Fund (2011) *The Future of Leadership and Management in the NHS: No More Heroes*. London: The King's Fund.

Watson C. (2018) *The Language of Kindness: A Nurse's Story*. London: Chatto and Windus.

Watson C. (2020) *The Courage to Care: A Call for Compassion*. London: Chatto and Windus.

Wible P. (2012) *Pet Goats & Pap Smears: 101 Medical Adventures to Open Your Heart & Mind*. Oregon: Pamela Wible Publishing.

Wigens I. (2006) *Communication in Clinical Settings*. Cheltenham: Nelson Thornes Ltd.

Winch S, Henderson A.J. (2009) Making Cars and Making Health Care: A Critical Review. *Medical Journal of Australia*, 191(1)**:** 28–29.

Womack J, Jones D. (2003) *Lean Thinking: Banish Waste and Create Wealth in Your Corporation*. London: Simon & Schuster UK.

Youngson R. (2012) *Time to Care*. New Zealand: Rebel Heart Publishers.

Why do I need to focus on my stress management in order to focus on compassionate care?

- Introduction
- Discussion – main points and evidence with case studies, exercises, aide mémoires and questions

  - What are the additional stressors of nursing through the COVID-19 pandemic?
  - What is stress and how can we identify when our stress levels are too high?
  - What particular stressors are there in different areas of practice?
  - How does compassion burnout relate to high stress levels?
  - Are my stress levels affecting my ability to be compassionate?

- Recommendations for leadership as individual practitioners, leaders and organisations

  - Focusing on stress management and compassionate care as individual practitioners and leaders
  - Focusing on stress management and compassionate care as organisations.

INTRODUCTION

This chapter will focus on stress management because we all experience stressful situations at home and work. It will focus on the links between compassion burnout and compassion fatigue, and stress management, and on the stressors that exist in different areas of practice. It will then discuss the nature of stress and how we can assess our stress levels, and whether stress is affecting our ability to be compassionate. There are better and worse ways to respond to stress and we need to increase our positive coping strategies, and reduce our negative coping strategies, to ensure that we stay as positive and as physically and emotionally healthy as possible. I will discuss these strategies in Chapter 4 where we focus on resilience. Chapter 3 will end by discussing leadership in relation to stress management and compassionate care, both as individuals and teams and within the organisations where we work.

DISCUSSION

Case study 3.1

Deepak's excellent care during the pandemic and his fears for his own health

Deepak could not remember ever feeling so stressed at work before, but then he had never had to nurse patients in a pandemic before. COVID-19 had turned everyday nursing care into alien surreal experiences which felt far from right. The personal protective equipment (PPE) was hot and uncomfortable and made every trip to the toilet, every drink and every food break into an immense challenge. So much so, that he and his colleagues were largely not prioritising these even when they were not too busy to do so. So at the end of each shift he was exhausted, hungry, dehydrated and desperate for the loo.

However, that appeared of no consequence alongside the extreme trauma of nursing men and women who were dying long before their time, in distress, without their loved ones being able to be with them. Neither he nor his colleagues had been prepared for that, and the distress being felt by the whole team was unbearable. In his unit they normally prided themselves on their end-of-life care and ensuring that every patient felt cared for with every attempt to meet their needs, physically, emotionally, culturally and spiritually. The team felt strongly about supporting families and friends when their loved one was dying. In this new pandemic world, they were really struggling to see every patient as an individual. Who were they, how did they normally spend their days, what were their interests and passions and who did they love? These were often unanswered questions, but they were trying so hard to build personal relationships. It was difficult to communicate through the PPE that they had to wear. Patients could not see their faces and although all the team put names on their gowns, and photos of what they looked like, he knew that many patients felt that robots and aliens, who were frightening to look at, were caring for them. Comforting a patient and holding their hand while wearing gloves did not feel very personal. He had to shout through his mask to get his voice heard, and it was difficult to use a soft tone and sound caring when shouting.

He had had to prioritise which patient to be with when they were dying, which went against everything he believed in. He had set up contacts between patients and family members using phones and tablets so that they could say goodbye to each other, and the conversations were heartbreaking to hear. How the fathers, mothers, wives, husbands, partners, siblings, daughters and sons at home coped with that at the time, and afterwards, he would never know. He sometimes had to take himself away from the situation and cry, and he knew that his colleagues were doing the same.

They had also had to care for their own colleagues who had contracted the dreadful virus and had died. He knew a little about these colleagues' lives, and how proud they were of their children, how much they were looking forward to retirement and having more time with their families. They had given so much to the NHS and now they had paid the ultimate sacrifice. He knew that he was of the age, gender and ethnic group who was most at risk of dying from the virus and he was putting himself in a situation which made him more vulnerable by coming to work to care for patients with the virus. He never doubted that he should carry on doing this, but it was very frightening to him, his family and friends. He knew he was not the only person to write letters to his loved ones in case he died. He had also made sure that his will was up to date and that plans were in place should he die. He had never needed to think like this before, and he was not of an age where he would usually think of his own death. Working in health care he had always understood the need to appreciate life and his own health, because he had known of tragic situations where death and illness had come very fast. However, that had always made him think positively and he had never really considered his own mortality. Being surrounded by death and critical illness, of people who had been well and active until a day or so ago, and who also never expected to die, had made him very aware of his own mortality. He was very scared, and he knew that others were too, but it was very difficult to talk of these feelings to others.

When he came through this pandemic, and he did try to think about when, not if, that happened, he knew that it would have had a huge impact on his physical health, but also his mental health too. It was not possible to care for and comfort colleagues who were deeply distressed at the time, and the team would usually have prioritised care of each other when a traumatic situation had just occurred. The amount of post-traumatic stress was immense. People who had survived critical illness, or whose loved ones had, those who had had to say goodbye over phones and tablets, those who had looked after so many people who were dying alone and in distress, those who had cared for dying colleagues, the list of traumatic situations went on and on. Where would all this stress go, and what sort of support would be available to help them to develop helpful long term coping strategies? He really hoped that there would be care available for the carers and that once stress levels returned to normal levels that they would all bounce back to their usual coping selves.

I am dedicating this chapter on stress management and how this impacts on our ability to be compassionate, to those who have cared for others through the COVID-19 pandemic because this has caused so much additional stress to everyone working in health care. Deepak, in our case study, is clearly very stressed by the challenges he is facing by nursing through the pandemic. He is worried about his own health, but he is also trying to give of himself personally when caring for people who are unexpectedly at the end of their lives. He is constrained by the PPE he is having to wear and is finding that his normal communication strategies are being compromised. He is also having to be the conduit between relatives and their dying loved ones who are not able to be together at this essential time. This goes against all he believes in; patients and their loved ones should be able to say goodbye face to face. All of this causes immense stressors, and this stress needs to be coped with somehow. I have written this case study using elements of lots of different things said to me, but three of my students have also written about their experiences of nursing through the pandemic, and their reflections are deeply moving.

Case study 3.2

Olivia's experience when caring for a patient dying alone

I will be discussing a patient who I was caring for and was dying without family members being able to be present during the COVID-19 pandemic.

The patient was 80 years old, and I went to perform mouth care. I decided to sit and stay with him for a while and spend some time with him. During this pandemic, patients are not able to have visits from their families, so this is a massive transition for that person and for the family who are not able to be there. Therefore, it is my role as the nurse looking after the patient to be an advocate for them and their families, to ensure that they are not alone and can receive empathy and compassion from me. It breaks my heart to see patients dying alone, with no loved ones holding their hands or telling them that they love them. I live and practice my nursing by the motto; "treat patients as you would treat your own family". And for me that means showing them that they matter by providing the care that they deserve.

I took the time to get to know some personal history about the patient; I personally like to know the person I am caring for, and to know their likes and dislikes, their hobbies, what their occupation is or was, if they are married and have children. I find it fascinating to know what their life was like before they got here, to hospital with me caring for them. They are more than just patients to me, they are people, who lived their life full of accomplishments that I feel honoured to know.

The patient was a pilot, was married for 60 years, had children and loved classical music, so I managed to find a radio station that played classical music and I played it whilst I sat with him. I read somewhere that when a patient is dying, the hearing is the last sense to go, and classical music is so peaceful yet full of bright sounds, and I think that this would have made the patient happy, and that makes me happy. I told them that I was playing their favourite music in a hope that this would provide comfort for them during this sensitive time, where I was privileged enough to be with them in their final moments. The Alberta hospice association (AHPCA) discusses the use of both music and touch as important therapies in end-of-life care (Trenerry-Harker, 2018). And it is very fulfilling to know that I individually thought of this myself and performed this for this patient.

I noticed his breathing becoming different – it was increasingly shallow and he was struggling to take breaths. I knew that he was coming to the end of his life, and I said to him; "it's ok Albert, I am here with you" whilst holding his hand and rubbing his chest. Even though I had gloves on for PPE, I was using therapeutic touch as a way of showing my empathy for what he was going through, and I wanted him to feel my warmth and concern for him (Roberts and Campbell, 2011).

Being a part of this experience was extremely fulfilling and heart wrenching. To witness this man take his last breaths and hold his hand was an honour that I will remember in my future nursing practice. I was able to tell his children that I was there, and I know that this must have been hard, as I was filling the role that they wish they could have done. However, I was able to tell them that I played his favourite music and held his hand. I was able to provide a sense of comfort for them that I know will help them grieve.

Case study 3.3

Megan's reflection on an episode of care during COVID-19

I arrived on to one of my shifts whilst working in the COVID-19 pandemic and I realised that one of my patients was very poorly and appeared to be in the dying process. I asked the on-call doctor to assess the patient and the decision was made to put the patient on our end of life care pathway, known as "Achieving priorities of care". The doctor rang the family to inform them of the situation but as the patient's family were all classed under the vulnerable category, they were not able to be with the patient whilst he was dying. This is a moment no family wants to ever be put through and I can only imagine how awful this must have been for them. To try and do something to help ease the pain, I arranged with the patient's granddaughter to drop a mobile phone off at the hospital entrance. I would facilitate them to be able to say their individual goodbyes, whilst I held the mobile phone up to the patient's ear as he became increasingly more unconscious. This was a long process that took over an hour and a half but thankfully each family member was able to say goodbye before the patient passed away. I then made the time to explain the process of what will happen next in terms of last offices, transfer to the mortuary, how to pick up the death certificate and how to go about planning the funeral. Whilst I feel so grateful that I was able to do this for the patient's family, I heard the pain, sadness and emotions the family expressed when talking to the patient that day. This made it a truly heart-wrenching process and one which I find difficult thinking about even two months later. Shedding tears under full personal protective equipment, including a face mask and a visor, was not easy. On this shift, my other patients were stable and did not need many nursing interventions, so I was able to provide this personalised compassionate care for the patient and his family. However, I am very aware that if my patient caseload that day was busier with other very acute patients, would I have been able to provide as high-quality person-centred care?

Even with COVID-19 changing the way hospitals are run, person-centred and compassionate care must still be seen as paramount in the last hours and days of life, not only for the patient but also for their family. This is possible through advocating for them and by communicating effectively with others (NMC, 2018). This truly is the essence of essential nursing care which when done well, provides such a positive impact. I learned from this situation that families feel a great sense of burden with the thought of their loved one dying alone. During this COVID-19 pandemic, this causes huge ethical and health care dilemmas which nurses never envisioned having to make in their careers. However, whilst families may not be able to physically be there at that time, there are ways we as nurses can be creative in ensuring families can still feel close to their loved ones. In this situation, using a mobile phone to hold up to the patient's ear whilst listening to their family members tell him how much he was loved, I felt I was fulfilling my role of a nurse to care compassionately and empathetically and to show kindness to both the patient and the family. On reflection, I also realised how important effective communication was in this situation, even more so than before. Every interaction had to be had over the phone due to COVID-19. The family did not know what was happening to their loved one, they relied on me to explain this to them. I found as I was able to communicate effectively to them, they knew the situation and what would happen. Whilst COVID-19 may stop some family members being there physically, we as health care workers can create ways to demonstrate creatively different compassionate solutions to help families feel connected and keep people safe.

As a student nurse about to qualify, I know the importance of ensuring I role model and lead good nursing practice to other colleagues and other more junior student nurses. I realised first hand from this experience the huge impact person-centred and compassionate care makes for patients and families; this is a situation I can use to teach others. I am also aware of the importance of communicating well in difficult situations, and this is a skill that has to be developed through experiences as a student nurse in preparation for qualifying.

When I become a practice supervisor and assessor after I qualify, I will use this example to teach other student nurses the importance we have as nurses for families. I hope I can inspire others to want to provide high-quality and effective care. A quote, a nurse I aspire to be like, once said to me was "patients and families may forget what you said and what you did, but they will never forget how you made them feel". This quote sums up this situation, what I have learned from this, and why it is so important I share my learning with others.

A postscript from this experience is a letter from the patient's family:

Dear Megan,

On Saturday 11th April, you sat with our grandfather whilst he sadly slipped away. We cannot thank you enough for being with him during a time we could not be. Your monumental efforts in obtaining his mobile phone and holding it to his ear so we could each say our goodbyes will never be forgotten. You were truly an angel that day, and knowing that we got to speak to him one last time, and tell him that we love him, makes the pain of loss just that little bit easier. A huge and heartfelt thanks from every family member you spoke with on that day. Thank you to all your colleagues for all that you are doing on the frontline.

These two examples of reflections from a second-year student nurse, and a nursing student who was about to qualify, demonstrate the exemplary care that was carried out for two patients at the end of their lives. Megan understands her leadership role in being a role model for other nurses, and using this experience to teach others when she is qualified, which is really important. However, both students are fantastic in my opinion and their reflections moved me to tears. We do not have feedback from the family in Olivia's experience, but In Megan's scenario there was feedback from the grandaughter which allows us to see how crucial the compassionate care given by Megan was to the whole family. They will remember this forever. In both the situations compassionate and proactive person-centred care shines through, and this is very impressive. Needing health care intervention during a pandemic is so distressing for families, and the patients themselves. Having to provide care in this way, when loved ones were not able to visit, goes against all we believe in, and people should not have to say goodbye like this. However, the feedback from Megan's patient's granddaughter is so important, and this reflects the feelings of the whole family. They will remember what happened for the rest of their lives, and they are appreciative of the "monumental effort" nurses go to in order to provide care. These scenarios truly reflect the art of nursing and the students have written about this so movingly. Superlative practice is demonstrated in both these reflections and the NHS is safe in their hands as future qualified nurses. They should be so very proud of what they did, and I am proud to know all of them, and to be involved in their nursing journeys.

What are the additional stressors of nursing through the COVID-19 pandemic

There is no doubt that nursing through the pandemic has created enormous challenges for health care practitioners in situations which they have never had to face before. Nursing with full PPE makes communication very difficult, as well as being very hot and uncomfortable. Patients being isolated from their loved ones, and vice versa, causes a great deal of anxiety, even when the person is only having an appointment and not terribly unwell. When a patient is in hospital the feelings of isolation from the outside world creates additional deep concerns, and they need help maintaining those close contacts with people they care about. Health care practitioners can be that communication conduit between patients and their family and friends, if the patient does not have a mobile phone, or is too unwell to use it. When a patient is dying this creates a situation that no nurse wants to be part of, because they need to make it possible for people to say goodbye using phones and tablets. This has been deeply emotional and incredibly upsetting for health care practitioners, however it is very much valued by family members who are not able to visit. All these issues are raised in the three case studies above. For nurses working in the community there has been an increased number of deaths at home, which is distressing. However, there has also been a marked increase in decomposed bodies needing autopsies due to not having been found earlier (While, 2022). People were much more socially isolated during the lockdowns, which was sad to see. However, dying alone, and with nobody knowing for some time, is something that should not happen to anyone. District nurses and GPs would be aware and distressed by this. Khanipour-Kencha et al (2022) highlight how anticipatory grief caused by the fear and grief of death before it takes place can cause physical, emotional, cognitive and spiritual issues for patients, families and health care practitioners. This anticipatory grief intensified during the pandemic, and this can cause sleep problems, nausea and loss of appetite, headaches, fatigue, amnesia, confusion as well as poor concentration, decision making and problem solving. Nyatanga (2022) agrees caring for patients at the end of their lives can increase the focus on our own death, and those of our loved ones. Death is inevitable but avoiding discussions about death does not help. Death anxiety, without resolution or exploration can have a negative impact on our wellbeing. Therefore, mental health support needs to be in place to help with the stress and to increase the resilience of all affected.

The stress of this kind of situation is being reported now and Ford's (2020) article on the negative impact on nurses' mental health draws on evidence from the *COVID 19 Are you OK? Campaign*. The 2020 survey found that 87% of respondents rated themselves as experiencing a "lot or a little more stress at work than usual", 90% said they were "a lot or little more anxious than pre outbreak", and over 50% of respondents said they were a "lot more anxious or stressed than usual". In the same study, nurses' main concerns and challenges were:

- worries about contracting the virus
- the health of family and friends
- lack of PPE
- dealing with death of patients who were alone due to social distancing
- failing to look after themselves, for example, missing breaks or not eating properly
- failing to provide effective care due to time or staffing pressures.

In an updated Nursing Times survey in March 2021, 44% of respondents described their mental health and wellbeing as "bad" or "very bad", which was a rise of 10% on the 2020 survey. In addition, 62% felt that their mental health was "worse" or "much worse" than it was in the first wave of the pandemic in Spring 2020. (Ford, 2021)

Other media reports backed up the fact that practitioners were really struggling in January 2021 due to the pandemic. They were physically and emotionally exhausted and ITUs were operating at over 200% capacity with patients suffering from COVID, and that was not taking into account ITU patients without COVID. High acuity care wards were also beyond capacity and working long shifts in full PPE added to the strain of working in such stressful circumstances. One study reported that nearly half of ITU staff were suffering from symptoms of PTSD, severe anxiety and were resorting to problem drinking (Greenberg et al, 2021). Professor Hugh Montgomery, chair of intensive care medicine at University College London is very clear about the stress on intensive care, and other health care colleagues. He says:

> Burnouts come in different forms. Sometimes it is just that the enthusiasm has gone, sometimes there is nothing left to give. There is also a moral burnout, when you have seen so much suffering that you can no longer empathise. Obviously, you cannot live the experience of every lost patient and their families because you would be completely destroyed over the course of a year. But you do have to have some heart left. And if you lose that ability to empathise, it extends to other parts of your life. It makes you so emotionally blunted that you can't feel anymore.
>
> (Carpenter, 2021)

In addition, health care practitioners are becoming ill themselves with COVID. A University of Glasgow study found that those working in health care roles were seven times more likely to have severe infections than non-essential workers (Demou and Katikireddi, 2020). If someone is admitted to ITU there can be severe mental health symptoms resulting from post-intensive care syndrome, as well as prolonged physical symptoms (McDonald and Clark, 2020a). The symptoms of long COVID can also be extremely debilitating and long term, (McDonald and Clark, 2020b) and these can make it difficult to return to work, which can create guilt, as well as insomnia, prolonged lethargy, anxiety and depression. People suffering from long COVID need specialist support (Maxwell, 2020), but some people in the early stages of the pandemic were never tested and therefore never diagnosed with COVID, but they are suffering with a range of symptoms, including cardiac, respiratory, neurological and mental health manifestations. (Maxwell, 2020). They need multidisciplinary help from clinical psychologists, physiotherapists and occupational therapists as well as nursing and medical input.

So, we need to consider that health care practitioners are also people in their own right. Many people were struggling in lockdown, and through the pandemic, with the restrictions and disruptions this caused to social life and to the anxieties people were feeling. Young people are particularly at risk of self-harm and psychological distress has increased in this age group since the start of the pandemic. This is particularly true amongst those with pre-existing mental health issues and those from lower income households (Patalay and Fitzsimons, 2020). Depression, which was always one of the most prevalent mental health disorders, has doubled to nearly one in five adults since the start of the pandemic (Pierce et al, 2020). This is particularly prevalent in those aged 16–39, those who are female, or have financial worries or a disability. In addition, personal wellbeing score and happiness and satisfaction levels fell. Levels of anxiety in January 2021 were the highest since April 2020 (ONS, 2021). We need to bear this in mind when supporting students in the health care environment, some of whom are young, and some have not been used to the health care environment, especially during a pandemic. In one study focusing on nursing students in placements during the pandemic they expressed the need to be heard, prepared and supported. The support of supervisors, preceptors and their nursing school was seen to be particularly important (Ulenaers et al, 2020). We also need to appreciate that many members of health care teams were also working outside their comfort zones. They could have been working without any warning in areas of practice which were unfamiliar to them, where they did not know where to find essential equipment and were not familiar with their team members each day. In addition, they could have been caring for patients with extremely high needs, who were in distress and there were no ways of totally alleviating that distress. This all added to high stress levels, and many members of staff were moved around from one ward to another, not knowing where they were going to be working on any given day.

Many nurses were struggling with nursing patients when their communication strategies were compromised because of using PPE. Tehranineshat et al (2019) state that compassionate care is reliant on three common themes. Firstly, effective verbal and non-verbal communication which involves kindness and building trust. Secondly, professionalism which includes clinical care, evidence-based practice and intuitive assessment of need. Lastly, continuous comprehensive care which includes adherence to moral values and meeting patients' needs and providing emotional support to patients and their loved ones. Brown (2020) says that that many of these themes are being compromised in caring for people through the pandemic. Nurses have no time to care for people as they want to, patients cannot see loved ones face to face and have to rely on virtual means of communication. In addition, they cannot use therapeutic touch to carry out tasks and promote comfort and alleviate psychological distress (Pedrazza et al, 2018) because they are using PPE. Using face masks also hinders communication through muffling speech, not being able to lip read and not allowing a more reassuring tone of voice because of needing to raise the voice. Smiling is often not visible with some PPE, and the use of social distancing, means that it is difficult for patients to determine who is caring for them, and sometimes even their gender. Ong (2020) points out that many women wear a niqab or burka, and maybe lessons can be learnt from women who often have their faces covered. However, in Ong's article the point is made by a woman who wears a niqab on a regular basis that wearing a mask feels hotter and more uncomfortable, and the fact that the mask fabric is thicker could cause more muffling of speech. Brown (2020) says that not being able to relieve distress through compassionate gestures and therapeutic touch can have a major impact on compassion satisfaction and cause compassion fatigue. As While (2021) says, touch conveys support, reassurance, care and compassion, and wearing PPE reduces the pleasure brought about by therapeutic touch. Therefore, nurses need to find new ways of demonstrating compassionate care which are acceptable to nurses and patients in their care.

Savitsky et al (2020), in looking at anxiety and coping strategies amongst nursing students in relation to COVID-19, found moderate anxiety was experienced by 42.8% and severe anxiety by 18.1%. In this study mental disengagement, through the use of alcohol, sedative drugs or excessive eating amongst people with higher anxiety levels was linked to being female, and also with being a parent. This was further increased by the lack of available PPE at work. It was suggested that respondents who had stronger self-esteem, and used appropriate humour, had significantly lower anxiety levels. So, exploring how to capitalise on the use of humour and higher self-esteem could be important.

In Wuhan where the pandemic first became prevalent Kang et al (2020a) cite similar issues:

- stress, anxiety and depressive symptoms
- insomnia
- denial, anger and fear combined with the high risk of contracting the virus with inadequate protection
- overwork, physical and mental exhaustion
- complex patient care
- discrimination and isolation and a lack of contact with families.

All these stressors could affect long term health status as well being very debilitating short term. It was suggested by Kang et al (2020a) that redeploying staff to other less intense care areas and shift patterns that allowed workers to rest, and also taking turns in high pressure roles could be helpful. In Wuhan 37% nursing and medical staff in the wake of the pandemic were suffering sub threshold mental health incidents, 34% had suffered mild disturbances, 22% moderate and 6% severe disturbances in terms of mental health (Kang et al 2020b).

Lam et al (2019) cite four themes in pandemics based on instabilities and vulnerabilities which could affect nurses' abilities to perform outbreak-response duties. These are:

- resource constraints – e.g. increased workload, insufficient beds and isolation rooms, shortage of staff made worse by increased sick leave
- threats of infection – working in higher risk areas, fear of transmission to families and a lack of confidence in PPE
- ubiquitous challenges – such as constant change in disease management, frequent changes in protocols leading to challenges in adoption and execution
- lingering uncertainties about patients' health status and ambiguous and confusing information.

These are all clearly very distressing situations to deal with and yet health care staff can feel that it is unprofessional to show their emotions, so they obscure their emotions at work (Hochschild, 2012) or "surface act" (Delgado et al 2017) which can increase the amount of their emotional labour (Graham et al (2020). So, it is important that practitioners can show their emotions if this is appropriate, and this can feel comforting to patients and their loved ones. Expressing how they feel to their colleagues is very important and having the opportunity to debrief and express their sadness after situations which have been distressing needs to be encouraged within the health care environment. A nurse has expressed her sorrow during the pandemic in the following poem:

"Why we're clapping" Chloe Kerwood (2020)

I'm sorry to the husband I spoke to on the phone,
frustrated as I tell she's 'critical but stable'
whilst you're forced to worry at home
I'm sorry to the consultant I couldn't hug when in tears,
after you said there is nothing more we could do,
facing the biggest challenge of your career
I'm sorry to my fellow colleagues,
that all I could do is just smile,
whilst knowing you are tired, upset and scared,
knowing this will haunt you for a while
I'm sorry for the patient that stirred and opened her eyes,
how frightened you must be feeling,
I promise this masked stranger is trying to keep you alive
I'm sorry to all my friends and family that asked me "you ok",
I just shrug and don't really reply,
I can't find any words to say
My biggest sorry of all is for the ones that lost their fight,
you weren't alone, I promise,

---

this stranger held your hand and sent you love whilst you drifted to the light
I'm sorry to the relatives you weren't allowed with your Mum, Dad, husband, wife, daughter or son,
but your unknown friend was there, holding their hands telling them how much they were loved by everyone.

(Reproduced with permission from Chloe Kerwood)

So, it is very clear that stress levels have been increased exponentially through the COVID-19 pandemic and certain strategies would appear to be suggested by the literature so far:

- More reliable availability of PPE
- Redeploying staff to less intense areas if this is possible
- Taking turns in higher pressure roles
- More preparation for areas which are unfamiliar and a long way out of comfort zones
- Shift patterns that allow staff to rest between shifts
- More available mental health support to help with anxiety, depression etc
- Strategies to help with insomnia and stress management, higher self-esteem and use of appropriate humour
- Debriefing after stressful shifts
- Preparing and supporting students
- Specialist support when suffering from long COVID.

Having looked at the specific challenges of the recent pandemic it is important to appreciate the impact of high stress levels on burnout in the wider context of health care practice.

Questions to ask yourself

Evaluating the impact of the COVID-19 pandemic on your stress levels.

- Have you been struggling through the pandemic and the lockdowns?
- How anxious have you felt since the pandemic started?
- Has your sleep been affected by your experiences through the pandemic?
- How stressed have you felt, and how have dealt with your stress?
- Has your work stress affected your home or social life?
- How depressed have you felt since the start of the pandemic?
- How would you assess your mental health since the pandemic started?
- How have you coped with caring for people with COVID?
- How difficult have you found it using PPE, in terms of the impact on you?
- How much do you think that wearing PPE has impacted on your communication with patients and colleagues at work?
- How have you helped patients to keep in touch with their loved ones?
- Has this communication with patients and their loved ones been very stressful?
- Have you had the opportunity to debrief after traumatic situations?

- Have you had to work in unfamiliar work environments, or outside your comfort zone?
- Where have you accessed support, and has this support been helpful?
- Has additional support been made available to you at work?
- Have you had support from family and friends? Has this been helpful?
- Is your team supportive, and could you do more to take a lead on your team being supportive for team members?

What is stress and how can we identify when our stress levels are too high?

Stress is caused when we are put under pressure for any reason. In his seminal text Selye (1946) describes how the body responds to stressors in terms of the General Adaptation Syndrome (GAS). The stages are alarm, the resistance stage and the stage of exhaustion. The alarm stage is when the body has a rapid physiological response to a stressor, followed by the body's mechanisms to counteract this shock. These responses are often referred to as "fight or flight" responses, where we are primed to fight an aggressor, or run away. The resistance or adaptation stage is when our bodies adapt to the stressor, and that can be when physical and psychological symptoms start to appear, or we start to use negative coping strategies, such as drinking too much alcohol or comfort eating. The exhaustion stage is when our natural resources have been used up and if we do not do something we become physically or mentally unwell. This stage is disabling and leads to long term health issues.

Stress is a word we use all the time, when we are discussing how we feel at any given time. However, we are usually referring to negative stress or distress, rather than the positive stress which is referred to as eustress. Clouston (2015) refers to the imbalance caused by too much to do, professionally or personally as burnout. Whereas the lack of stimulation and engagement she refers to as rust-out, others refer to this as boreout. It is easy to forget that we can become stressed when we are understimulated and bored, and that people perceive levels of stimulation very differently. What is too much stimulation for some, is too little for others.

Work overload can be a potential source of stress. The Yerkes-Dodson Law and the inverted U hypothesis (Sutherland and Cooper, 1992) describe the relationship between the amount of work and health and performance. However, it is interesting to note that although work overload can make us tense, more likely to make mistakes, have low self-esteem and create insomnia, having too little work to do can make us bored, apathetic, suffer from low morale and make us more likely to go off sick. It is only at the middle of the curve, where we have sufficient work but not too much, that we are at our optimal work performance and are creative, calm, motivated and experience high energy levels. So positive stress, or eustress, is good for us, whereas negative stress presents itself as distress and that is bad for us.

So firstly, it is very helpful to understand when we are more at risk of higher than usual levels of stress. The Holmes and Rahe (1967) Social Readjustment Rating Scale helps to identify stressful life events. Some stressors are positive like holidays, marriage and positive changes in circumstances. Others are much more negative such as bereavement, problems at work or being fired from work, personal injury or illness, or relationship difficulties. Many stressors are identified, all of which have a score. Identifying the overall score can be helpful in identifying when the amount of change in our life has reached an unhealthy level, where the chances of suffering from stress related illnesses is much more likely. A high score on the scale indicates a major life crisis and 79% of people fall ill in the following year if this is the case. However, it is important to note that over 20% of people with a score as high as this do handle these life changes well, and do not appear to suffer illness at this stage. Personality can be an important factor here and certain personalities do appear to be able to deal with change and pressure in their lives. The rating scale can be used by us to try to control the amount of change we are voluntarily introducing to our lives, so that we are less likely to suffer from stress. So, if we are going through a very difficult time, with a major bereavement likely or just experienced, or relationship difficulties which are very difficult to cope with, it might not be a good idea to increase our stress through more change. So, changing our job or planning a big holiday or moving house, might not be a good idea at this time, even if these are positive moves in the long run. However, it might not be possible to avoid other changes. For example, if a relationship breaks down then moving away from the joint property might be inevitable, and moving job might also be necessary. It is all a matter of controlling the controllable, where possible, to try to keep the amount of change down as much as possible when there is a lot of other change happening in life. So, it might be helpful to assess the life events in your life (Questionnaire 3.1) to see how much change this amounts to, and the potential effect on your health. You might want to assess yourself again at times of change in the future, or just on a regular basis, so that you are aware of any negative impact that could result from more change in your life.

QUESTIONNAIRE 3.1 What life changes increase your stress?

(adapted from The Holmes Rahe Life Stress Inventory, 1967)

Life Events	Score rating
Death of partner	100
Divorce	73
Separation from partner	65
Being imprisoned *or* admitted to an institution *or* death of a close family member	63
Major personal injury or loss	53
Marriage	50
Being fired from work	47
Marital reconciliation or retirement	45
Major health or behaviour change of family member	44
Pregnancy	40
Sexual difficulties *or* gaining a new family member *or* major business change	39
Major change in finances (+/-)	38
Death of a close friend	37
Changing to a different line of work	36
Major change in number of arguments with a partner (+/-)	35
Taking on a mortgage	31
Foreclosure on mortgage/loan	30
Major change in responsibilities at work (+/-) *or* children leaving home *or* troubles with in-laws	29

Outstanding personal achievement	28
Partner starting/finishing work **or** leaving/starting school	26
Major change in living conditions (new home/building work, deterioration)	26
Changes in personal habits (dress, associations, smoking cessation)	24
Difficulties with manager at work	23
Major changes in work conditions/hours **or** new accommodation **or** new school	20
Changes in recreation **or** church activities	19
Changes in social activities	18
Taking on a loan	17
Changes in sleeping habits	16
Change in number of family get-togethers (+/-) **or** eating habits	15
Vacation/holidays	13
Major public holidays	12
Minor law violations (parking fines etc)	11

If there is more than one change in each category add the score for each change experienced.

Add up the points for anything that has changed for you in the past year to assess your score.

- Less than 150 – indicates a relatively low amount of life change and you have a low risk of stress induced health problems
- 150–300 – you have a 50% chance of major stress induced health problems in the next 2 years
- 300+ – you have an 80% chance of stress related problems in the next 2 years

Score	Chance of stress related problems

Having thought about how susceptible we are to stress, due to the amount of change that we are coping with, it is important to think about our symptoms of stress physically, emotionally, behaviourally and cognitively. Recognising symptoms of stress is the first step in addressing areas of stress and developing helpful strategies to reduce the impact of stress on our health. The following questionnaire (Questionnaire 3.2) can be helpful in thinking about the severity of our symptoms, and the impact these have on our lives.

QUESTIONNAIRE 3.2 Stress symptom questionnaire

Stress symptom questionnaire

How is your level of stress?

Stress can manifest itself in lots of different ways, physically, emotionally, behaviourally and cognitively. These symptoms can also be indicators of compassion burnout and exhaustion. Try to think of how these symptoms manifest themselves in your life and score the extent to which you are affected by these:

5 = All of the time
4= Most of the time
3= Sometimes
2= Occasionally
1= Very occasionally
0= Never

Physical symptoms:

Digestive problems (diarrhoea, nausea, sickness, poor appetite, indigestion)

5	4	3	2	1	0

Symptoms and impact on your life:

Cardiac and respiratory symptoms (palpitations, dizzy spells, hyperventilation, breathing problems, worsened asthma symptoms)

5	4	3	2	1	0

Symptoms and impact on your life:

Aches and pains (headaches, migraines, backache, unexplained pain, muscle tension)

5	4	3	2	1	0

Symptoms and impact on your life:

Sexual problems (lack of libido, impotence, pain on intercourse, fear of intercourse)

5	4	3	2	1	0

Symptoms and impact on your life:

Emotional symptoms:

Feeling less control over emotions (mood swings, feeling helpless, trapped, powerless, lack of enthusiasm, loss of control and/or freedom)

5	4	3	2	1	0

Symptoms and impact on your life:

Anxiety problems (feeling irritable, agitated, angry, resentful, tense, anxious, panicky, restless, unable to relax, being oversensitive, feeling overly vulnerable to danger)

5	4	3	2	1	0

Symptoms and impact on your life:

Depression problems (feeling tearful, depressed, lack of feelings of hope, pleasure or joy, lack of pleasure in activities you usually enjoy, low energy levels, isolating yourself, tiredness and fatigue)

5	4	3	2	1	0

Symptoms and impact on your life:

Difficulty in personal relationships (feeling underconfident in social situations, difficulty in initiating new relationships or building and maintaining current relationships, feeling suspicious of others, distancing yourself from others)

5	4	3	2	1	0

Symptoms and impact on your life:

Self-esteem issues (low self-esteem, low self confidence, feeling like everyone copes better than you do, taking a victim blaming approach to how you cope with situations when they were really challenging, low feelings of personal accomplishment)

| 5 | 4 | 3 | 2 | 1 | 0 |

Symptoms and impact on your life:

_____

_____

_____

_____

Behavioural symptoms:

Sleep problems (inability to get to sleep or stay asleep, early morning waking, napping during the day, waking suddenly in a state of anxiety, excessive fatigue and tiredness)

| 5 | 4 | 3 | 2 | 1 | 0 |

Symptoms and impact on your life:

_____

_____

_____

_____

Negative coping strategies (drinking, smoking or eating excessively, excessive use of other substances, prescription/over the counter/recreational drugs, caffeine)

| 5 | 4 | 3 | 2 | 1 | 0 |

Symptoms and impact on your life:

_____

_____

_____

_____

Work based problems (avoiding particular clients or colleagues, dread of going to work, less empathy to others who are having problems, frequent time off sick, resentment towards your employer or others, work and home life blending together, feeling unable to fulfil your usual role, feeling insecure about your job security without good reason)

| 5 | 4 | 3 | 2 | 1 | 0 |

Symptoms and impact on your life:

_____

_____

_____

_____

Cognitive symptoms:

Concentration and memory problems (difficulty in concentrating and focusing, concentration span issues, forgetfulness, memory lapses, making more mistakes or being less organised than usual)

5	4	3	2	1	0

Symptoms and impact on your life:

Decision making problems (difficulty in making decisions, poor judgement, difficulty in thinking clearly)

5	4	3	2	1	0

Symptoms and impact on your life:

Being very critical of others (being cynical about the motives of others, being overly critical about how others behave, lack of usual objectivity about situations, motives, behaviour of others)

5	4	3	2	1	0

Symptoms and impact on your life:

Next, we need to be able to recognise the importance of having a balance in all areas of our lives. If we have a total health balance we have:

- Social health – through contact with family and friends.
- Intellectual health – through intellectual stimulation, discussion and interest in activities outside work.
- Physical health – through activities like making sure that we make time to have breakfast, relaxing before lunch and sufficient physical activity.
- Emotional health – through laughter, showing affection to others, satisfying sexual relationships, enjoying music etc.

So, this questionnaire (Questionnaire 3.3) should help us determine how much balance there is in our lives, and whether we need to create a better balance through introducing new activities, or cutting back on those which are having too much influence on our time and inbuilt resources.

QUESTIONNAIRE 3.3 Health balance questionnaire

- What do you do already?
- What would you like to increase in your life?
- Think about ways to create a better balance between work, home and play, and between these different aspects of your life.
- All the specific suggestions are for your consideration only. Some of the bullet points will not be appropriate for you. The important point is to think about the balance between the four areas of health. You might come up with your own suggestions which are more central to your life.

Activity	Do already	Do more
Physical health		
• Plan regular exercise during your week		
• Take the opportunity to increase your exercise during the day when possible, for example walking upstairs rather than taking the lift		
• Walk briskly for a short burst of time		
• Take a walk before bedtime		
• Go for a swim		
• Take part in fun activities – dance, swim, walk, sing, play sports		
• Eat regularly		
• Eat healthily		
• Sit down and enjoy a really good breakfast		
• Take time to relax after a busy morning and enjoy your lunch		
• Plan to take time to really enjoy your supper		
• Eat calmly and in a relaxed way		
• Seek medical help when you are ill		
• Take time off sick when you are unwell		
• Take all your annual leave entitlement		
• Go away on holiday		
• Take mini vacations and day trips		
• Spend time away from phones, computers, social media		
• Wear clothes that you like		
• Get enough sleep		
• Any suggestions….		

Activity	Do already	Do more
Emotional health		
• Look for things to make you laugh out loud		
• Allow yourself to cry		
• Spend time really enjoying music		
• Watch a film or television for pure enjoyment		
• Think about ways to decrease your stress levels		
• Read for pleasure – short stories, magazines, books, poetry		
• Take time to express your caring and affection for friends or family		
• Take time to be sexual		
• Tell yourself how well you have done when something was not easy		
• Think about what situations, places, activities, things and people you find comforting and then actively think of ways to experience these more		
• Practice saying no sometimes and think about in what situations you might need to do this more		
• Practice receiving back from others – time, praise, gifts etc		
• Listen to your thoughts and notice your beliefs, attitudes, values and thoughts		
• Do something where you are not the expert or in charge		
• Make quiet times in your life		
• Take a break during the day		
• Any other suggestions….		

Activity	Do already	Do more
Social Health		
• Spend time with people whose company you enjoy		
• Stay in contact with important people in your life, however far away they live		
• Think about being in contact with *all* of your family (if appropriate)		
• Entertain people at your home		
• Spend time with children or animals		
• Spend time outside and enjoy the feeling of being outside		
• Think about what is meaningful to you and find ways to explore these activities more		
• Contribute time or money to causes you believe in		
• Find a spiritual or community connection		
• Take time to chat with work colleagues		
• Give and receive support from others		
• Any other suggestions…		

Activity	Do already	Do more
Intellectual health		
• Feel genuinely stimulated intellectually by your job		
• Enjoy a good discussion with friends		
• Become involved with interests outside your job		
• Reread favourite books, watch again programmes and films that you enjoy		
• Be curious about things		
• Develop a new hobby		
• Write in a journal or a diary		
• Focus on times when you feel positive and happy, and spend time doing these things more		
• Any other suggestions….		

So, it is crucial to work out how much change is happening, or imminent, in our lives, and what symptoms we have of high stress and how much balance we have in our lives. Being more aware of all these parts of our lives can help us to understand when our stress levels are getting too high. A natural result of this could be that our ability to be compassionate to patients in our care could be compromised.

Questions to ask yourself

Assessing change, stress symptoms and amount of balance in your life

- Have you come to any conclusions about the impact of life changes on your life?
- Do you think that you need to reduce change in your life, if so in which areas?
- Having completed the stress symptom questionnaire how does stress cause symptoms in your life?
- Are your stress symptoms in one particular area of health? Is there anything you can do to address these symptoms?
- Have you come to any conclusions about whether you have sufficient balance in your life?
- What areas do you need to focus on, and what activities will you be thinking about introducing into your life?
- How will you make space for these additional activities, and how will you reduce other aspects of your life to create a greater balance?

What particular stressors are there in different areas of practice?

Working in health care environments can be inherently stressful, whether practitioners have been working in the same area for some years, or if they have just moved to working in that area of practice. In the same way working with patients who have specific needs can be stressful, whether we are doctors, occupational therapists, physiotherapists, speech and language therapists, qualified nurses, health care assistants or students of any of those professions. So, I wanted to look at whether different areas of practice create particular stressors for those working there, or whether there are common denominators in many areas of practice. I have read a large range of papers focusing on doctors, therapists and nurses, and a few articles focus on those working in education and management. The areas of practice were as diverse as district nursing and health visiting in the community, to those working with people with learning disabilities or mental health issues. I have included articles focusing on nurses and doctors caring for burns sufferers, renal patients and those at the end of their lives. I also researched articles focusing on those working in high acuity care such as theatres, emergency departments and intensive care. The articles spanned all age groups from paediatrics to older age, and the articles were written from the perspectives of those working in a range of countries from here in the UK and Ireland, to France, Belgium, The Netherlands, Greece, Portugal, Israel, Australia, Canada and the USA. The issues were surprisingly similar, and they focused around the culture of the environment, the needs and attitudes of the patients in their care and the impact and coping strategies of the practitioners themselves.

Maslach et al and Maslach et al (1996 and 2001) found that people who experience emotional exhaustion, depersonalisation and a reduced sense of personal accomplishment are at the greatest risk of burnout, although emotional exhaustion has been identified as the hallmark of burnout.

Poncet et al (2007) found that a third of staff working in intensive care in their study in America were suffering from severe burnout syndrome. This has been more than backed up by evidence from practitioners working in intensive care and other settings in the UK in extremely high emotionally demanding care necessary during the COVID-19 pandemic. This is unsustainable and exhausting work, physically and emotionally, and there will be a price to pay in relation to post traumatic stress disorder. This could affect practitioners for years if sufficient resources are not available very quickly to support staff on an ongoing basis. Without this we will lose many highly experienced health care professionals, which will have a huge financial cost to their professions and the country, as well as creating an enormous personal cost to those involved, and their loved ones. Haik et al (2017) focused on those caring for burns sufferers in Israel; they found that compassion fatigue and vicarious trauma was leading to an increase in depression, reduced carer satisfaction and reduced physical and mental quality of life. In addition, stress was causing problems at home due to less free time and work/home disputes. Without a supportive workplace culture, debriefing opportunities and psychological support health care practitioners would be unable to deal with the stress involved within their working lives. I will be discussing Post Traumatic Stress Disorder (PTSD) and secondary stress, or vicarious stress, in greater detail later.

When reading the research papers, the types of patient who were highlighted as potentially causing additional stress to practitioners were primarily patients with high dependency needs, or who were reaching the end of their lives. This was particularly the case if the death was unexpected or if their lives were being cut short long before their time. Renal patients, or those with chronic and long-term needs, were often challenging due to their high stress levels, and sometimes their unrealistic demands and expectations. However, cancer care staff experienced considerable occupational stress, and this was true in many different countries. The main cause of burnout was a very heavy workload and palliative care staff were at particularly high risk. However, Martins Pereira et al (2016) compared the burnout in palliative care with that of ITU staff and found that ITU staff had over double the chance of burnout in comparison with palliative care staff. Girgis and Hansen (2007) focused on oncologists and palliative care physicians in Australia and found that higher exhaustion levels were found in those with direct patient contact. Also, that staff without direct social contact were more likely to suffer from depersonalisation, also those early in their careers with low patient contact. Both these categories of staff scored high on personal accomplishment and professional efficacy which could be seen as mitigating factors for burnout. However, Girgis and Hansen (2007) also found that low personal accomplishment was most likely associated with low patient contact, whilst emotional exhaustion was highest in people with high levels of patient contact. High cynicism was associated with those longer in their careers and was also related to factors impacting on their home lives such as problems with arranging leave.

Organisational culture was responsible for high levels of stress amongst health care practitioners. This could be in relation to the pressure from challenging targets, or a lack of adequate equipment. However, poor staffing levels, work overload and long working hours were the cause of a great deal of stress, with no choice of working hours, or last-minute changes in shift patterns, frequently cited as stressors. This is not really surprising because a lack of control over work and poor working conditions create many problems with work/life balance and in relationships with loved ones. Work demands such as demanding environments and unmanageable time pressures, and expectations which are impossible to achieve being frequently cited as areas of concern. However, low organisational commitment, and poor organisational environments with unsupportive management created a great deal of stress according to many studies. Availability of mentorship, supervision and protected hours for CPD were found to be helpful strategies for supporting individuals within high stress environments (Cedar and Walker, 2020). However, strategies to enhance staff satisfaction, and individuals feeling valued by their peers and superiors, and communication between members of the MDT, and good team working were also perceived as very important in helping to reduce stress levels (Kompanje, 2018 and McKinley et al, 2017). Greater social contact with colleagues, more opportunities for laughter, when appropriate, and collaborative approaches between MDT team members were perceived as very important. Positive team spirit, regular team meetings and opportunities to discuss challenging situations and debrief from traumatic events were perceived as particularly crucial. Conflicts and psychosocial bullying were perceived as key determinants of burnout, and symptoms of this could be views and opinions being ignored or undervalued, escalating to more overt signs of harassment and bullying. This will be discussed again in Chapter 4 with a focus on resilience. Conflict prediction, prevention and de-escalation strategies, initiatives to decrease bullying and increase awareness of this (Wunnenberg, 2020), team empowerment, and problem solving were all perceived as important strategies to focus on. (Martins Periera, 2016, Lahana et al, 2017).

Kompanje (2018) identified three interlocking syndromes in relation to stress:

- **Professional wear syndrome or burnout** leading to emotional exhaustion. This is characterised by high work demands, repeated exposure to traumatic events which leads to decreased job satisfaction and depression. This can be helped by supportive workplace environments, peer and psychological support, management awareness of burnout, supervision, debriefing and education opportunities.
- **Boreout syndrome or labour boredom** characterised by a lack of challenge and repetitive tasks combined with limited education, innovation and career progression opportunities which results in a low sense of accomplishment. This can be helped by access to professional development opportunities.
- **Compassion fatigue syndrome and depersonalisation** which can be characterised by a loss of compassion towards patients and negative and cynical attitudes towards them, combined with heightened stress levels and anxiety. This

can be helped by training in self-care and compassion, and initiatives to maximise compassion satisfaction, combined with a focus on staff wellbeing and on the positive impact of roles. A focus on communication strategies, emotional intelligence and emotional management, resilience and self-compassion can be helpful.

- **Combination of all three syndromes** which is characterised by demotivation, absenteeism, loss of efficiency and increased errors. This can be helped by stress management, resilience, positivity, self-care, mindfulness, reflective practice and cognitive problem-solving strategies. Focusing on vicarious trauma and coping with grief and loss are also helpful strategies.

These syndromes would be a potential risk in all health care professionals in all areas of practice, in all countries, and in practitioners working with all age groups, in hospital and in community settings.

Edmonds et al (2012) review a one-day care giver programme which focuses on vicarious trauma and loss, coping with grief, coping and self-care strategies. Participants, many of whom were experiencing high levels of burnout, found that positive changes to cope with emotional exhaustion appeared to have long term benefits. The table below (Table 3.1) sums up the findings of our literature search in terms of area of practice, areas of concern and strategies, particularly focusing on organisational culture, areas of patient care and personal impact.

The way that different areas of practice can cause different stresses has now been discussed, and also how these can be manifested differently in terms of burnout. Burnout, bore out and compassion fatigue, or a combination of all three syndromes, can be a result of different aspects of our working lives (Kompanje, 2018). Individual coping strategies, different areas of practice and organisational culture strategies can be used to address all these areas of burnout. Consequently, a combination of approaches to address personal and organisational stressors, as well as the specific demands of our practice areas in relation to patient needs, can be the most effective in reducing workplace stress. I have summed up the impact on health care professionals of both the culture of the organisation, and specific patient care needs, as well as the personal impact on the individual themselves, in Figure 3.1 (see below).

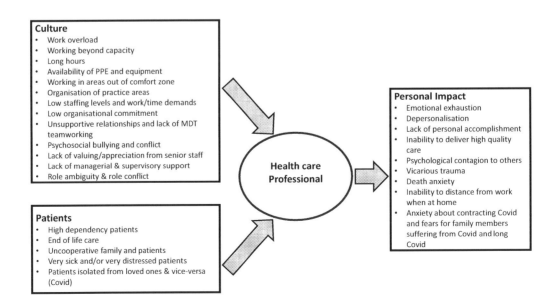

Figure 3.1 Causes of stress

Table 3.1 Areas of concern and potential strategies in relation to specific areas of practice

Causes	Reference	Areas of practice	Area of concern	Strategies
Culture				
Targets	Jones 2014 Dermody and Bennett 2008 Murphy 2004	Renal UK Renal Renal NI	Pressure from targets	
Equipment	Jones 2014 Dermody and Bennett 2008 Murphy 2004	Renal UK Renal Renal NI	Adequate equipment	Adequate equipment (Jones 2014), Dermody and Bennett (2008) Murphy (2004)
Organisation of practice areas	Girgis and Hansen 2007 Adriaenssens et al 2015	Oncology Australia ED Netherlands	Poor access to/cover for leave linked to high cynicism Poor organisational culture, lack of quality assurance, understaffing	Choosing own days off (Poncet et al 2007) Management which supports empowering leadership, best care, healthy engaged staff (Adriaenssens et al 2015) Organisational culture that reflects shared values, especially round the 6Cs (Bewick, 2019 HV) Realistic understanding and correct values, planned staff breaks, participation and autonomy incentives (Lahana et al, 2017, LD Greece)
Working hours	Embriaco et al 2007 Girgis and Hansen 2007 Kompanje 2018	ICU France Oncology Australia ICU UK	Long working hours Health fatigue Heavy workload in EOL care linked strongly to burnout	Decreased working hours and greater flexibility (Girgis and Hansen 2007 palliative care Australia)
Staffing levels and work overload	Jones 2014 Dermody and Bennett 2008 Murphy 2004 Girgis and Hansen 2007 Kompanje 2018 Poulsen et al 2014	Renal UK Renal Renal NI Oncology Australia ICU UK OT Australia	Workload too heavy Low staffing levels and poor skill mix Unrealistic demands/expectations Few hours to rest Stress in relation to tasks	Improved staffing levels, reduction of clinical load, access to and cover for leave (Girgis and Hansen 2007)

(Continued)

Table 3.1 (Continued) Areas of concern and potential strategies in relation to specific areas of practice

Causes	Reference	Areas of practice	Area of concern	Strategies
Culture				
Work/time demands	Adriaenssens et al. 2017 Lambert and Lambert 2001 Kompanje 2018 McKinless 2020 Hannafin et al 2020	Managers Netherlands International ICU UK DNs UK PHNs Ireland	Work/time demands High job demands Work overload Repetitive tasks Time pressures, too much expected, work environment too demanding	Control over work (Adriaenssens et al, 2017). Protected hours for training, better working conditions, longer rest periods, strategies to increase satisfaction (Kompanje 2018)
Low organizational commitment	Embriaco et al 2007 Lambert and Lambert 2001 Kompanje 2018	ICU France International ICU UK Paediatrics USA	Poor ITU organisation Poor working conditions	Supportive management focusing on staff (Lambert and Lambert 2001, Jones 2014, Dermody and Bennett 2008) Murphy 2004). Availability of mentorship and supervision (Cedar and Walker, 2020 palliative care UK). Protected hours for training, better working conditions, longer rest periods, strategies to increase satisfaction (Kompanje 2018). Financial rewards, valuing individuals, improved communication between staff, team working (McKinley et al 2017)
Psychosocial bullying	Embriaco et al 2007 Poncet et al 2007 Martins Pereira 2016 Wunnenberg 2020 Waddington 2016 Adrienssens et al 2015	ICU France ICU USA Palliative care Portugal Nurse educators USA Nurse education HE UK ED Netherlands	Conflicts and these are key determinants of burnout Prevalent in nurse education – being excluded, opinions ignored, high workload Toxic HE environments compound crisis in compassionate care Interpersonal conflicts	Conflict prevention strategies and team empowerment (Poncet et al 2007, Martins Periera 2016, Lahana et al 2017, LD Greece). Strategies to include problem solving, seeking social support, predicting and de-escalation. Also, initiatives to decrease bullying and increase awareness of this (Wunnenberg, 2020). Critical appreciative enquiry, narrative approaches which reveal and rectify failures of compassion. Courageous conversations to challenge dysfunctional organisational systems and processes. Leadership development programmes which include the application of skills of compassion in organisational settings (Waddington, 2016)

MDT liaison	Embriaco et al 2007 Haik et al 2017 Lambert and Lambert 2001 Adrienssens et al 2015	ICU France Burns Israel International ED Netherlands	Communication in team Inability to reach physicians Poor relationships with doctors	More social contact with colleagues (Embriaco et al 2007) collaborative approach with medical staff (Adrienssens et al 2017 and Lambert and Lambert, 2001).
No time for laughter	Poulsen et al 2014	OTs in Australia	Especially in those under 10 years' experience mixed with inability to say no	Encouraging distancing from work when at home. Managers to be aware of risk of burnout when staff cannot recover at the end of each shift. Encouraging self-care, resilience, stress management and coping strategies, and times to appreciate and maximise humour opportunities
Unsupportive relationships	Adriaenssens et al 2017 Lambert and Lambert 2001 Embriaco et al 2007 Poncet et al 2007 Jones 2014 Dermody and Bennett 2008 Murphy 2004 Girgis and Hansen 2007 Adrienssens et al 2015	Managers Netherlands International ICU France ICU USA Renal UK Renal Renal NI Oncology Australia ED Netherlands	Unsupportive relationships Poor relationships with supervisors Lack of appreciation from senior staff Dissatisfaction with management Little recognition & acknowledgement Lack of managerial support Poor communication with managers, poor relationships with doctors	More appreciation from managers, improved teamwork (Embriaco et al 2007, Girgis and Hansen 2007), positive feedback (Poncet et al 2007) Training in communication (Poncet et al, 2007). Promoting relationships with colleagues and managers and greater teamwork, staff recognition policies, positive reappraisal, strengthening of collaboration (Lahana et al, 2017 LD Greece). Organisational support, regular team meetings, supervision, detecting signs of chronic stress eg work overload, value conflict (Gosseries et al, 2012 neuro nurses, Belgium). Greater professional autonomy, good team spirit, peer and social support, good communication and coaching around innovation and quality assurance. Importance of reducing repetitive exposure, creating time out and counselling and support in anticipatory coping skills (Adrienssens et al, 2015)

(Continued)

Table 3.1 (Continued) Areas of concern and potential strategies in relation to specific areas of practice

Causes	Reference	Areas of practice	Area of concern	Strategies
Culture				
Patients				
High dependency	Jones 2014 Dermody and Bennett 2008 Murphy 2004 Kompanje 2018 Gosseries et al 2012 Rodger and Atwal 2018	Renal UK Renal Renal NI ICU UK Brain injury Belgium Theatre	Chronic care of patients and high need and severely ill patients Persistent vegetative state, brain injury and disorders of consciousness Perioperative death devastating and long lasting if no support	More on principles and practice of palliative care in ITUs and more education in intensive care and palliative (Martins Pereira, 2016 ITU, Portugal)
End of life care Death anxiety and/or vicarious trauma	Embriaco et al 2007 Lambert and Lambert 2001 Poncet et al 2007 Girgis and Hansen 2007 McKinless 2020 Forbes 2019 Evans 2019 Nyatanga 2016 Rodger and Atwal 2018	ICU France International ICU USA, UK and Portugal Oncology Australia and Canada DNs UK HVUK HV UK Palliative nursing UK Theatres	Dealing with death and dying Parental stress Support re Sudden Infant Death Syndrome Dealing with death causes death anxiety leading to vicarious trauma Perioperative death	Better management of end-of-life care (Poncet et al, 2007) Training in self-care and coping with death competence (Sanso et al, 2015) Training re psychosocial needs of dying patients and families (Slocum-Gory et al 2011) Liaison with chaplaincy services and understanding of multi faith issues and pastoral care (Cedar and Walker, 2020). More on principles and practice of palliative care in ITUs and more education in intensive care and palliative care (Martins Pereira, 2016) Programme focusing on vicarious trauma, coping with grief and loss, self-care and coping strategies (Edmonds et al, 2012) Training re sudden infant death (Forbes, 2019). Importance of debriefing, education, peer support, morbidity and mortality meetings, emotional intelligence/resilience (Rodger and Atwal, 2018)
Uncooperative family and patients	Lambert and Lambert 2001 Jones 2014 Dermody and Bennett 2008 Murphy 2004 Girgis and Hansen 2007	International Renal UK Renal Renal – NI Oncology Australia	Unrealistic demands – renal leading to physical and verbal abuse Demanding patients	Better support and relationships (Jones 2014 Dermody and Bennett 2008, Murphy 2004)

104

Personal impact

Professional wear syndrome or boreout Emotional exhaustion	Kompanje 2018 McKinless 2020 Adriaenssens et al 2015 Ray et al 2013 Haik et al 2017 Maslach et al 1996 and 2001 Girgis and Hansen 2007 Medland et al 2004 Lambert and Lambert 2001	ICU UK DNs UK LD Greece ED Netherlands Physios Greece MH Canada Burns Israel International	Type of work and long working hours Compassion fatigue causing reduced job satisfaction, retention, Job demands, exposure to traumatic events Low person/job match Burnout reduces care of MH patients Increased depression, reduced satisfaction, problems at home and work/home disputes. Particularly in EOL direct patient care and greater in those with most patient contact Burnout occupational hazard of working in oncology emotional injury. Unfamiliarity with situations and inability to deliver high quality care	Supportive workplace which encourages psychological support, debrief support, peer support networks, access to supervision and support, management awareness of burnout and educational provision etc (Haik et al, 2017, Girgis and Hansen 2007 pall care, Australia, Lahana et al, 2017). Clinical supervision (Fischer et al, 2013). Improved mental health amongst staff will enhance patient care, high person/job match, promoting higher compassion satisfaction (Ray et al, 2013) Importance of support from colleagues, normalizing grief and bereavement, ongoing support and education (Medland et al, 2004)
Labour boredom or boreout syndrome Low sense of accomplishment	Kompanje 2018 Maslach et al and 1996 2001 Girgis and Hansen 2007	ICU UK All areas Oncology Australia, USA All areas	Lack of challenge, loss of interest in work, repetitive tasks, limited progression in illness, lack of training/ innovation in tasks Highest in those with less patient contact	Access to professional development (Girgis and Hansen, 2007)
Compassion fatigue syndrome Depersonalisation and emotional dissonance	Kompanje 2018 Bakker et and Heuven 2006 Maslach et al 1996 and 2001 Girgis and Hansen 2007 Panagopoulou et al 2006	ICU UK Paediatric doctors Palliative care Canada HV	Loss of compassion towards patients, causing increased anxiety, stress and reduced productivity, sense of incompetence, difficulty in continuing to do the work Negative/cynical attitudes to patients	Training in self-care (Sanso et al, 2015 Palliative care, USA, Kompanje 2018) and nurturing family, social support, adequate rest and time with families. Also increasing personal resilience, confidence in providing compassionate care, mindfulness and stress reduction (McKinley et al 2017)

(Continued)

Table 3.1 (Continued) Areas of concern and potential strategies in relation to specific areas of practice

Causes	Reference	Areas of practice	Area of concern	Strategies
Culture				
	Kompanje 2018 Poulsen et al 2014 McKinless 2020	Nurses and police officers Netherlands All areas Oncology Australia Physicians Greece Oncology Australia ICU UK OTs Australia LD Greece DNs UK	Particularly those with less social contact Higher in those with least patient contact Highest in those earlier in their careers and junior doctors. Danger of role modelling and psychological contagion to less experienced residents, medical students and other staff. Inability to distance from work when at home. Life dominated by work Decreased family life Inability to distance from work when at home. Dissonance between real feelings and those needed to show creates increased cynicism, low energy, emotional exhaustion and dissonance and low quality service and psychological distress.	Training programme to maximise compassion satisfaction and minimise burnout (Slocum-Gory et al, 2011) Focus on staff wellbeing and positive impact of role (Bewick, 2019) Hidden curriculum should not include promotion of detachment. Help with coping with stressful situations, time management, interpersonal skills training and focusing on burnout, communication skills and emotional management (Panagopoulou et al, 2006). Ongoing education re sharing of feelings & normalising experiences and stress coping strategies (Lahana et al 2017). Healthy behaviours, emotional intelligence and emotional resilience, effective caseload and staffing management, Organisations to promote healthy behaviours, self-care and self-compassion which increases resilience (McKinless, 2020). Suppressing negative emotions is stressful so promoting positive emotion e.g., problem solving, alleviation of pain, enhancing morale, reducing anxiety and despair, determining whether staff should express their true emotions to reduce emotional dissonance (Bakker and Heuven 2006)
Combination of 3 syndromes (above)	Kompanje 2018	ICU UK and Portugal Palliative care UK Neuro nurses Belgium	Cause demotivation, absenteeism, loss of efficiency and increased errors	Stress management and burnout prevention workshops and training (Poncet et al 2007). Resilience training focusing on positive relationships, positivity, accepting some things are out of our control. Also, on strategies around self-care, mindfulness, reflective practice, Schwartz rounds (Cedar and Walker, 2020, Martins Pereira et al, 2016) Relaxation, cognitive strategies, communication skills, social support, problem solving and resilience (Gosseries et al 2012)

As can be seen in Figure 3.1 the impact on the practitioner can be immense and this is not acceptable. During the pandemic we have been in extraordinary times and practitioners have had to rely on resources that they did not know they had. However, if during the period when the pandemic is abating slightly these human sacrifices are not valued, then people will leave the professions, or be unable to recover. Strategies need to be put in place to support those who have been affected so deeply by the traumatic situations they have witnessed. Time needs to be given to recovery and revisiting how relationships with patients can, and should, be supported, as well as time for CPD, team building and stress management. The following section discusses more about high stress levels and how burnout can be manifested and avoided.

How does compassion burnout relate to high stress levels?

Chapter 2 already discussed how burnout is prevalent in health care environments, and how we can start to recognise burnout in ourselves. Burnout is the prolonged response to chronic emotional and interpersonal stressors at work and it is often characterised by exhaustion, cynicism and inefficiency (Maslach et al, 2001). It is not always clear about cause and effect, whether job dissatisfaction causes burnout or vice versa, but it is clear that high stress levels can cause burnout which can then impact on our ability to be compassionate. Work engagement is a sign of job satisfaction, and this can have a potential impact on burnout. In Dall'ora and Saville's (2021) extensive literature review of 91 studies the conclusion drawn was that individual targeted support strategies like encouraging mindfulness and resilience could be less effective than fixing more endemic organisational problems. Peer and social support from loved ones and friends can also be strong mitigating factors in relation to reducing the incidence of burnout.

Burnout starts with extreme tiredness, which depletes our emotional energy. When this tiredness is chronic this leads to emotional exhaustion. Symptoms of burnout are emotional exhaustion, cynicism and depersonalisation. These together with feeling a lack of professional effectiveness, efficacy and worthlessness can lead to increased absenteeism, less efficiency at work and health problems for us personally (Abidi et al 2014). Exhaustion and disengagement are different from other short-term consequences of mental strain. Exhaustion is primarily linked to mental fatigue whereas disengagement is primarily linked to a feeling of satiation and experiencing a sense of monotony. Monotony is the result of repetitive tasks which causes fatigue, and satiation is emotional rejection of repetitive tasks. Mental fatigue is the temporary impairment of mental and physical efficiency. Burnout is the long-term consequence of mental strain, and addressing mental strain in its early stages may prevent burnout (Demerouti et al 2002).

Bakker and Costa (2014) say that chronic burnout can be mitigated by cycles of losses and gains. The **Cycle of losses** relates to our daily job demands which can cause incremental daily exhaustion due to daily job demands which are self-undermining. The **Cycle of gains** relates to our daily job resources and incremental daily engagement and daily job crafting, or honing our professional skills. Employees with high levels of chronic burnout are not only more likely to end up with the loss cycle of daily job demands. They are also less likely to profit from the gain cycle of daily job resources, in terms of daily work engagement and daily job crafting. Job crafting involves modifying aspects of our job to improve the fit between characteristics of our job, our own abilities, and our needs and preferences. Job crafting is a helpful "bottom up" personal strategy which helps us to optimise our work environment to help us stay engaged. So, burnout strengthens the "loss" cycle and weakens the "gain" cycle. We need to be able to help change our working conditions and enhance our ability to be healthy at work. Organisations should identify, and try and reduce, job demands such as role ambiguity and role conflict, as well as identify job resources that focus on work engagement and helping individuals cope with their work demands. Employers should also help employees with job crafting and adapting the work environment to themselves. They should also help employees to focus on recovery activities such as social activities with friends, and low effort activities for example reading, music and internet surfing. In addition, employees should be encouraged to engage in physical activities, for example sport, exercise and dancing, because they could promote the next day's work engagement. Bakker et al (2012) say that people who have more proactive personalities are more likely to craft their jobs and therefore increase their structural and social job resources and increase their job challenges. People who craft their work roles are more likely to be engaged and have vigour, dedication and absorption at work, and colleagues are more likely to rate their performance more highly. Therefore, if we are more proactive we will adjust our own work environments which helps us to perform at a higher level and stay engaged.

Gruman and Saks (2011) also say that in order for employees to feel engaged they need to feel psychologically safe, and not feel at risk of damage to their self-image or career. They also need to feel meaningful, valuable, and that they matter. Finally, they need to feel psychologically available, in terms of what they feel able to bring to their roles, so physical and emotional energy are important. Gruman and Saks (2011) says that factors which can promote engagement are:

- Job design and a good fit between the role and employees' skills, needs and values.
- Coaching and social support which fosters psychological safety, meaningfulness, optimism and resilience through supervisor support and encouragement.
- Transformational leadership which promotes challenge, a feeling of control, autonomy, performance feedback and participation in decision making.
- Training again around self-efficacy, hope, optimism and resilience.

So, who is most at risk of burnout? Opinions vary here to some extent, but the following factors seem to have some relevance:

- Males (Bhagavathula et al, 2018) – higher levels of depersonalisation and cynicism (Maslach et al, 1996)
- Those who are unmarried (Bhagavathula et al, 2018)
- Less experienced employees (Bhagavathula et al, 2018)
- Younger employees (Maslach et al, 1996)
- Women – higher levels of exhaustion (Maslach et al, 1996)
- Those who are more highly educated (Maslach et al, 1996)
- Those who have an external locus of control, rather than feeling that they are to some extent in charge of their own destinies
- Those with ineffective or passive coping strategies
- Those with low self-esteem.

Links between burnout and post-traumatic stress disorder (PTSD) were explored by Mealer et al (2009). The huge impact of working through the COVID-19 pandemic and the PTSD that appears to be a long-term consequence of this, has already been discussed. Mealer et al (2009) state that individuals with PTSD will almost always have symptoms of burnout and this has a dramatic impact on work and home environments and social lives, as well as on an individual's perceptions. PTSD and symptoms such as anxiety, depression, nightmares and severe panic attacks can be triggered by what feels like futile care and caring for people who are dying. The high incidence of mortality in practice areas where patients with COVID were being cared for would be examples of both these types of care. Many patients suffering from COVID were not expected to die at that age, and they were previously well. Patients could become severely unwell very fast, and in many cases, interventions were known to be unlikely to be effective, and that probable death would follow. This was incredibly stressful for those providing the care. In the past PTSD was mainly focused on people who had been exposed to a single catastrophic event. However, in hospital and community environments health care practitioners are often exposed to repeated sub-catastrophic stressors which could also lead to PTSD. Individual strategies are unlikely to be sufficient when people are experiencing PTSD and burnout. Improved communication and support groups and debriefing after traumatic events could be much more helpful. In addition, it is essential to increase awareness of PTSD, and the manifestations of both PTSD and the combined impact of PTSD and burnout. Greater awareness would decrease the risk of substance abuse, suicide and individuals leaving their profession. Strategies to improve working environments and job satisfaction are also very important (Mealer et al, 2009). Figley (2002) also says it is important to focus on self-soothing, stress management and desensitisation strategies such as CBT and Eye Movement Desensitization and Reprocessing (EMDR) to alleviate secondary traumatic stress. EMDR uses lateral eye movements as an external stimulus when briefly focusing on traumatic memories, but hand tapping and audio stimulation can also be used (https://www.emdr.com/what-is-emdr/).

In order to determine Secondary Traumatic Stress (STS), which can be a result of experiencing the trauma of others, practitioners need to be closely monitored. After a single traumatic event, such as a terror incident, there can be support put in place to support practitioners involved in the treating and caring for victims of these events. It is important that this also takes place after more everyday occurrences. A student of mine became very upset at a review meeting with her practice assessor and myself about the death of a patient in her care. This patient was only 49 and she was well known to nursing staff because of her various comorbidities. This student was very distressed, and the practice assessor and I did our best to comfort her. The practice assessor was in the room with her, but I was at a distance because virtual meetings only were possible as the pandemic was limiting access to the hospital. She was very embarrassed but clearly gained comfort from us both. I tried to reassure her that being upset is normal, and it is more worrying when we are not upset at unusual and upsetting situations like this. The next day she told me that her husband had died 14 years ago, and she had not been able to visit him in hospital when he died. The trauma of her nursing situation had not been appreciated at the time, and as she said the unresolved feelings about her husband's death had also contributed to this. The importance of opportunities to debrief with peers, and gain mutual support, should never be underestimated. Symptoms of STS in practitioners can include (Bride et al, 2004):

- Feeling emotionally numb
- Sleeping problems
- Feeling jumpy

- Feeling discouraged about the future
- Being easily annoyed
- Having trouble concentrating
- Memory gaps
- Expecting something bad to happen
- Disturbing dreams about work with patients
- Wanting to avoid working with some patients.
- Avoiding people/places that remind them of working with patients
- Not wanting to work with patients when they did intend to
- Being reminded of work with patients upsets them
- Reliving the trauma experienced by patients
- Heart pounding when thinking about work with patients
- Having little interest in being around others
- Being less active than usual
- Feeling discouraged about the future.

It is very important that practitioners have access to support because STS impairs the ability to help patients, and STS has a strong negative impact on the practitioners themselves.

It is important to recognise that in order to be burnt out, we need to be 'burning' in the first place (Korunka et al, 2010). Therefore, the implication is that we strongly like and are committed to our job. Therefore, engagement, enthusiasm and interest in our job is a necessary pre-cursor to burnout. This does not happen overnight, it is a prolonged and slow process, and burnout usually begins at an early stage of emotional exhaustion. This can lead to withdrawal from patients, colleagues and our role in general, and can cause a cynical attitude towards our role and our patients. This results in emotional exhaustion which can lead to depersonalisation. Korunka et al (2010) identify key stages of the burn out process:

1. High workload, high job stress and high job expectation. Job demands exceed the job resources. Therefore, our job no longer fulfils our expectations.
2. Physical/emotional exhaustion. Chronic exhaustion can be due to the result of higher energy levels being needed to carry out all tasks of the role. Sleep disturbances can add to this, and we can be more susceptible to headaches and other physical pain. In addition, we can suffer from emotional exhaustion, and experience fatigue even when thinking about work.
3. Depersonalisation/cynicism/indifference. For example, apathy, depression and boredom, negative attitude towards our job, colleagues and patients, withdrawal from the role and its challenges and reduced work effort.
4. Despair/helplessness/ aversion. This can be in relation to ourselves, other people and other aspects of our lives. Feelings of guilt and insufficiency can then result.

Korunka et al (2010) cite the following causes of burnout:

- Job characteristics
- Workload and time pressures
- Work demands and work hours
- Role conflict and role ambiguity
- Lack of resources
- Lack of support from supervisors and co-workers.
- Lack of job autonomy and control.

So if we think that we could be suffering from burnout it might be a good idea to ask ourselves the following questions:

Quick "burnout test"

- Do I feel emotionally drained by my work?
- Do I feel tired when I get up in the morning and have to face another day on the job?
- Have I become less interested in my work since I started this job?
- Have I become less enthusiastic about my job?
- Have I become more cynical about whether my job contributes anything?
- Do I doubt the significance of my work?

If you answer yes to any of the previous questions, it would be a good idea to seek support and question what is causing these symptoms. If they are not new thoughts for you, or if they precede the pandemic, you might need to question whether you are still happy in your current role. If they have been caused by the pandemic, a change of work environment might still be worth thinking about, but maybe some counselling, and other strategies which I will discuss in Chapter 4, might help you with what could be a relatively temporary problem.

Schaufeli and Enzmann (1998) sum up signs of burnout at individual, interpersonal and organisational level:

Four types of **individual** level signals of burnout:

1. *Affective* – depressed, changing mood, tearfulness, increased tension or anxiety, emotional exhaustion.
2. *Cognitive* – powerlessness or feeling trapped, sense of failure, poor self-esteem, guilt, suicidal ideation, inability to concentrate, forgetfulness, difficulty with complex tasks.
3. *Physical* –headaches, nausea, dizziness, muscle pain, sleep disturbance, ulcer and gastro-intestinal disorders, chronic fatigue.
4. *Behavioural* – hyperactivity or impulsivity, increased use of caffeine, tobacco, alcohol and prescribed or illicit drugs, abandoning recreational activities, compulsive complaining or denial.
5. *Motivational* – loss of zeal, loss of idealism, resignation, disappointment, boredom.

Four types of **interpersonal** level signals of burnout:

1. *Affective*: Irritability, over sensitivity, increased anger, lower emotional empathy with patients.
2. *Cognitive*: Cynical and dehumanising perception of patients, negative and pessimistic view of patients, labelling patients in derogatory ways.
3. *Behavioural*: Violent outbursts, increased violence and aggressive behaviour, aggressiveness towards patients, interpersonal marital and family conflict, social isolation and withdrawal, responding to patients in a mechanical manner.
4. *Motivational:* Loss of interest, indifferences, lack of respect for patients.

Four types of **organisational** level signals of burnout:

1. *Affective*: Job dissatisfaction.
2. *Cognitive:* Cynicism and work role, distrust in management; peers and supervisors.
3. *Behavioural:* reduced effectiveness, poor work performance, reduced productivity, turnover, increased sick leave/absenteeism, over dependency on supervisors, increased accidents.
4. *Motivational:* loss of work motivation, resistance to going to work, low morale.

Again, questioning whether we have any of these signs of burnout will enable us to take active measures to address these serious burnout issues. We need to do this for the sake of ourselves, our patients and our friends and loved ones before even more challenging problems develop. Kearney et al (2009) also sum up the signs of individual and team burnout, and the strategies which could mitigate against these. They were focusing on physicians, but the same applies to all health care professionals (see Table 3.2).

Table 3.2 Individual and team symptoms of burnout and strategies to address burnout (Kearney et al, 2009)

Individual symptoms of burnout	Team symptoms of burnout	Strategies to address burnout
• Overwhelming physical and emotional exhaustion • Feelings of cynicism and detachment from the job • A sense of ineffectiveness and lack of accomplishment • Overidentification or overinvolvement • Irritability and hypervigilance • Sleep problems, including nightmares • Social withdrawal • Professional and personal boundary violations • Poor judgement • Perfectionism and rigidity • Questioning the meaning of life • Questioning prior religious beliefs • Interpersonal conflicts • Avoidance of emotionally difficult clinical situations • Addictive behaviours • Numbness and detachment • Difficulty in concentrating • Frequent illness – headaches, gastrointestinal disturbances, immune system impairment	• Low morale • High job turnover • Impaired job performance with decreased empathy and increased absenteeism • Staff conflicts	• Mindful meditation • Reflective writing • Adequate supervision and mentoring • Sustainable workload • Promotion of feelings of choice and control • Appropriate recognition and reward • Supportive work community • Promotion of fairness and justice in the workplace • Training in communication skills • Development of self awareness skills • Practice of self-care activities • Continuing educational activities • Participation in research • Mindfulness-based stress reduction for the team • Finding meaning in care taking place for the team

It is important for us to assess whether our personal burnout is linked to burnout which can be endemic in the team we work in. If this is the case we might need to think about our personal strategies, and then take a lead in helping our team to recognise the stressors that are causing burnout for many of those working there. If staff absence and turnover is high, then our joint resources are depleted by understaffing and an underskilled workforce, leading to an even greater impact on morale, team spirit and individuals working in the team. Team strategies can then be helpful, but we need to recognise when organisation-wide measures need to be taken, and how we can escalate our concerns to higher management levels. Having discussed how high stress levels can lead to burnout I will go on to discuss resilience strategies in greater detail later in Chapter 4. However, I will now focus on how high stress levels and burnout have an impact on our ability to be compassionate.

Are my stress levels affecting my ability to be compassionate?

In order to be compassionate, we need to be able to cope with our own emotions and find a way to cope with the personal and professional stressors in our lives in a way that enables us to be able to give of our ourselves to others. If we are suffering from compassion fatigue we are not able to do this, and it is important to recognise the early signs of burnout, which can be easily missed. These can be:

- Loss of confidence
- A change in how we socialise with others at work
- A change in general behaviour
- Lack of care at work
- Physical illness.

I have already discussed the physical manifestations of stress, and physical illness like headaches, gastrointestinal symptoms can be an indicator of increasing stress levels. However, changes in our general behaviour, and not wanting to spend time with others, or changes in how we communicate with others, at home or at work, can be important indicators of stress. We might have less confidence than before, and question our abilities at work, but we also might lower our standards and take less care, or become less motivated in our care of patients.

El-Bar et al (2013) say that compassion fatigue causes patient dissatisfaction, compromises patient safety and increases the chances of medical and care errors. They state the importance of focusing on compassion fatigue, particularly through education and early intervention. These can focus on:

- Treatment programmes and focusing on wellbeing and building resilience
- Incorporating resilience into on-going continuing education.

Also more specifically focusing on:

- Work life balance
- Attending to spiritual needs
- Regular professional supervision
- Personal self-care strategies
- Awareness of goals
- Organisational culture of support and respect. (El-Bar et al, 2013)

Chapter 4 will discuss resilience but understanding the reasons for our high stress, and what resilience strategies might be helpful is key to addressing compassion fatigue and burnout. We also need to work in environments where we feel valued and supported, and that needs to be at a team and organisational level.

Smajdor (2013) has a slightly different perspective and says that they believe that it can be damaging for health care practitioners to feel too much compassion because they might become deeply distressed by their experiences. This might put them at risk of burnout and compassion fatigue and that they might become desensitised to patient distress. They go on to say that good health care workers will ensure that the presence or absence of compassion does not interfere with their care. They say that hiring nurses on the basis of their compassion is not the answer to systematic failings in the NHS. In response to the findings of the Francis Report (2013) they say that Mid Staffordshire would not have been staffed entirely by individuals who lacked compassion. The report (Francis, 2013) contained accounts of nurses feeling distressed, depressed and helpless. The point is that if they lacked compassion, they would not be suffering so much distress, so their ability to be compassionate was not totally compromised by their poor working environment. I would agree with the majority of these points, and fully support the fact that nurses in Mid Staffordshire were under incredible amounts of stress, and were not being supported by their organisation. I do not however agree with the fact that we can be too compassionate, and that distress caused by our experiences can lead to desensitisation. In fact, in my opinion working in a culture where becoming desensitised is the norm can be at odds with our personal and professional values and this can be much more likely to bring about compassion fatigue. We need to work in positive organisations who care about us, and access support and care for ourselves, which will be discussed more in Chapter 4.

The King's Fund 2020 in The Courage of Compassion (West et al, 2020) say that major causes of stress at work are:

- Work pressures (high workload, complexity of care, low staffing levels, high staff turnover, dissatisfaction).
- Moral distress (being prevented from delivering high quality care, going against moral compass which undermines integrity, self-worth and wellbeing).
- Pay issues (struggling to pay for food, housing costs and utilities).
- Education and entry onto the nursing and midwifery professions. Highly stressful for newly qualified care professionals, feeling apprehensive, unprepared and being treated like students, continual monitoring and little autonomy.
- Work schedules (long working hours, shift work and impact on home/work life balance and working additional unpaid hours. This impacts on personal safety, increases the likelihood of occupational accidents, absenteeism and turnover).
- Discrimination (from patients and relatives particularly to minority ethnic staff which impacts on stress and physical health).
- Bullying, harassment and abuse (physical violence, emotional abuse from patients, colleagues and senior staff combined with hierarchical management cultures and disempowerment). (West et al, 2020)

Work pressures, and work scheduling issues have been discussed. Chapter 4 will discuss moral distress, how conflict between what we believe our care should be and what is reasonably possible, creates stress. There is no doubt that many health care practitioners have real financial issues which cause immense pressure. This needs to be addressed urgently but it is difficult to see how pay levels will be improved in the future. If practitioners are having to work additional paid or unpaid hours this increases the chances of errors being made. This will be discussed next, as well as issues in relation to bullying and harassment.

White (2018) says that medical errors in the USA are responsible for 100,000–200,000 deaths per year. In this study, 55% of physicians reported symptoms of burnout. 10% also reported they had made at least one major medical error in the previous 3 months. Physicians with burnout had more than twice the odds of self-reported medical errors after adjusting for other factors. Rates of medical errors tripled in medical work environments, even in those ranked as extremely safe, if the physician working on the unit had high levels of burnout. Having checklists to avoid mistakes and better teamwork is probably insufficient in their opinion, there needs to be an organisational, holistic and systems-based approach to create high quality health care. Halbesleben et al (2008) says that when there are higher levels of burnout there are lower incidents of near misses reported. Reports of near misses are essential to organisations as they are markers of larger problems and suggest future harm. It is understandable though that practitioners who are under pressure, already feel that they are struggling, and therefore they do not want to highlight times when they perceive themselves as failing. In this way it can be seen that burnout can cause organisational issues, but also that organisational issues can cause burnout through overly critical or unsupportive management practices. Health care practitioners need to feel that they are being supported, and that the organisation will work with them to avoid future errors. However, often there is a victim blaming approach to near misses and errors in judgement, and this does not lead to transparency and increased reporting. This actually leads to covering up of situations where organisational measures could have been taken to increase staffing or resources, or enhance training and problem solving.

This point about under reporting of errors can link to workplace bullying and employee workplace colleague abuse. Popp (2017) says that this can involve:

- Having zero empathy for patients or colleagues.
- Those targeted are often those who are more intelligent and more respected.
- There can be increased gossiping about other people.
- This can involve negative comments and encouraging others to do the same.
- Also not challenging negative comments made about others.
- People who are targeted could suffer from long term effects on their careers, their mental wellbeing, their self-esteem and their physical health.

All this stress caused by workplace bullying can increase levels of cortisol which may increase the chance of raised blood pressure and coronary heart disease. Also, high levels of stress can impair memory, thinking and problem solving and can cause panic attacks, reduced self-confidence and physical illness. If we are being bullied we need to keep evidence, for example emails. We also need to consider leaving that post if necessary, because it is better to leave with our mental health intact, so that we can be successful elsewhere. Some people do not recognise bullying, and people who are malignant forces, because this behaviour is incomprehensible to them. Therefore, having friendship from those who can stay rational in these situations is vital. It is also important to access self-help advice, personal coaching and help from human resources personnel. It is essential to resist self-blame, which is really difficult to do in the circumstances.

We need to understand that zero-empathy **individuals** lack a conscience, enjoy inflicting pain on better qualified employees and gain satisfaction in bringing down a well-regarded colleague. Zero-empathy **organisers** direct stealth attacks with the intention of increasing stress, reducing colleagues' social status and creating conditions to increase the chances of them leaving the workplace. They find pleasure and satisfaction in causing distress and anguish to the extent that colleagues become physically ill, resign or in extreme circumstances commit suicide. They are lacking in social intelligence and conscience and are incapable of expressing shame or remorse (Popp, 2017). People like this need to be identified in the workplace, and organisations need to support those who are at risk from them and support them. They also need to discipline those who have zero empathy, and who are bullying others. It is essential that all employees know that bullying and harassment will not be tolerated, and that they can escalate concerns and that they will be heard, and action will be taken as appropriate.

Anasori et al (2019) say that workplace bullying significantly predicts the potential for emotional exhaustion. Personal resilience strategies can mitigate against this, although in their study mindfulness was not reported to be a significant factor in moderating the effect of workplace bullying and resultant emotional exhaustion. Anasori et al (2019) also agree that organisations need to define and clarify what constitutes workplace bullying, and identify enforceable policies to deal with bullying and encourage employees to report this. Organisations also need to promote healthy and friendly work environments which mitigate against abusive behaviours, and make these practices unacceptable (Anasori et al, 2019).

Chapter 4 will focus more on strategies to address stress and burnout, but it would be useful for you to assess the extent to which you are suffering from burnout and the questionnaire below is designed to help you to assess the extent of your:

- Psychological distress
- Emotional exhaustion
- Depersonalisation and cynicism
- Personal accomplishment and efficacy.

Try to think of your own strategies which will help you to address areas of burnout that you have identified for yourself, and then plan for how you can integrate these strategies into your day-to-day life (Questionnaire 3.4).

QUESTIONNAIRE 3.4 To what extent are you experiencing burn out?

To what extent are you experiencing burn out?
(based on elements of Maslach's Burnout Inventory (1996) and Kessler's Psychological Distress Scale (2002)

How much does each statement apply to you?	*Consider what this means*				
Read each statement and decide how strongly the statement applies to you. Score yourself 1–5 based on the following guide: 1 = none of the time 2 = a little of the time 3 = some of the time 4 = most of the time 5 = all of the time	Ring the number that shows how strongly the statement applies and think about what it means in relation to your emotional wellbeing and your role.				
How are you feeling generally?					
I am feeling worn out for no good reason	1	2	3	4	5
I feel hopeless	1	2	3	4	5
I feel restless and agitated	1	2	3	4	5
I feel unhappy and depressed	1	2	3	4	5

I feel that everything is an effort	1	2	3	4	5
I feel sad and nothing cheers me up	1	2	3	4	5
I feel worthless	1	2	3	4	5
I feel constantly under pressure	1	2	3	4	5
I am losing confidence in myself	1	2	3	4	5
I feel reasonably happy, all things considered	1	2	3	4	5
I feel as if I play a useful part in things	1	2	3	4	5
I feel capable of making decisions	1	2	3	4	5
I am able to enjoy my day to day activities	1	2	3	4	5

How are your feelings showing themselves at work?

I feel emotionally drained and used up at the end of my work day	1	2	3	4	5
I feel tired when I get up and feel daunted by another day at work	1	2	3	4	5
I find it difficult to concentrate	1	2	3	4	5
I find it hard to be empathetic towards patients in my care and understand their feelings	1	2	3	4	5
I feel as if I treat patients as impersonal objects	1	2	3	4	5
I worry that my job is making me emotionally hard	1	2	3	4	5
I think that patients should take more responsibility for their health and I am blaming them more than I did					
I feel more cynical about whether what I do makes a difference	1	2	3	4	5
I can create a relaxed atmosphere with my patients	1	2	3	4	5
I can help solve problems that my patients have	1	2	3	4	5
I feel energetic when I am at work	1	2	3	4	5
I really enjoy my job and am enthusiastic about my work	1	2	3	4	5
I feel that I can make effective decisions at work	1	2	3	4	5
I feel that I am good at my job	1	2	3	4	5

How burnt out do you feel?

I enjoy my job and do not think I have any signs of burnout	Yes/no
I sometimes feel under stress and tired but I do not feel burn out	Yes/no
I definitely feel as if I am burning out and feel physically and emotionally exhausted at times	Yes/no
The symptoms of burn out will not go away and I feel very frustrated at work	Yes/no

I feel completely burnt out and do not know how much longer I can go on. I need to make some changes and maybe seek help	Yes/no

Consider your results and identify one or two actions you can take immediately to reduce your level of burnout

Action 1 Psychological distress:

Action 2: Emotional exhaustion:

Action 3: Depersonalisation and cynicism:

Action 4: Personal accomplishment and efficacy:

Another questionnaire I have devised also focuses on your compassion fatigue and strategies in relation to your personal and professional life (Questionnaire 3.5). This questionnaire, like all the others, is for you to carry out privately, so that you can be as honest as possible. Again, try to think about possible strategies to address any areas that you are not happy with.

QUESTIONNAIRE 3.5 Assessment of compassion fatigue and strategies

Assessment of your current feelings in relation to your personal and professional life

Please read each statement and circle the term that best fits your response and please use the spaces provided to comment in response to the prompts.

I feel stressed by the demands of my role at the moment						
Very strongly agree	Strongly agree	Agree	Neither agree nor disagree	Disagree	Strongly disagree	Very strongly disagree

Please comment further if you would like to:

I feel positive about my professional role						
Very strongly agree	Strongly agree	Agree	Neither agree nor disagree	Disagree	Strongly disagree	Very strongly disagree

Please comment further if you would like to:

I do not feel as if I can make a real difference in my work situation

Very strongly agree	Strongly agree	Agree	Neither agree nor disagree	Disagree	Strongly disagree	Very strongly disagree

Please comment further if you would like:

My stress at work is primarily due to caring for patients

Very strongly agree	Strongly agree	Agree	Neither agree nor disagree	Disagree	Strongly disagree	Very strongly disagree

Please comment further if you would like to:

My colleagues add significantly to my stress at work

Very strongly agree	Strongly agree	Agree	Neither agree nor disagree	Disagree	Strongly disagree	Very strongly disagree

Please comment further if you would like to:

My employer/manager causes me additional stress

Very strongly agree	Strongly agree	Agree	Neither agree nor disagree	Disagree	Strongly disagree	Very strongly disagree

Please comment if you would like to:

I feel that my work/life balance is generally good.

Very strongly agree	Strongly agree	Agree	Neither agree nor disagree	Disagree	Strongly disagree	Very strongly disagree

Please comment further if you would like to:

My home life helps with the stress I experience at work

Very strongly agree	Strongly agree	Agree	Neither agree nor disagree	Disagree	Strongly disagree	Very strongly disagree

Please comment further if you would like to:

I feel able to be compassionate towards my patients

Very strongly agree	Strongly agree	Agree	Neither agree nor disagree	Disagree	Strongly disagree	Very strongly disagree

Please comment further if you would like to:

I feel able to be compassionate towards my colleagues

Very strongly agree	Strongly agree	Agree	Neither agree nor disagree	Disagree	Strongly disagree	Very strongly disagree

Please comment further if you would like to:

I feel valued within my working environment

Very strongly agree	Strongly agree	Agree	Neither agree nor disagree	Disagree	Strongly disagree	Very strongly disagree

Please comment further if you would like to:

I feel as if I have good coping strategies to combat stress at work

Very strongly agree	Strongly agree	Agree	Neither agree nor disagree	Disagree	Strongly disagree	Very strongly disagree

Please comment further if you would like to:

I feel that I have strategies to make a positive difference at work

Very strongly agree	Strongly agree	Agree	Neither agree nor disagree	Disagree	Strongly disagree	Very strongly disagree

Please comment further if you would like to:

I feel that I have strategies to make a positive difference to my health and wellbeing

Very strongly agree	Strongly agree	Agree	Neither agree nor disagree	Disagree	Strongly disagree	Very strongly disagree

Please comment further if you would like to:

Overall, I feel satisfied with my working environment.

Very strongly agree	Strongly agree	Agree	Neither agree nor disagree	Disagree	Strongly disagree	Very strongly disagree

Please comment further if you would like to:

Any further comments:

Having completed this questionnaire now try to focus on the questions below in order to ascertain the extent to which you are experiencing burnout and where your specific areas of concern lie. Then you can start to work out strategies that can address these areas.

Questions to ask yourself

Assessing your level of burnout.

- Do you feel bored or inadequately stimulated in your work area?
- Do you feel stressed on a daily basis by your patients, team or organisation?
- Do you feel despairing or hopeless?
- Do you feel emotionally exhausted?
- Do you feel cynical or disengaged from your patients?
- Are there ongoing conflicts in your team or evidence of bullying or harassment?
- Do you constantly feel that your team is overworked?
- Do you feel at risk of PTSD or secondary or vicarious trauma due to experiences in your practice area?
- Do you often have to care for patients who die unexpectedly?
- Do you feel that your patients are highly stressed or have unrealistic demands or expectations?
- Do you have support in your team and from your managers?
- Is your organisation committed to supporting you?
- Are you usually able to access CPD?
- Do you have access to supervision?
- Do you feel socially connected to your team?
- Do you enjoy working where you do?
- Do you still feel enthusiastic about your role?
- Do you think that what you do is significant and makes a difference?

RECOMMENDATIONS FOR LEADERSHIP AS INDIVIDUAL PRACTITIONERS, LEADERS AND ORGANISATIONS

Once we have thought about our own stress levels, and identified our personal and professional stressors, we need to think about our leadership role in terms of helping others with their stress levels and maximizing their ability to be compassionate. As can be seen in Figure 3.2 (below) there are many negative manifestations of stress which we need to recognise in others, as well as ourselves, because these can all contribute to burnout.

McCormack and Cotter (2013) highlight factors which can lead to burnout as being:

Individual and socio-demographic factors:

- Age and years of experience – younger workers can be more likely to suffer from emotional exhaustion and depersonalisation maybe because of a lack of person/job fit so older workers are more suited to their roles. Also, they have not had as much training and education, or maybe the maturity to handle certain stressors. However, less experienced practitioners might not be necessarily younger, but could still be vulnerable to burnout.
- Personality – for example, workaholics, enthusiastic high achievers, perfectionists who have less boundaries between work and home might be more susceptible to burnout. People who have elements of neuroticism which includes negative emotions, emotional instability and acute responses to stress are more vulnerable to burnout. This is also true of passive introverted and more negative personalities. Hardy personalities who are committed, feel in control of their circumstances and see change as a challenge can find stressful situations less threatening. These will be discussed more in Chapter 5.
- Locus of control – People who feel that they are in control of their circumstances, rather than that their lives are controlled by others and external forces, are less susceptible to burnout.
- Marital status – longer stable relationships have been found in some studies to reduce burnout.
- Gender – women can view themselves as more emotionally exhausted and burnt out, whereas men can report more depersonalization.

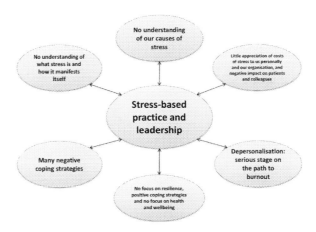

Figure 3.2 Alleviation of stress in practice and taking a lead on stress management (Chambers and Ryder, 2019, p 82)

- Work – home crossover – conflict between the demands of home and work can cause stress and sickness and absence.
- Expectations – unrealistic expectations of the job can cause a reality shock which can contribute to burnout.

Environmental and organisational factors:

- Workload – including excessive demands and pressures and overload.
- Underwork – not feeling sufficiently challenged or stimulated.
- Type of work – teachers and health and social care practitioners can be vulnerable due to the nature of their work.
- Physical environment – too much noise, poor lighting, noxious substances, poor air quality and crowding can lead to burnout. However, being exposed to infected patients or substances, hazardous situations and situations that can make people feel vulnerable can also be a cause of burnout.
- Conflict – interpersonal conflict with colleagues, patients, families and a lack of social support from colleagues diminishes job satisfaction and causes burnout.
- Role conflict and role ambiguity – competing and incompatible demands or a lack of clarity, uncertainty and unpredictability within the role.
- Control – a lack of job autonomy and control over the role.
- Social support – a lack of support and appreciation can lead to emotional exhaustion and depersonalisation.
- Reciprocity – a lack of two way investment in the role whether from patients or employers leads to exhaustion, depersonalisation and reduced personal accomplishment.
- Social comparison – feeling that people are not doing as well as colleagues.
- Leadership style – a lack of trust in managers and not being able to identify a leadership style, or a transactional and directive leadership style are linked to burnout. Transformational leadership which motivates and inspires workers tends to reduce work related stress.

It is important that as leaders in care that we recognise these personal identifiers as being significant in predicting high stress levels. We cannot change some of these factors, although we can help individuals to feel more in control of their environments. However, managers and leaders can help to create a positive work environment where there is less role conflict, and more social support and more positive leadership styles to help to address burnout and the environmental and organisational factors highlighted by McCormack and Cotter (2013).

Focusing on stress management and compassionate care as individual practitioners and leaders

Clark and Clarke's bio-psycho-pharmaco-social model (2014) highlights the facts that these domains are inextricably linked and impact on each other, and environmental factors should be considered too. For example, social factors can mediate against physical and psychological stressors, and conversely side effects of some medication can impact on sleep and diet. The different domains are:

- Biological considerations – sleep, exercise, diet, nutritional supplements, yoga etc
- Psychiatric considerations – mental health problems and risks, engagement with hobbies and interests, access to support resources

123

- Pharmacological considerations – medication concordance, side effects of medications, levels of alcohol intake, use of illicit drugs, nicotine and over the counter medications
- Social considerations – avoiding loneliness and connecting with others, meeting for exercise, social activities and work, virtual meetings with family and friends, addressing concerns about the health and welfare of friends and family
- Environmental considerations – access to outside space and indoor ventilation, separate areas for home and work when working from home or home schooling, level of cleanliness, reduction of household chores and clutter in the home.

It could be helpful to identify areas of concern by developing a personalised map to visualise aspects of burnout, and then to develop a personal management plan to address these (While and Clark, 2021).

I have identified self-care and team strategies in Figure 3.3 which I think are helpful to us as individuals in order to address our stress levels, and to help colleagues with their stress (see below).

Focusing on stress management and compassionate care as organisations

I have then identified cultural and educational strategies which could be helpful in reducing stress in our workplaces (Figure 3.4). It might be helpful to identify which of these strategies could be helpful in your own practice area.

The COVID-19 pandemic has undoubtedly added immense stress to those working in health care. In addition to all the personal and organisational self-care strategies above, one piece of research also stressed the importance of available COVID-19 testing resources and availability of PPE. In addition, exercise classes and access to psychological support, including counselling, crisis resolution sessions and wellbeing workshops were found to be helpful (Murashiki et al, 2021).

I hope that you have found it helpful to think about what causes stress in your personal and professional life, and how this could impact on your ability to provide compassionate care. The COVID-19 pandemic has had a major impact on health care environments and has caused a great deal of stress to patients, families and health care practitioners, and it is important to acknowledge this, and where stress levels have been too high. Different stressors exist in different areas of practice and these also need to be acknowledged. High stress levels are a strong predictor of burnout, and this could lead us to be less compassionate than we would be in different circumstances. Chapter 4 will discuss how resilience can help us to manage our stress, and what strategies could be useful in helping us to do this.

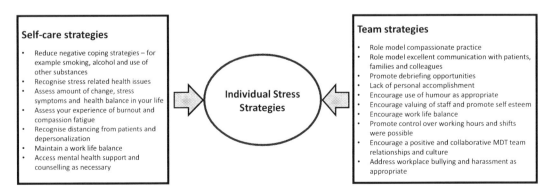

Figure 3.3 Individual and team stress strategies

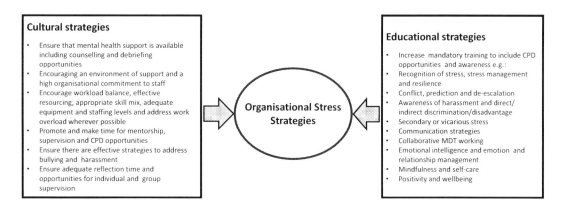

Figure 3.4 Organisational stress strategies

REFERENCES

Abidi A, Mangi R, Soomro H, Chandio F. (2014) A Meticulous Overview on Job Burnout and its Effects on Health. *International Journal of Management Sciences*, 3(9): 683–94.

Adriaenssens J, De Gucht V, Maes S (2015) Determinants and Prevalence of Burnout in Emergency Nurses: A Systematic Review of 25 Years of Research. *International Journal of Nursing Studies*, 52(2**)**: 649–61.

Adriaenssens J, Hamelink A, Van Bogaert P. (2017) Predictors of Occupational Stress and Well-Being in First Line Nurse Managers: A Cross-Sectional Survey Study. *International Journal of Nursing Studies*, 73: 85–92.

Anasori E, Bayighomog S, Tanova C. (2019) Workplace Bullying, Psychological Distress, Resilience, Mindfulness and Emotional Exhaustion. *The Service Industries Journal*, 40(1–2): 65–89. https://doi.org/10.1080/02642069.2019.1589456 (Accessed 12/9/23).

Bakker A, Costa P. (2014) Chronic Job Burnout and Daily Functioning: A Theoretical Analysis. *Burnout Research,* 1(3): 112–19.

Bakker A, Heuven E. (2006) Emotional Dissonance, Burnout and In-Role Performance Among Nurses and Police Officers. *International Journal of Stress Management*, 13(4): 423–40.

Bakker A, Tims M, Derks D. (2012) Proactive Personality and Job Performance: The Role of Job Crafting and Work Engagement. *Human Relations*, 65(10): 1359–78. https://doi.org/10.1177/0018726712453471 (Accessed 12/9/23).

Bewick J. (2019) Newly Qualified Health Visitor: Staff Well-Being and Delivering an Effective Service. *Journal of Health Visiting*, 7(1): 12–13.

Bhagavathula A, Abegaz T, Belachew S, Gebreyohannes E, Gebresillassie B, Chattu V. (2018) Prevalence of Burnout Syndrome Among Health-Care Professionals Working at Gondar University Hospital, Ethiopia. *Journal of Education and Health Promotion*, 7(145): 1–7.

Bride B, Robinson M, Yegidis B, Figley C. (2004) Development and Validation of the Secondary Traumatic Stress Scale. *Research on Social Work Practice*, 14(1): 27–35.

Brown A. (2020) Will COVID-19 Affect the Delivery of Compassionate Nursing Care? *Nursing Times*, 116(10): 32–35.

Carpenter L. (2021) PTSD. Burnout. Grief. What the ICU Doctor Diagnosed – for his Colleagues and Himself. *The Times Magazine 13th March 2021*.

Cedar S, Walker G. (2020) Protecting the Wellbeing of Nurses Providing End-of-Life Care. *Nursing Times*, 116(2): 36–40.

Chambers C, Ryder E. (2019) *Supporting Compassionate Health care Practice.* Abingdon: Routledge.

Clark L, Clarke T. (2014) Realising Nursing: A Multimodal Biopsychopharmacosocial Approach to Psychiatric Nursing. *Journal of Psychiatric Mental Health Nursing*, 21(6): 564–71.

Clouston T. (2015) *Challenging Stress, Burnout and Rust-Out: Finding Balance in Busy Lives.* London: Jessica Kingsley Publishers.

Dall'ora C, Saville C. (2021) Burnout in Nursing: What Have We Learnt and What Is Still Unknown? *Nursing Times*, 117(2) 43–45.

Delgado C, Upton D, Ranse K, Furness T, Foster K. (2017) Nurses' Resilience and the Emotional Labour of Nursing Work: An Integrative Review of Empirical Literature. *International Journal of Nursing Studies*, 70: 71–88.

Demerouti E, Bakker A, Nachreiner F, Ebbinghaus M. (2002) From Mental Strain to Burnout. *European Journal of Work and Organizational Psychology*, 11(4): 423–41.

Demou E, Katikireddi V. (2020) *Health care Workers 7 Times as Likely to Have Severe COVID-19 as Other Workers*. University of Glasgow. https://www.gla.ac.uk/news/headline_766731_en.html (Accessed 12/9/23).

Dermody K, Bennett P. (2008) Nurse Stress in Hospital and Satellite Haemodialysis Units. *Journal of Renal Care*, 34(1): 28–32.

Edmonds C, Lockwood G, Bezjak A, Nyhof-Young J. (2012) Alleviating Emotional Exhaustion in Oncology Nurses; An Evaluation of Wellspring's "Care for the Professional Caregiver Program". *Journal of Cancer Education*, 27(1): 27–36.

El-Bar N, Levy A, Wald H, Biderman A. (2013) Compassion Fatigue, Burnout and Compassion Satisfaction Among Family Physicians in the Negev Area – a Cross-Sectional Study. *Israel Journal of Health Policy Research*, 2(1): 31.

Embriaco N, Papazian L, Kentish-Barnes N, Pochard F, Azoulay E. (2007) Burnout Syndrome Among Critical Care Health care Workers. *Current Opinion in Critical Care*, 13(5): 482–88.

Evans R. (2019) Finding a calm balance. *Community Practitioner*, 92(3): 40–43.

Figley C. (2002) Compassion Fatigue: Psychotherapists' Chronic Lack of Self Care. *Journal of Clinical Psychology*, 58(11): 1433–41.

Fischer M, Mitsche M, Endler P, Mesenholl-Strehler E, Lothaller H, Roth R. (2013) Burnout in Physiotherapists: Use of Clinical Supervision and Desire for Emotional Closeness or Distance to Clients. *International Journal of Therapy and Rehabilitation*, 20(11): 550–58.

Forbes L. (2019) Support for Professionals After Trauma. *Journal of Health Visiting*, 7(1): 16.

Ford M. (2021) Lack of "Safety Net" Risking Nurses' Mental Health. *Nursing Times*, 117(4): 6–7.

Ford S. (2020) COVID-19 Negative Impact on Nurse Mental Health *Nursing Times*, 116(5): 6–7.

Francis R. (2013) *Report of the Mid-Staffordshire NHS Foundation Trust Public Inquiry.* London: The Stationary Office.

Girgis A, Hansen V. (2007) *Prevalence and Predictors of Burnout with COSA Oncology Workforce.* Clinical Oncological Society of Australia and Cancer Australia: The University of Newcastle Australia.

Gosseries O, Demertzi A, Ledoux D, Bruno M, Vanhaudenhuyes A, Thibaut A, Laureys S, Schnakers C. (2012) Burnout in Health care Workers Managing Chronic Patients with Disorders of Consciousness. *Brain Injury*, 26(12): 1493–99.

Graham Y, Fox A, Scott J, Johnson M, Hayes C. (2020) How a Pandemic Affects the Mental Health of the Nursing Workforce. *Nursing Times*, 116(8): 20–22.

Greenberg N, Weston D, Hall C, Caulfield T, Williamson V, Fong K. (2021) Mental Health of Staff Working in Intensive Care During COVID-19. *Occupational Medicine*, 71(2): 62–67.

Gruman J, Saks A. (2011) Performance Management and Employee Engagement. *Human Resource Management Review*, 21(2): 123–36.

Haik J, Brown S, Liran A, Visentin D, Sokolov A, Zilinsky I, Kornhaber R. (2017) Burnout and Compassion Fatigue: Prevalence and Associations Among Israeli Burn Clinicians. *Neuropsychiatric Disease and Treatment*, 2017(13): 1533–40.

Halbesleben J, Wakefield B, Wakefied D, Cooper L. (2008) Nurse Burnout and Patient Safety Outcomes: Nurse Safety Perception Versus Reporting Behavior. *Western Journal of Nursing Research*, 30(5): 560–77.

Hannafin S, Cosgrove A, Hannafin P, Brady A, Lynch C. (2020) Burnout and its Prevalence Among Public Health Nurses in Ireland. *British Journal of Community Nursing*, 25(8): 370–75.

Hochschild A (2012) *The Managed Heart: Commercialization of Human Feeling*, Oakland, CA: University of California Press.

Holmes T, Rahe R. (1967) Social Readjustment Rating Scale (SRRS). *Journal of Psychosomatic Research*, 11(2): 213–18.

Jones C. (2014) Stress and Coping Strategies in Renal Staff. *Nursing Times*, 110(10): 22–25.

Kang L. plus 14 authors (2020a) Impact on Mental Health and Perceptions of Psychological Care Among Medical and Nursing Staff in Wuhan During the 2019 Novel Coronavirus Outbreak: A Cross-Sectional Study. *Brain, Behavior and Immunity*, 87:11–17.

Kang L plus 14 authors (2020b) The Mental Health of Medical Workers in Wuhan, China Dealing with the 2019 Novel Coronavirus, *Lancet Psychiatry*, 7(3): E14.

Kearney M, Weininger R, Vachon M, Harrison R, Mount B (2009) Self-Care of Physicians Caring for Patients at the End of Life: "Being Connected... A Key to My Survival". *JAMA*, 301(11): 1155–64.

Kessler R.C., Andrews G, Colpe L, Hiripi E, Mroczek D, Normand S, Walters E, Zaslavsky A. (2002) Short Screening Scales to Monitor Population Prevalences and Trends in Non-Specific Psychological Distress. *Psychological Medicine*, 32(6): 959–76.

Khanipour-Kencha A, Jackson A, Bahramnezhad F. (2022) Anticipatory Grief During COVID-19: A Commentary. *British Journal of Community Nursing*, 27(3): 114–17.

Kompanje E. (2018) Burnout, Boreout and Compassion Fatigue on the ICU: It is Not About Work Stress, But About Lack of Existential Significance and Professional Performance. *Intensive Care Medicine*, 44(5): 690–91.

Korunka C, Tement S, Zdrehus C, Borza A. (2010) *Burnout: Definition, Recognition and Prevention Approaches.* BOIT: Burnout Invention Training for Managers and Team Leaders. https://www.bridgestoeurope.com/wp-content/uploads/2020/03/BOIT_theoretical_abstract_2705.pdf (Accessed 12/9/23).

Lahana E, Papadopoulou K, Roumeliotou O, Tsounis A, Sarafis P, Niakas D. (2017) Burnout Among Nurses Working in Social Welfare Centers for the Disabled. *BMC Nursing*, 16(1): 15.

Lam S, Kwong E, Hung M, Pang S, Chien W. (2019) A Qualitative Descriptive Study of the Contextual Factors Influencing the Practice of Emergency Nurses in Managing Emerging Infectious Diseases, *International Journal of Qualitative Studies on Health and Well-being*, 14(1): 1626179.

Lambert V, Lambert C. (2001) Literature Review of Role Stress/Strain on Nurses: An International Perspective. *Nursing and Health Sciences*, 3(3): 161–72.

McCormack N, Cotter C. (2013) *Managing Burnout in the Workplace: A Guide for Information Professionals*, Oxford: Chandos Publishing.

McDonald G, Clark L. (2020a) Mental Health Impact of Admission to the Intensive Care Unit for COVID-19. *British Journal of Community Nursing*, 25(11): 526–30.

McDonald G, Clark L. (2020b) COVID-19: It Happens to Nurses Too – A Case Study. *British Journal of Community Nursing*, 25(12): 594–97.

McKinless E. (2020) Impact of Stress on Nurses Working in the District Nursing Service. *British Journal of Community Nursing*, 25(11): 555–61.

McKinley T, Boland K, Mahan J. (2017) Burnout and Interventions in Pediatric Residency: A Literature Review. *Burnout Research*, 6(3): 9–17.

Martins Pereira S, Teixeira C, Carvalho A, Hernandez-Marrero P, In Palln. (2016) Compared to Palliative Care, Working in Intensive Care More than Doubles the Chances of Burnout: Results from a Nationwide Comparative Study. PLOS ONE, 11(9): 1–21. doi:10.1371/journal.pone.0162340 (Accessed 12/9/23).

Maslach C, Jackson S, Leiter M. (1996) *The Maslach Burnout Inventory Manual (3rd ed).* Palo Alto, CA: Consulting Psychologists Press.

Maslach C, Schaufli W, Leiter M. (2001) Job Burnout. *Annual Review of Psychology*, 52: 397–422.

Maxwell E. (2020) Living With the On-Going Effects of COVID-19 – Gathering the Evidence. *Nursing Times*, 116(11): 18–19.

Mealer M, Burnham E, Goode B, Rothbaum B, Moss M. (2009) The Prevalence and Impact of Post Traumatic Stress Disorder and Burnout Syndrome in Nurses. *Depress Anxiety*, 26(12): 1118–26.

Medland J, Howard-Ruben J, Whitaker E. (2004) Fostering Psychological Wellness in Oncology Nurses: Addressing Burnout and Social Support in the Workplace. *Oncology Nursing Forum*, 31(1): 47–54.

Murashiki D, Ollis L, Shanahan P. (2021) Which Wellbeing Resources are Helpful in Managing Stress During COVID-19? *Nursing Times*, 117(8): 21–24.

Murphy F. (2004) Stress Among Nephrology Nurses in Northern Ireland. *Nephrology Nursing Journal*, 31(4): 423–31.

Nursing and Midwifery Council (NMC) (2018) *The Code: Professional Standards of Practice and Behaviour for Nurses, Midwives and Nursing Associates* [Online]. Available at: https://

www.nmc.org.uk/globalassets/sitedocuments/nmc-publications/nmc-code.pdf. (Accessed 3 June 2020).

Nyatanga B. (2016) Death, Anxiety and Palliative Nursing. *British Journal of Community Nursing*, 21(12): 636.

Nyatanga, B. (2022) Reflecting on Caring and Death Anxiety During the Pandemic. *British Journal of Community Nursing*, 27(3): 144–46.

Ong S. (2020) How Face Masks Affect our Communications. *BBC Future* 9th June 2020. https://www.bbc.com/future/article/20200609-how-face-masks-affect-our-communication (Accessed 24/06/21).

ONS (2021) *Coronavirus and the Social Impacts on Great Britain 2021*. Office for National Statistics.https://www.gov.uk/government/statistics/coronavirus-and-the-social-impacts-on-great-britain-10-september-2021 (Accessed 12/9/23).

Panagopoulou E, Montgomery A, Benos A. (2006) Burnout in Internal Medicine Physicians: Differences Between Residents and Specialists. *European Journal of Internal medicine*, 17(3): 195–200.

Patalay P, Fitzsimons E. (2020) *Mental Ill-Health at Age 17 in the UK*. University College London. https://cls.ucl.ac.uk/wp-content/uploads/2020/11/Mental-ill-health-at-age-17-%E2%80%93-CLS-briefing-paper-%E2%80%93-website.pdf (Accessed 12/9/23).

Pedrazza M, Berlanda S, Trifiletti E, Minuzzo S. (2018) Variables of Individual Difference and the Experience of Touch in Nursing. *Western Journal of Nursing Research*, 40(11): 1614–37.

Pierce M, Hope H, Ford T, Hatch S. (2020) Mental Health Before and During the COVID-19 Pandemic: A Longitudinal Probability Sample Survey of the UK Population. *The Lancet Psychiatry*, 7(10): 883–92.

Poncet M, Toullic P, Papazian L, Kentish-Barnes N, Timsit J, Pochard F, Chevret S, Schlemmer B, Azoulay E. (2007) Burnout Syndrome in Critical Care Nursing Staff. *American Journal of Respiratory and Critical Care Medicine*, 175(7): 698–704.

Popp J. (2017) Social Intelligence and Explanation of Workplace Abuse. *Journal of Workplace Rights*, 7(2): 1–7.

Poulsen A, Meredith P, Khan a, Henderson J, Castrisos V, Khan S. (2014) Burnout and Work Engagement in Occupational Therapists. *British Journal of Occupational Therapy*, 77(3): 1–9.

Ray S, Wong C, White D, Heaslip K. (2013) Compassion Satisfaction, Compassion Fatigue, Work Life Conditions and Burnout Among Frontline Mental Health Care Professionals. *Traumatology*, 19(4): 255–67.

Roberts K, Campbell H. (2011). *Using the M Technique as Therapy for Patients at the End of Life: Two Case Studies. International Journal of Palliative Nursing*, 17(3) 114–18.

Rodger D, Atwal A. (2018) How to Mitigate the Effects of Peri-Operative Death on Nursing Staff. *Nursing Times*, 114(8): 26–29.

Sanso N, Galiana l, Oliver A, Pascual A, Sinclair S, Benito E. (2015) Palliative Care Professionals' Inner Life: Exploring the Relationships Among Awareness, Self-Care, and Compassion Satisfaction and Fatigue, Burnout, and Coping with Death. *Journal of Pain and Symptom Management*, 50(2): 200–07.

Savitsky B, Findling Y, Ereli A, Hendel T. (2020) Anxiety and Coping Strategies Among Nursing Students During the COVID-19 Pandemic. *Nurse Education in Practice*, 46:102809.

Schaufeli W, Enzmann D. (1998) *The Burnout Companion to Study and Practice: A Critical Analysis*. London: Taylor & Francis.

Selye H. (1946) The General Adaptation Syndrome and the Diseases of Adaptation. *The Journal of Allergy and Immununology*, 17(4): 231–47.

Slocum-Gori S, Hemsworth D, Chan W, Carson A, Kazanjian A. (2011) Understanding Compassion Satisfaction, Compassion Fatigue and Burnout: A Survey of the Hospice Palliative Care Workforce. *Palliative Medicine*, 27(2): 172–78.

Smajdor A. (2013) Reification and Compassion in Medicine: A Tale of Two Systems. *Clinical Ethics*, 8(4): 111–18.

Sutherland V, Cooper C. (1992) *Understanding Stress: A Psychological Perspective for Health Professionals (Psychology and Health Series, vol 5)*. London: Chapman & Hall.

Tehranineshat B, Rakhshan M, Torabizadeh C, Fararouei M. (2019) Compassionate Care in Health care Systems: A Systematic Review. *Journal of National Medical Association*, 111(5): 546–54.

Trenerry-Harker K. (2018). *Therapeutic Touch in End of Life Care.* AHPCA. https://ahpca.ca/therapeutic-touch-end-life-care/ (Accessed 12/9/23).

Ulenaers D, Grosemans J, Schrooten W, Bergs J. (2020) Clinical Placement Experience of Nursing Students During the COVID-19 Pandemic: A Cross Sectional Study. *Nurse Education Today*, 99:104746.

Waddington K. (2016) The Compassion Gap in UK Universities. *International Practice Development Journal*, 6(1): 10.

West M, Bailey S, Williams E. (2020) *The Courage of Compassion: Supporting Nurses and Midwives to Deliver High-Quality Care.* London: The King's Fund.

While A. (2021) Touch: Knowledge and Considerations for Nursing Practice. *British Journal of Community Nursing*, 26(4): 190–93.

While A. (2022) Assuring Good Deaths at Home. *British Journal of Community Nursing*, 27(3): 150.

While A, Clark L. (2021) Management of Work Stress and Burnout Among Community Nurses Arising from the COVID-19 Pandemic. *British Journal of Community Nursing*, 26(8): 384–89.

White T. (2018) *Medical Errors May Stem More from Physician Burnout than Unsafe Health Care Settings.* Stanford Medicine Press Release July 8, 2018. https://med.stanford.edu/news/all-news/2018/07/medical-errors-may-stem-more-from-physician-burnout.html (Accessed 12/9/23).

Wunnenberg M. (2020) Psychosocial Bullying Among Nurse Educators: Exploring Coping Strategies and Intent to Leave. *Journal of Nursing Scholarship*, 52(5): 574–82.

How can I increase my resilience?

- Introduction
- Discussion – main points and evidence with case studies, exercises, aide mémoires and questions

  - What is resilience and why is this crucial for compassionate care?
  - What is the impact of our values on our levels of moral distress?
  - What strategies can we use to manage our anxiety?
  - How can I predict and de-escalate conflict?
  - Why is it so important to care for ourselves in order to keep our stress levels manageable?
  - What strategies could I use to manage my stress and increase my resilience to maximise my ability to be compassionate?

- Recommendations for leadership as individual practitioners, leaders and organisations

  - Focusing on resilience and compassionate care as individual practitioners and leaders
  - Focusing on resilience and compassionate care as organisations

INTRODUCTION

This chapter will focus on resilience, because this is fundamental to individuals working in ways that they can bend and not break in relation to life and work pressures. It will start by defining what resilience is, and why this is crucial for compassionate care. Our personal and health care practice values and beliefs are really important to us, and the moral distress brought about when these are compromised will then be discussed. It then touches on anxiety, and how this can increase our distress and make it difficult to be as resilient as we normally would be. We need to be able to care for ourselves in order to care for others, and I will discuss what this means, and how we can be effective in our care of ourselves when we are working in stressful environments. Conflict in relationships, and in the workplace, is endemic and we need to be able to predict, as well as resolve, conflict and the chapter will discuss strategies to help us to do this with patients and colleagues, because this can really challenge us in our professional roles. We all need to work on strategies to increase our own natural resilience in order to deal with the challenges in our lives. Again, the format will be:

- Case study
- Discussions – main points and evidence with case studies, exercises, aide mémoires and questions
- Recommendations for leadership as individual practitioners, leaders and organisations

DISCUSSION

Case study 4.1

Vanessa's experience of reading emails to an end-of-life patient

During the COVID-19 pandemic many restrictions were in place regarding visitors to the wards. I recently supported a gentleman who was suffering from the virus and was quite unwell. He had come in with multiple illnesses as well as suffering a stroke. He was not able to have family to visit due to the risk of them catching the virus, as he was on high flow oxygen, which is classed as an aerosol generated procedure, as is the use of regular nebulisers. The patient was also actively coughing which was also a cause for airborne transmission.

The Patient Advice Liaison Service (PALS) provided a way for patient relatives to send their loved one's emails; they would print them out and laminate them so they could be read out and were wipeable to comply with infection control measures. The patient had been in the cubicle for several weeks and he had a few emails sent up from the PALS department from his friends and family. I applied the necessary personal protective equipment (PPE) such as gown, gloves and FFP3 mask and visor for the protection of myself, the patient and my colleague. When I went in to reposition him with my colleague, I explained that he had these emails and asked if he would like me to read them out to him once we had finished getting him more comfortable. He nodded, as saying more than a few words left him breathless.

When my colleague left the room, I read out the emails, many from close friends and his family, which were dated from a few weeks ago. I explained this to the patient as he was aware of his deterioration, and the emails at the time said how they were glad the patient was getting better. I apologised to the patient that these were not read out at the time and explained that there was no excuse. I went on to read a long email from his daughter and it was evident that they had not spoken for a long time. She lived in Scotland and in the email stated that once he was better, and as COVID allowed, she would love for them to meet up again as when they had met up a few years earlier they appeared to get on well. This was clearly quite an emotional email for the patient to listen to and I found this emotional too.

Once I had read the emails I asked the patient if he would like some time alone with his thoughts; he nodded. I de-gowned from all my PPE, washed my hands and left the room. I needed to take a moment to myself after this incident as I found it quite emotional. I spoke with the nurse in charge regarding a reply to the daughter from us or a family member, so that his daughter could be updated if the patient consented. They said this would be allowed and would be arranged in the morning. I also asked that on the ward safety briefing they discuss the importance of reading out these notes and emails to patients, as I feel this gentleman could have possibly had the chance to speak to his daughter, or at least hear her on the phone, before he became too unwell to do so. This is unfortunately what happened, he was very near the end of his life and to my knowledge he did not get the opportunity to speak with her.

I think this is a very important lesson to be learnt and going forward I have ensured on each shift that every patient has their letters, notes and emails read out to them as soon as they arrive on the ward.

Vanessa clearly demonstrates her excellent compassionate nursing care in this case study. Her sensitivity and care of this patient would have been such a comfort to him, and knowing his daughter had been in contact was also so important. Vanessa is right that there is no excuse not to have helped him to access the emails that had been sent to him. Relationships are complex and major inroads can be made into challenging situations even at the end of people's lives. She recognised this and provided feedback for the handover meeting to ensure that others understood the need for this, and she was a caring patient advocate in doing so. She will also take this learning forward for the future. Being compassionate in this scenario involved resilience for Vanessa because she found this very distressing. Her personal and nursing moral values had been compromised because the emails should have been read to him long before this. She had to take time away from the situation after she had been with this patient, and it was important for her to acknowledge the need to do this. This demonstrated clear self-awareness and emotional intelligence, in understanding the need for self-care, before she carried on with other patient care.

Case Study 4.2

Jodie's experience of being an advocate for a patient who was critically unwell

Working on a surgical ward there is always the possibility of post-surgical complications, and as a renal ward we are separate from all general surgeons and doctors, We have specialists who work closely with our patients and are on hand to provide assistance either personally or through the use of their surgical teams. Renal transplant patients have treatment plans prewritten for simple adjustments to be made based on doctors' and nurses' judgements, with a set of instructions of what steps to take following any concerns.

During the coronavirus breakout the transplant ward became a green secure area. No staff were to go on or off the ward throughout their shift and no other people were to enter the ward. At the beginning of a new shift, we took a handover of a patient who was four days post transplantation. The handover detailed how just two days earlier this patient had an episode of chest pain. However, it resolved quickly, with no tests showing anything of concern and no changes. We noted this as something to be aware of and continued with our usual regular observations, as well as spending time with this patient, as it had been a traumatic time and he was an older man missing home.

That day the patient had an initial set of observations recorded but later I noticed the patient had a vague look on his face and approached him quickly whilst calling for my mentor to assist, he said he was feeling strange but had no other symptoms, so we transferred him back to his bed and I started patient monitoring in terms of an ECG and the doctor was asked to attend as a matter of urgency.

The patient looked scared, and although there was a lot of PPE equipment between us, I wanted this patient to know we were with him every step. I told him we would not leave him and by now you could see he was in pain and his fists were clenching. It was important for me to change how I communicated with him and for him to see my eyes to know I was genuine, and tactile hand holding, when possible, showed we were still there.

The doctor arrived at the ward quickly. However, she refused to enter the ward as she had failed to have her COVID swabbing as required and felt it was too unsafe. I took her the patient's notes, including ECGs, to compare and his drug chart for anything that was required. I pleaded with the doctor to view this patient in person as I felt she needed to understand the seriousness of his situation, but again this was declined. Returning to the patient we administered the medication we were told to give but as we were not happy with her response we called again, and again she refused to come to see the patient. I then called the on call surgeon's mobile number which is generally only to be used in the event of a possible transplant, or for the doctor to use if they need to advise. However, I felt the doctor was not providing adequate care so as an advocate for my patient I felt it was necessary. I just felt fear for my patient and anger on his behalf.

The surgeon did not stay long on the phone but he assured me this patient would be assessed immediately and that allowed me to give real reassurance to the patient that I had spoken to the surgeon and someone was coming, I took a new recording on the ECG as the patient seemed to be getting worse and the pain was becoming more severe but before I had the chance to put out the cardiac call the same doctor arrived who had previously refused to view the patient. It took just one glance for her to gauge just how serious this event was and the cardiac team were called immediately. When the cardiac team arrived, he was assessed and taken directly to the cardiac catheterisation lab for treatment.

The surgeon I had called arrived on the ward. He was shocked at the behaviour of the doctor and changes were implemented to ensure nothing like this happened again. I learnt a lot about speaking up and having the confidence to go higher when I felt the need. I was surprised that I managed it with such ease, and experiences that day pushed me into overcoming boundaries that I know I would never question again.

The surgeon gave me feedback on how refreshing it was to have a student out of their comfort zone challenge seniors for the good of the patient. I was there when the patient returned to the renal department following a stent insertion, and he said he would never forget how I got him through by not leaving his side and he was so happy to be returning to be my patient as he knew he was in good hands.

I will take this forward for my final stage of nursing and I hope to influence other students to be bold and go with their judgement in each situation and always challenge where needed and never be afraid to speak up for your patient.

Jodie was incredibly impressive in her practice. To go above the doctor and contact the consultant was far from easy. Her assessment was taken very seriously in terms of how ill the patient was and her assessment was fully vindicated by how quickly the situation progressed. She was such a strong advocate for the patient in her care and it was so good to see how impressed the consultant was about her approach. Her communication skills were clearly excellent and much appreciated by the patient in her care and she should be very proud of all that she did in this extremely challenging situation, and she learnt a great deal from this experience. Jodie would have felt very stressed and worried about the patient in her care, yet she showed real resilience in managing her stress and keeping her patient calm, whilst she challenged the need for a doctor to come to his bedside to assess him.

Case Study 4.3

Abbie's experience of breaking down barriers to communication

During my time on placement I was assigned to a COVID positive ward. During this time, we faced many challenges, changes and worries. Communication became challenging due to the necessity of wearing masks or visors and having to keep a two metre distance in the bays. Face masks conceal the volume of voices as well as covering half of the face meaning facial expressions are also compromised (Knollman-Porter and Burshnic, 2020). I therefore often resorted to telling my patients that I was smiling. I personally found it hard to read people wearing masks and could empathise with my patients who were no doubt scared during their time in hospital due to the vast media coverage about the ongoing increase in mortality rates for those who contracted the virus.

One patient struggled with communication due to being hard of hearing. She would normally rely on facial expressions and lip reading but the wearing of masks meant she was unable to. This caused her a lot of distress and began affecting her mood. Previous experience of working with patients who are hard of hearing had already given me evidence of what works well to break the communication barriers in relation to having a conversation, so I started there. I collected a white board and pen. I began the conversation with writing down; "Hi I am Abbie, I am a student nurse and will be looking after you today". I awaited her response which at first was just a simple "Hi Abbie". I then proceeded to ask "if this was an easier way to communicate or is there anything else she would prefer". She explained this is easier but she really misses the face to face interaction and flowing conversation. At this point I was stuck on what I could do to help improve this. As the shift went on I continued thinking about how I could help improve this patient's stay in hospital. Due to having COVID she was unable to see family or friends and I could imagine she felt very alone at this time. We had been bought an iPad so patients could Facetime their family and friends. I realised this could be a way of communicating virtually with my patient. I took the iPad into the bay; I had connected to it with my phone (my number would remain confidential due to the iPad set up) and explained using the white board that I would be on the screen once I had my phone again and was in an area where I was allowed to remove my mask. Once I was in the staff room, I removed my mask and said hello and she instantly smiled, she was able to lip read and partially hear what I was saying due to the speaker being closer than I was able to be. We had a 15–20-minute conversation which allowed me to understand her individual needs better. I explained we would not be able to do this all the time but if she feels she needs this specific one to one contact to please ask and we will arrange this. I was unable to get the patient to fully engage just using the white board but was able to achieve this better through the iPad.

After I had spoken with my patient, I handed over to the nurse in charge about how this has helped my patient and to please hand over that this is another way we can communicate with her and with any other patients having a similar issue. I also wrote it in the notes for the consultant's team who were also struggling with how to effectively and clearly communicate with this patient. By handing this over and writing in the notes I had made sure that everyone was aware of this option and the benefits it had to the patient. This follows the NICE guidance for patients with COVID in relation to documenting any specialist needs the patient may need including specific adjustments\considerations for those with physical impairments.

I have taken away from this experience that sometimes it takes thinking outside the box to break down what the barrier is. In this instance the barrier was the patient being unable to hear and lipread and see facial expressions due to masks. I could write down what I needed to communicate but I still would not be able to assess her emotional needs. So, the next step was how I could do this without a mask and remain safe. Using the ideas from community-based care within a hospital setting worked well. The video consultation meant I could assess my patient's emotional needs as well as understand any other needs she had without putting myself, or other members of my team, at risk. I also reflected on the positive outcome of breaking down communication barriers and how this enabled me to meet the needs of the patient whilst under my care.

Abbie's reflection is also very impressive, and very moving to read. She demonstrated excellent communication skills, but also her proactive and forward-thinking innovative practice with this patient who felt so alone and isolated would have made such a difference. She also shared this knowledge and exemplary practice with the rest of her team and could use this experience to coach others. Abbie demonstrated her innovative thinking and person-centred care when caring for a patient who had COVID, which also shows her resilience in challenging circumstances.

The reflections of all these students' show innovation, leadership, excellent practice and being an advocate for patients in their care. These were all written during a time when they were facing immense challenges due to the pandemic, and yet they demonstrated their continued commitment to excellent care, which were all examples of resilience in practice.

What is resilience and why is this crucial for compassionate care?

So, what is resilience? Resilience is a person's capacity to recover quickly from setbacks and withstand the negative effects of adversity. In other words, coping and adapting to negative or stressful circumstances in life. The ability to adapt to changing circumstances and function normally, is referred to as allostasis. Allostatic load is caused by becoming worn down by the cumulative biological burden of adapting to life's circumstances. This is often the point of onset or exacerbation of disease, or even death (Ewen and Kinney, 2014). Karatsoreos and McEwen (2013) refer to this as "bending but not breaking". Sometimes past adversity, trauma or stress can lead to maladjustment, but at other times it can lead to greater resilience. For example, people who have never suffered illness, pain or ill health, might become used to this and consider that these happen to others, but not to them. So, when they do encounter ill health in older years, they can lack the resilience to cope with health issues. We all need to learn to bend, but not break.

There are two schools of thought; one that resilience is a personality trait, characterised by perseverance and self-reliance, or that it is a developmental process which takes place through exposure to adversity, and that vulnerability and resilience are at the opposite ends of a continuum (Atkinson et al, 2009). Charney (2004) incorporates both perspectives by saying that personal qualities and the ability to thrive in the face of adversity is important. However, resilience can also be learnt and personal characteristics such as our individual temperament, family bonds and external support systems are important. We need to be able to seek support from others, be optimistic, have some sort of faith or belief that stress can be strengthening, and actively strive towards our personal goals. Mealer et al (2012) found in their study that characteristics found in Charney's model of resilience (2004) were prevalent in ICU nurses, and this resilience reduced posttraumatic stress syndrome and burnout symptoms, as well as symptoms of anxiety and depression. Smith et al (2008) highlight that the Brief Resilience Tool is a useful tool in assessing the ability people have to bounce back from stressful events. This self-reporting tool measures how quickly we recover from stressful events, and how easy it is for us to bounce back. This is seen as important in predicting how we might respond to future stressors. Post-traumatic growth can be a result of coping with adversity. This can mean that we are stronger and have an increased capacity to prevail. So, we can have better relationships with others, a greater sense of belonging and greater compassion. Additionally, we can have a greater sense of purpose and pleasure and appreciation for life. Calhoun and Tedeschi's (2014) model of post-traumatic growth shows that distress through post-traumatic growth can create connections between events and greater wisdom.

Snyder (2014) says that resilience is a healthy reaction to trauma or loss, and it is possible to feel sad and upset, and suffer from sleep disturbances and other symptoms of stress, whilst maintaining psychological and physical functioning and healthy emotions over a period of time. Snyder (2014) says that a hardy personality and salutogenesis are important components of resilience. We have discussed in Chapter 2 how a hardy personality involves having a locus of control over our lives, a sense of commitment and having a strong sense of purpose, and being able to challenge situations that are not right in our opinion. Hardiness (Kobasa, 1979) is associated with higher levels of resilience (Connor and Davidson (2003) and involves being committed and having a sense of coherence where things make sense to us, seeing change as a challenge and having an internal locus of control. Salutogenesis allows us to focus on our health and wellbeing and to manage our stress, health, resilience and coping. In our case studies Vanessa, Jodie and Abbie felt able to challenge situations where patient needs were not being met. They were able to demonstrate hardiness, salutogenesis and resilience when they were under pressure, and were able to be strong advocates and end the day feeling like they had accomplished what needed to be done in very challenging circumstances. This is true resilience in practice,

There are different interpretations of resilience competence but they include much the same elements.

Snyder (2014, p129) describes the components of resilience as being:

- Realistic optimism – optimism combined with reality
- Flexible and accurate thinking
- Empathy and connection
- Self-efficacy – I can do this
- Impulse control and self-regulation
- Emotional awareness and emotional intelligence.

We need to think about whether any of these are particular challenges for us and then take action to further develop these traits if necessary.

Grant and Kinman (2013) also state that resilience includes four competencies:

- The ability to reflect and solve problems
- The ability to persist at times of frustration, regulate our moods, empathise and remain hopeful (emotional intelligence and emotional literacy)
- Being socially confident, assertive, and being a good communicator. This also includes the ability to resolve conflicts and having emotional resilience in the workplace (social competence)
- Having social connections and networks (social support).

Grant and Kinman (2014 and 2020) carry on their work by highlighting the importance of a systematic approach which involves resilient individuals, resilient teams, emotionally literate leaders and organisational resilience. The underlying competencies are:

- Emotional literacy, or emotional intelligence
- Reflective thinking skills, focusing on self-reflection, empathetic reflection and reflective communication. This involves knowing what we are doing and why, understanding others' cultural and religious perspectives and being open to challenge and discussion.
- Empathy
- Social competence and confidence
- Social support
- Supervision and organisational support
- Coping skills and flexibility
- Self-compassion and self-care
- Mindfulness and relaxation
- Thinking skills and cognitive behavioural techniques.

So, again we need to think about the components of resilience identified by Grant and Kinman (2014 and 2020) and see whether any of these are areas that we might want to focus on. Are we working in resilient teams and organisations with resilient leaders and, if not, how do we increase our own resilience to make up for any deficits?

Adamson et al (2014) focused on resilience in social workers and identified the importance of individual resources, context and mediating factors:

- Individual resources – attributes, personal history and sensitising experiences, moral and ethical code, beliefs and spirituality, self-awareness and self-protection
- Contextual issues – organisational structures, political and legal frameworks
- Mediating factors – work-life balance, developmental learning, coping behaviours and relational skills, supervision and peer support, professional identity, knowledge, education and theory.

Hunter and Warren (2014) identified issues in relation to resilience in midwives and discussed the importance of understanding the challenges to resilience, and how to manage and cope with them, by building self-awareness and protection of themselves and becoming as resilient as possible.

The American Psychological Association (2014) identify steps on the road to resilience:

- Make connections with others in your life
- Avoid seeing crises as insurmountable problems
- Accept that change is a part of living
- Move towards your goals
- Take decisive actions
- Look for opportunities for self-discovery
- Nurture a positive view of yourself
- Keep things in perspective
- Maintain a hopeful outlook
- Take care of yourself
- Learn from your past
- Stay flexible
- Seek help and continue your journey through life.

One of the problems that raises concerns about resilience is that the very term "bouncing back" implies a reset to business as normal and the speed of perceived trajectory is that this will happen very fast. This is not always the case; sometimes people do not return to normal and PTSD can mean that situations can impact us long term. In addition, we might gradually return to our usual coping patterns, but this might take longer than for others. This could enable others to see us as coping less well, and in nursing circles we all can expect ourselves to be seen as "copers" all the time. It is alright for others to find life difficult, but not us. We need to give ourselves time to recover from challenges, and how fast we recover is not necessarily a matter of personal choice. Breslin (2023) discusses the innate strands of privilege which mean that some people have a greater safety net than others. This safety net can involve some individuals having greater social support, financial support and positive experiences than others. Without this safety net are we simply setting ourselves, and others, up to fail. Further to this, resilience can be perceived as a victim blaming strategy, blaming individuals for a perceived lack of resilience, when organisations need to take responsibility for their own systemic issues which cause employees to become more stressed and less able to cope. As individuals we need to give ourselves more space to recover and recognise that if we recover faster that others simply cannot do this. We need to appreciate how our own positive experiences, social and family networks and financial buffers give us advantages that others do not have. Then we need to speak out and help our teams and organisations to put structures and strategies in place to support staff who are understandably struggling with the environment in which they work.

Beddoe et al (2013) in their research on resilience in social work practitioners identified three influences which support resilience in individual practitioners:

- Factors which reside in the individual
- Factors which reside in the organisation
- Factors which relate to the educational preparation of the practitioners.

I have tried to sum up the previous points in Table 4.1 below:

Having discussed resilience the discussion now considers a major challenge to our moral values which is caused by moral distress.

Table 4.1 Individual, organisational and educational resources to increase resilience

Individual Resources	Organisational Strategies	Educational preparation
Hardiness – change as a challenge, internal locus of control, sense of coherence	Clinical and restorative supervision	Allow space to explore personal attributes Adapting to change, perseverance and flexibility
Optimism and hope Realistic optimism	Peer support	Build resilience knowledge base
Coping mechanisms e.g. problem solving, reframing the problem cognitive restructuring and seeking support	Professional development opportunities and encourage seeking help when required.	Encourage creative thinking and cognitive strategies
Cognitive behavioural approaches e.g. preparing and rehearsing for potential situations	Organisational culture based on strengths and resilience building culture	Foster peer support and reflective supervision
Dispositional goal orientation e.g. maximising competence and motivation	Appraisals to encourage a sense of purpose and striving towards personal and professional goals	Coaching and mentorship preparation
Self-efficacy and self-reliance and positive view of self. Strong valuing of practice	Valuing of the profession	Develop the "big" picture in relation to professional identity and how this fits into the organisation
Competence and knowledge e.g. time management and organisational skills and solid knowledge base	Encourage staff support, team relationships, and team learning and a sense of belonging	Foster team resilience
Work-life balance	Value members of staff as individuals with home lives	Develop coping strategies and the importance of maintaining work life balance, external support and family bonds
Subjective wellbeing e.g. relationships outside work and self-identify separate from work role and pleasure and appreciation of life.	Focus on self-compassion and self-care, wellbeing, mindfulness and relaxation.	Demonstrate professional leadership, coaching, role modelling, teamworking and motivation of others
Emotional competence e.g. emotional intelligence (EI)	Encourage social competence and confidence	Create coping strategies, conflict resolution, regulation of moods and EI
Reflection and empathy	Encourage group supervision to increase empathy and connection in relation to adverse incidence and good practice	Focus on reflection, accurate thinking, challenging care decisions

What is the impact of our values on our levels of moral distress?

Case Study 4.4

Jo's personal reflection about nursing through the COVID pandemic

As much as I hoped that it would amount to nothing, there was a part of me that diligently followed the government's daily updates and epidemiology reports concerning COVID 19. It quickly transpired that the coronavirus was not merely a virus that would have minimal impact. Sure enough, what started as an epidemic, with pandemic potential, soon evolved into a global pandemic that, as we now know, would change the world as we knew it. We could not, at that moment, slow the virus's progress. We could not stop it. We were not in control.

Opting-in dilemma

When the email dropped into my inbox asking me to consider opting into a critical care unit, I felt conflicting emotions. To consider anything other than opting in was not an option. I remember discussing the potential ramifications of the virus with doctors and staff, shortly before the change to the opt-in calling. I recall detailing how, if student nurses were sent into clinical practice, it would be an excellent learning opportunity to develop our skills. I was certain that the university would not put us in danger.

Now the COVID-19 placements have come to end, I stand by that assertion. I remember thinking to myself, "I am a future nurse. I have a professional responsibility and duty of care to my patients". I also realised, however, that I had a duty of responsibility to my family. Aside from being a student nurse, I have a son and daughter. I think my decision to opt in hit my family. My 19-year-old son's shoulders weighed heavily with the countless "what ifs" he had played over and over in his mind.

Quite simply, my son was worried that I would die in clinical practice and was scared that I would one day go to work and never come home. As the news headlines began to report that nurses were dying on the "front line", I received calls and messages from my extended family forbidding me to go into clinical practice.

A part of me felt excited at the prospect of getting to witness, firsthand, what nursing in a pandemic meant. A part of me felt selfish and guilty for wanting to opt in, but a greater part of me knew that I was learning to nurse during a pandemic. When I reflect on this, I want to do humanitarian work as a nurse in the future, as I am from a military background. As I explained this to my son he was coming around to the idea and feeling increasingly reassured and comforted.

But news of close relatives' illnesses and a friend's death exacerbated the situation, and the fragility of life hit me. This death confirmed one thing: coronavirus spares no one. A few days later, I sat at my desk and wrote goodbye letters. You know, just in case. The experience allowed me the opportunity to feel useful and it gave me purpose.

November 2020 marked my return to practice as a student nurse, though lockdown continued. Returning to practice also helped me rationalise what COVID-19 meant on the ground. In a harsh contrast to the controversial and dramatised media reports, it was reassuring to witness, first-hand, how the hospitals were coping and what coronavirus meant practically and logistically on a day-to-day basis.

The hospital had, seemingly overnight, altered and I remember thinking how the accident and emergency department adjusted to hot, amber, and cold areas for patients at the front of the hospital in the event of trying to separate patients with symptoms, and those without, whilst helping the sick and injured in their hour of need.

As far as my clinical placement was concerned, I could not have asked for a better team, environment or experience. Doctors, nurses, physiotherapists, health care support workers, domestic staff and even the patients themselves seemed to appreciate how we must be feeling and welcomed us with (socially distant) open arms. There was a great sense of companionship felt across the board and between disciplines. At times there was a very real sense of collective anxiety, but even this seemed to do nothing other than to bring the team closer together.

I learnt a great deal clinically, for example, the different types of light and heavy PPE, working with non-invasive ventilation and other different clinical equipment and, without doubt, I developed professionally as a nurse. My COVID-19 journey has been an overwhelmingly personal one. This journey has, I feel, impacted upon and enhanced my clinical and professional development, but it has also allowed me the opportunity to grow emotionally.

Knowledge gained:

Enhanced infection control procedures can be taught and learned. Interventions and treatments can be taught and learned. What cannot be taught, though, is how we, as individuals, will react emotionally and physically to the unseen burden of a pandemic. I include my patients in this. The fluidity and constant evolution of the virus meant that we were all learning about its impact at the same time.

It was a learning curve for all nurses and patients in the thick of it together. There were occasions when my team and I, simply did not have the answer to a patient's or relative's questions and, as I was quickly reminded, honesty and transparency were (as they always have been) the most reliable tools of our practice (NMC, 2018). Deep down, our patients or relatives have a greater respect for the nurse who admits that they do not have an answer right now but that they will endeavour to find out. If, of course, an answer exists.

Since the beginning of my nurse training, I have kept a reflective journal. There is something rather emotional about seeing past experiences I had gone through, and my thoughts and feelings at that point in time. During this period, I had done a lot of reflective writing too, maybe in the desperate attempt to make sense of what I had witnessed, or what I had learned.

My entries taught me about not just the ability to survive a clinical placement in a pandemic, but also how to survive, more profoundly, as a human being. There were family and friends who were not able to say goodbye. There were anxious relatives on the end of a phone wanting to see and touch their loved ones. Compassion had been deprived of the one thing that lies at its heart: the ability to make a connection with loved ones. Often, we were the bridge between the two. It was the responsibility of the frontline staff to allay fears and anxieties, reassure if possible, and keep those channels of communication open and hope alive.

I feel extremely proud and privileged to have been able to complete a clinical placement during the COVID-19 pandemic. It is no overstatement to say that we have witnessed, first-hand, history in the making and it is a story we will tell for many years to come, if not for the rest of our lives.

Unfortunately, in February of this year I contracted COVID-19, and this is putting an impact on my wellbeing. I am aware of the support groups available to assist on days I struggle, my mentor has been very supportive and encouraging, allowing breaks when need be. My line managers have been supportive of the change to my wellbeing.

I have continued to demonstrate a holistic person-centred approach to patients being mindful of the restrictions in place. I have continued to work collaboratively with my patients, families/carers, and colleagues during these difficult times.

I have adapted to the changing work situation regarding the trust-wide COVID-19 contingency management plan.

I have tried to ensure that my wellbeing is maintained by trying to rest, eat healthily, exercise and also seek support from colleagues, my supervisor, and family/friends. This experience has definitely made me more resilient.

The COVID-19 crisis has certainly helped me to improve my knowledge of infection control measures, health and safety requirements and the treatment and prevention of illness. I have been involved in trying to help patients to stay well, both mentally and physically, by reinforcing social distancing, handwashing and staying at home, when they cannot be with their relatives (a very difficult situation).

I have also been encouraging, with my mentor and other colleagues, and have used coping strategies to continue to provide safe care.

Jo was struggling to reassure her son and her wider family, at the same time as coping with the challenges of working in a very busy Emergency Department. She then contracted COVID and unfortunately was still suffering from symptoms many months later. It is so clear how her courage and resilience has developed throughout the pandemic, but also how she has been supported by her colleagues in the wider care team, including, physiotherapists, domestic staff and medical and nursing colleagues, as well as in many cases, patients. Jo's reflection on her journey is inspiring and humbling and her resilience shines out throughout.

Compassion fatigue and moral distress contribute to burnout. Compassion fatigue is often internally driven. Moral distress is the result of external circumstances where actions are invasive and futile, not in the patient's best interests and do not alleviate suffering.

Compson (2015) says that there can be a "values mismatch" where individuals want to help others but are unable to, with "compassion satisfaction" where individuals want to help and can do so. This enables translation of moral choices into moral action. The inability to help others puts people at risk of compassion fatigue. This relates to moral distress when you are unable to translate your moral choices into moral action. So, in Jo's case her moral values did translate into moral action and her compassion satisfaction was undimmed, despite the incredible stressors of nursing though the pandemic. In fact, it could be said that she would have suffered more distress if she had not acted in line with her moral values and moral imperatives. However, these values can vary from person to person, and we need to have a level of spiritual intelligence which involves offering compassion and our wealth of knowledge alongside accepting and encouraging others to recognise different cultural norms, values, beliefs and views (Nyatanga, 2020). This is very challenging when we are, for example, being put at risk as a result of someone else's health choices. Another of my students, also working in a busy emergency department was very distressed by having to care for a patient who had travelled to her area in lockdown from a geographical area which had a higher level of COVID. He had come into a green area of ED and was refusing to wear a mask despite having very apparent symptoms of COVID. The student felt a sense of moral outrage on behalf of her patients, colleagues, her family members and herself because of his behaviour.

Caouette and Price (2018) say that compassion is a moral motivation, and this plays an important role in the life of a virtuous person. However, compassion might be a strong motivator for us but we do not always feel the motivation to be compassionate, or alleviate someone's suffering, in some cases. We might feel a sense of moral outrage, rather than empathy, or a sense of moral duty which is not tied in with any shared feelings or any ability to identify with the person who is suffering. Also, we might not be able to act on our compassion and alleviate the sufferer's distress. We all have a level of self-interest, and the authors give an example of whether we would want to stop to help someone who has fallen if this was going to make us late for an important interview, even if we are intrinsically morally motivated. So, although there can be challenges involved in feeling and acting in a compassionate manner in all circumstances, being altruistic is an important part of being morally virtuous.

Nolan (2020) discusses the damage caused by moral injury, and explains that this is not burnout or PTSD, although there are similarities. He says that burnout can be seen as a result of personal failure to maintain resilience, and that more access to self-help strategies can be effective in increasing resilience. Burnout, PTSD and moral injury can cause anxiety, despair, depression, social isolation and suicidal ideations. However, moral injury is an injury to the person's conscience, which causes a moral disorientation, "or trauma wrapped up in guilt", or a betrayal of what is considered to be right. This violation of deeply held moral beliefs causes guilt and shame and self-condemnation, where it is difficult to move on to self-forgiveness. During the pandemic many health practitioners had to restrict visiting of loved ones to dying patients which has created moral injury to those involved. So, in the case study Jo had to cope with the impossible dilemma of feeling a need to be part of the pandemic health care workforce and care for patients, as well as understanding the fears of her son and her family who were concerned for her safety. Their concerns were very valid considering Jo was at increased risk of illness due to her ethnicity and her work in a busy Emergency Department where she was caring for patients with COVID. She was also needing to reconcile the needs of families and patients who wanted to be together, when this could not be possible due to reducing COVID risks. Nolan (2020), as a hospice chaplain, says that chaplains can be instrumental in ameliorating the impact of moral injury. As he says, they are already based in intensive care units, EDs and hospices, and they can help those who are suffering from moral injury at any early stage before this sets in strongly. They can help people to feel accepted, forgive themselves and make sense of their conflicted experience. As he says, "no health care worker should have to cry alone".

Bradshaw (2009) discusses the moral virtues of compassion as having virtuous intention and practices and doing "the morally right thing even when no one is watching" (p466). Jarvis (1996) in their seminal text says that moral virtues include patience, kindness and cultivating unselfishness. The education of character, and the character of the nurse, is as important as the knowledge they possess. Bradshaw (2009) says that there is a move towards trying to measure techniques that appear to represent compassion, such as smiling and the use of warm words, so that they can be ticked and audited. This "McDonaldisation" of saying and doing the right thing can be merely a façade and a pretence and can actually be a parody of true compassion if this is divorced from virtue. This fakeness would be a travesty for genuinely caring nurses and would also be a cause of moral distress for them.

Selecting and recruiting nurses and nursing students based on the principles of values-based recruitment is a move towards ensuring that nurses have the characteristics and moral values necessary to be compassionate. Health Education England developed a values-based recruitment framework (HEE, 2016) which included a system of scenario tests and interview questions to assess whether candidates have the right values to be a nurse, partly as response to the poor care highlighted in the Francis Report (2013) in Mid Staffordshire. This was intended to be used with all university nursing students, and the expectation was that patients and members of the public would be involved in the process (Lintern, 2014).

However, defining, measuring and incentivising compassion might not improve care and compassion, particularly if the problem lies with inadequate resourcing

(Smajdor, 2013). Time and effort could be diverted away from providing excellent nursing care to time consuming tick box type measurement of outcomes and perceived values, to the detriment of actually providing care in line with nursing values.

Kristjansson et al (2017) in their research into virtuous nursing practice found that respondents, who were qualified nurses or nursing students, rate honesty and kindness as being the most important character strengths of nurses. Other strengths were identified as teamwork, fairness, leadership and judgement. They make the following recommendations:

- They stress the importance of moral role modelling at the heart of nurse education, and avoiding mindlessly following rules and standards of practice, which focus mainly on outcome measurement and not on individualised patient care.
- More inclusion of theoretical ethical aspects of virtues and values in nurse education.
- Recruiting nursing students based on their moral character and monitoring the development of this through student training.
- Ensuring that the ethical core of nursing is more explicit in CPD for qualified nurses.
- Mentorship being enhanced in relation to morals and values.
- Professional bodies need to influence curricula to ensure that there is a strong focus on values and the moral dimensions of nursing.

Leiter et al (2010) highlight the importance of having the capacity to influence our work environments in line with our core values. This involves decision making, participation, organisational justice (fair treatment where legitimate concerns are not treated with indifference or the self-interest of powerful others) and supervisory relationships. Together control and fairness describe an employee's capacity to develop a responsive, supportive work life.

Nurses who really care, are the nurses you want to be nursed by. Radcliffe (2020a) talks movingly about the death of his friend who was a nursing tutor, who ended his life being nursed by three of his former students. One of these nurses was on the brink of leaving the profession because someone told her that nurses should not get upset when patients were dying, his friend had said that if he was ever ill he hoped that he was nursed by someone like her. Unfortunately, in his final days this was the exact situation he was in, and the nursing care was exceptional right up to the end. Radcliffe (2020a) describes the care his friend received as beautiful and says how "transcendant and life affirming being brilliant at nursing is" (p 15). This is when a nurse's moral values shine through at their exceptional and wonderful best. Radcliffe (2021a) in another article makes the point that kindness, as a moral value, is more common than we think, it just does not make the news as much as bad actions do. Small acts of kindness are everywhere, and this has been particularly notable during the pandemic, and maybe we need to realise that humans are usually kind, despite what social media and negative news stories would tell us.

The University of Sussex partnered with BBC Radio 4 to carry out a large research project focused on increasing understanding of the role that kindness plays in our lives. Psychologists were researching what prompts us to act kindly and what prevents us from being kind, and how kindness is viewed within society at large. The kindness questionnaire will enable exploration concerning the most common acts of kindness, whether kindness is perceived as a weakness, and whether this is valued in the workplace. In addition, the role that kindness plays in wellbeing, mental health and personality. and how this connects to compassion and empathy will be explored (www.sussex.ac.uk/broadcast/read/55933).

Questions to ask yourself

Resilience and moral distress

- How resilient do you think that you are? Do you feel that you can bend without breaking? How can you help others to do the same?
- Do you seek support when you need it? Is support available at work, if so, what might be helpful? If not, what should you do to encourage this in your team?
- How much control do you have in your personal and professional life? Have you got more potential for influence than you think?
- Are you realistically optimistic? Could you think more positively or could you lower your expectations on what is possible so you are not disappointed?
- Do you have sufficient access to coaching, supervision and CPD? If not, what could you do about this?
- Are there any ways that you could increase team learning, teamworking and team support?
- Are you always able to practice in line with your moral values? If you feel that there is tension there can you think of what might help?
- Are there patients and patient situations who challenge your moral values and create moral injury or moral distress? How do you cope with that?
- To what extent do you help others to cope with a mismatch in values or moral distress? Could you do more to help?
- Do you feel that you are able to nurse compassionately and in line with your moral values? If not, what would help with this?

Having thought about our resilience and moral distress we need to think about how we manage the inevitable anxiety in our lives. Anxiety can be debilitating and create other health problems, so we need to think about strategies that might be helpful.

What strategies can we use to manage our anxiety?

Milne and Munro (2020) state that anxiety disorders are the most prevalent of psychiatric illnesses and generalised anxiety disorder (GAD) is the most common manifestation of anxiety. Causes of anxiety can include stress and trauma, environmental factors and inherited genetic causes. Symptoms can be psychological and physiological and can cause immense trauma and distress to the sufferer and their families and loved ones. Physical symptoms can include insomnia, palpitations, shortness of breath, headaches, nausea, sweating and trembling. Psychological symptoms include restlessness, a sense of dread, difficulty concentrating, irritability, avoidance of some situations and isolating oneself and constantly feeling on edge (www.nhs.uk/conditions/generalised-anxiety-disorder. Treatments can include self-help strategies; these can include Cognitive Behavioural Therapy (CBT) which encourages individuals to question negative or anxious thoughts. The use of apps has been highly effective in helping with self-help strategies and the identification of triggers. CBT is based on the concept that our thoughts, feelings, physical sensations and actions are interconnected, and that negative thoughts and feelings can trap us in a vicious cycle. CBT aims to help you deal with overwhelming problems in a more positive way by breaking them down into smaller parts (https://www.nhs.uk/mental-health/talking-therapies-medicine-treatments/talking-therapies-and-counselling/cognitive-behavioural-therapy-cbt/overview/).

Health care practitioners need to have awareness of anxiety and simple self-help measures. In the UK it is estimated that 8.2 million people are suffering from anxiety at any given time (Fineberg et al, 2013). Milne and Munro (2020) go on to say that anxiety creates a large degree of impairment mentally and physically. This causes a high use of health care services and work absences which has a large financial impact on individuals and society at large. Anxiety is a normal response to stressful triggers and perceived threats but when this takes over our lives this can be a sign of an anxiety disorder. Common quality of life issues can be impaired and there can be a reduction in social or work functioning. There can be increased comorbidities and other disorders and an increased risk of suicide (Hoge et al, 2012). GAD manifestations involves ongoing anxiety, worry and tension, which are not attributed to a direct environmental trigger (Alladin, 2015, Rhoads and Murphy, 2015). Prolonged stress and occupational stress, particularly in response to workload, tasks and job insecurity, is also considered to be the most likely cause of anxiety in working people. This causes extreme distress and has a negative impact on the productivity of organisations. (Fan et al, 2015).

Anxiety can be a nameless dread or fear without a target, or it can attach itself to an object or a situation. We need to have some anxiety in order to keep ourselves safe. If we feel anxious but feel that we have the ability to deal with the situation this can cause an arousal of anxiety, or a stress alert, and we might be able to use strategies to deal with this stressor. So, if we have high abilities we can cope with high challenges. Our cortisol levels rise during the night and our melatonin levels are falling during the early hours. This can result in early morning waking and waking up feeling worried, but not sure why. We cannot escape these worries because they are internally driven and inside ourselves. Carrying on looking inwards and excessive talking about ourselves and catastrophising and thinking the worse makes this much worse. I have put together a list of possible strategies (Table 4.2) that could be helpful. It is really a matter of knowing what might work for you and experimenting with different resources and strategies.

Table 4.2 Anxiety resources and strategies

Cognitive approaches

- Learning more about anxiety can help you to keep your anxiety levels as low as possible.
- This can also help you to develop strategies to spot episodes of panic at their earliest stages, or minimise their effect on you.
- Read about different anxiety disorders and options for treatment.
- Try to stop catastrophising and constantly worrying about what might happen, and ways in which things could go wrong. Try to contain your worry to certain times of the day when you think about your problems in a strategic way. Try to focus on best possible outcomes too.
- Learn techniques to manage your symptoms of anxiety.
- Think about using CBT strategies and maybe focus on psychotherapy approaches for specific phobias.
- Work out the things that trigger panic for you, track your moods and set goals.
- Learn meditation and mindfulness techniques and apply these to your life.
- Think about ways to reduce your negative thinking and increase your positive thinking.
- Join networks that put you in contact with others who struggle with anxiety.
- Ask for a referral to someone who can help you with your anxiety.
- Look for resources online, find helpful self-help books and maybe download apps that can help you.

Websites

- www.nopanic.org.uk – resources to help with health anxieties
- www.mind.org.uk – treatments and self-help resources for anxiety and panic attacks
- www.anxietyboss.com – articles and treatment options
- www.anxietycoach.com – self-help guide for people with anxiety with information and strategies to help
- www.anxiety.org – overview of risk factors, causes and treatments
- www.socialphobia.org – helps understanding of social anxiety disorder
- www.anxietysocialnet.com – for people struggling with anxiety
- www.childanxiety.net – information for parents, teachers and professionals to help children who suffer from anxiety
- Action for Happiness https://www.actionforhappiness.org/coping-calendar – coping calendar to promote the importance of keeping calm, staying wise and being kind
- Action for Happiness https://www.actionforhappiness.org/how-to-be-happy
- University of Cambridge – Five ways to beat anxiety during the COVID-19 Pandemic. From the Department of Public Health and Primary Care at the University of Cambridge https://www.cam.ac.uk/research/news/opinion-five-ways-to-beat-anxiety-and-take-back-control-of-your-life-during-the-covid-19-pandemic
- Shout. Free text service for anyone wanting immediate support for their mental health. https://www.giveusashout.org/
- Calm. Helpline and webchat. https://www.thecalmzone.net/help/get-help/.

Apps

- *Mood track diary* which helps to track and graph mood patterns and triggers
- *Pacifica* which helps reduce stress and anxiety with mood tracking, goal setting, relaxation and through peer support
- *Happify* which works on overcoming stress and negative thoughts and helps to train our mind towards happiness
- *Headspace* which has easy meditation and mindfulness exercises
- *Calm* which helps us to reduce anxiety, sleep better and feel happier using meditation, breathing and relaxation techniques
- *Breathe2relax* which includes stress management tools and practice exercises to help learn stress management tools
- *Catch-it* which looks at problems differently and turns negative thoughts into positive ones to improve mental health
- *SAM (Self-help for anxiety management)*
- *Mindshift* (particularly for younger people) Bit.ly/MindMHApps
- *Feeling Good* – Improves thoughts, feelings, self-esteem and self-confidence using the principles of cognitive therapy
- *My Possible Self* – Pick from ten modules to learn how to manage fear, anxieties and stress, and take control of your thoughts, feelings and behaviour
- *Stress and Anxiety Companion* – Guided breathing exercises, relaxing music and games made to help calm the mind, and handle stress and anxiety on the go
- *Reflectly* – Simple personal journaling app, mood tracker and daily gratitude journal for self-care

- *Cove* – Create music to reflect emotions like joy, sadness and anger to help express how you feel
- *SilverCloud* – An eight-week course to help manage stress, anxiety and depression at your own pace
- *Thrive* – Use games to track your mood and teach yourself methods to take control of stress and anxiety
- *Ten Percent Happier* – Get better at feeling good with guided meditations, videos, talks and sleep content
- UCLA Mindful – With this easy-to-use app, you can practice mindfulness anywhere, anytime with the guidance of the UCLA (University of California, Los Angeles) Mindful Awareness Research Centre.

Psychoeducation resources

- What is anxiety? Bit.ly/WhatAnxiety information sheet
- What is anxiety? Overview Bit.ly/AnxietyFlowchart
- Fight-or-flight Response fact sheet Bit.ly/FightFlightR.

Progressive Muscle Relaxation

- Information sheet Bit.ly/ProgressiveMuscle
- Progressive Muscle Relaxation Script Bit.ly/ProMuscleRelaxation.

Breathing Exercises

- Breathing Retraining information sheet Bit.ly/RetrainBreathe
- Deep Breathing information sheet Bit.ly/BreathingDeep.

Self-help psychological approaches

- Mindfulness, yoga, meditation and prayer
- Zen thinking and focusing on the art of simple living
- Aromatherapy or acupuncture
- Listening to music, breathing and relaxation strategies.

Lifestyle adjustments

- Reducing caffeine, alcohol and smoking
- Drinking herb or Earl Grey tea
- Consider trying St John's Wort
- Seek advice on pharmacological therapy, including beta blockers, benzodiazepines.

The APPLE approach

This is a self-help tool which could help many of us to start to reduce our anxiety. This approach focuses on:

- Acknowledging – noticing and acknowledging uncertainties
- Pausing – not reacting as usual and not reacting at all, just pausing and breathing
- Pulling back – telling ourselves it is the anxiety of depression talking, and this is only a thought or feeling. We do not have to believe everything we think, thoughts are not statements of fact

- Letting go – letting go of the thought or feeling, it will pass, we do not need to respond to it. Imagine it floating away in a bubble or a cloud
- Exploring – exploring the current moment, because right now all is well. Focusing on our breathing and the sensations of breathing, and the ground beneath us. Focusing on what we can see, hear, touch and smell. Then shifting our attention to something else, or something we need to do, or what we were doing before the worry occurred and focusing mindfully on this with full attention. (www.getselfhelp.co.uk).

The 3 Ds approach

- Drop – what does not need to be done
- Delay – what can be put off until later
- Delegate – what can be carried out by someone else.

The 3 Rs approach

- Remove – removing stressors
- Reduce – reducing stressors to manageable portions
- Reconsider – changing our mindsets to manage our emotions and encourage more effective coping strategies.

The 3 Cs approach

- Catch it – recognise negative thoughts early
- Check it – consider the evidence for these thoughts and challenge these
- Change it – change the thought to something more positive.

Aloufi et al (2021) discuss stress, anxiety and depression in nursing students and have carried out a systematic review on a broad range of international research articles. Helpful approaches in relation to stress, anxiety and depression symptoms were evaluated to be:

- Mindfulness-based stress reduction programmes based on meditation
- Stress coping programmes focusing on mindfulness meditation
- CBT
- Emotional intelligence interventions
- Stress management training programmes helped with depression
- Mindfulness training with physical education helped with depression
- Music therapy helped with depression
- Interpersonal relationship programmes helped with depression
- Biofeedback training strategies were helpful in relation to stress and anxiety but less helpful in terms of depression
- Emotional Freedom Technique (EFT) which involves light tapping at acupuncture pressure points was helpful to some extent with anxiety
- Guided reflection helped with anxiety
- Progressive muscle relaxation helped with anxiety
- Stress management programmes helped with anxiety
- Mindfulness combined with humour helped with anxiety.

The authors suggest that nursing educationalists should consider including prevention of stress, anxiety and depression strategies and mindfulness-based interventions in nursing curricula. Health care employers should also consider facilitating workplace learning around these areas to support the mental health of nursing students, and other staff would benefit as well.

Anxiety is not right or wrong, it is part of being human. We all have anxieties and phobias; it is when they take over our lives that we need to take action to reduce the debilitating affect that they can have on us and the choices we make. Healthy anxiety keeps us safe and makes us take action to ensure that we, and our loved ones and others, are safe. So, we need to focus on paying attention to the here and now in a mindful way, so that we are less ruled by our anxieties but approach them in a reflective way to see whether they have any validity. We can then make changes if we feel that they are needed. Coping with our anxiety is particularly important when we are coping with conflict, which is incredibly stressful to deal with, particularly when it is part of our life day after day. So, the next topic focuses on conflict and on strategies that can be helpful.

How can I predict and de-escalate conflict?

Conflict is a constant reality in health care and nursing. Conflict is "an interactive process manifested by incompatibility, disagreement or dissonance within or between social entities" (Rahim, 2011, p 16). Conflict has different dynamics, but it is:

- Inevitable in any group that has been together for any period of time. Teams are made up of imperfect people.
- Different people have different viewpoints, ideas, opinions and needs and there can be just enough difference to create misunderstandings.
- We also tend to have different attitudes, values, beliefs and goals.
- Conflict is not a constant process and it can vary from time to time.

There are many issues that can lead to conflict, and these are highlighted in Table 4.3 (below).

Table 4.3 Reasons and antecedents leading to conflict

- Complex organisations - Differing role expectations - Communication problems - Decision making issues - Competition over resources - Unclear job boundaries - Personality differences (Labrague and McEnroe-Petitte, 2017) - Lack of clear boundaries - Conflicts of interest - Lack of clear communication and misunderstandings - Dependence on one person - Increased number of organisational tiers - Too many people making decisions - Difficulty in gaining consensus if team numbers are too large - Strict rules and regulations - Unresolved prior conflicts (Rungapadiachy 1999)	Also: - Disagreement on how things should be done - Incompatible goals - Personal, self or group interest - Tension, stress, long hours and overwork - Power and influence issues - Personality clashes or conflict - Previous experiences which make people look for trouble or act defensively - Papering over but not solving previous challenging situations - If someone loses they could feel a sense of loss which makes future conflict more likely - If conflict is suppressed without resolution it makes future conflict more likely - A person might not have intended to cause conflict and they might not be aware that it is happening. Accidental conflict can be avoided

Weeks (1992) says that conflict is inescapable and is "an inevitable result of our highly complex, competitive and often litigious society" (Weeks, 1992, p. ix). We have different ideas, opinions, priorities and needs, and the conflicts that can arise can cause anything from minor inconvenience through to extreme anxiety. This can cause long term damage to our confidence, relationships, work environments and potentially our communities. Resolving conflict takes a lot of time and effort but trying to predict or deescalate conflict speedily alleviates distress and leaves more time to spend on more positive activities which we should be spending time doing. Weeks (1992) says that the ingredients of conflict are diversity and difference. This includes different needs, perceptions, power, values, principles, feelings and emotions and the internal conflicts inside us all.

Conflict can be positive or negative and positively handled conflict can:

- Result in greater creativity, new ideas and innovation
- Create higher morale, commitment, and performance
- Stimulate interest
- Create a forum for discussion
- Increase cohesiveness and develop better relationships
- Promote change
- Provide a means to work together.

So, in our work teams it is a good idea to think about:

- What is the advantage of working in a team
- What makes a team function well
- What is an effective team
- Effects of team development – positive and negative
- Team roles
- Why don't teams work
- The negative impact of conflict on teams.

However, unresolved or negatively handled conflict leads to organisational and team issues, as well as feelings that can be difficult to resolve (see Table 4.4 below):

Table 4.4 Organisational and team issues and feelings relating to conflict

Organisational	Team issues	Feelings
• Disruptions in work • Lower staff performance • Absenteeism, sickness and staff attrition • Wasting resources • Reduced morale • Increased stress and burnout. • This also leads to poor patient outcomes	• Waste of time which diverts attention away from important issues • May damage morale • May cause polarisation of views • Reinforces differences in values and beliefs • Produces regrettable behaviours • Reduces team effectiveness and teamworking	• Getting angry is a waste of time • They won't understand me • I am afraid of the consequences • Confrontation is unprofessional • They will argue back

So it is imperative that we have just enough friction to generate creativity, but not enough to damage working relationships, self esteem and self-confidence. Conflict can be physical or verbal and can be obviously aggressive or passively aggressive. Rungapadiachy (2008) uses the characters in The Simpsons to explain different categories of behaviour, see Table 4.5 below.

Table 4.5 Categories of aggressive behaviour (Rungapadiachy, 2008, p 106)

Types of aggression	Explanation	Example
Physical-active-direct	Physical assault	Bart punches Lisa
Physical-active-indirect	Using a 3rd party to assault someone	Homer hires Bart to beat up Lisa
Physical-passive-direct	A non-violent act that is aimed at preventing another reaching their goal	Bart locks Homer in the toilet
Physical-passive-indirect	Non-involvement that causes disruption	Homer refuses to move during a sit in at the plant
Verbal-active-direct	Making a derogatory comment towards someone	Bart swears at Lisa
Verbal-active-indirect	Making derogatory comments about A to B	Bart expresses negativity about Lisa to Marje
Verbal-passive-direct	Remaining silent when questioned	Homer refuses to respond to Bart

Some of the attitudes that can be hardest to address are the less overt behaviour and you might recognise some of the scenarios below:

- Don't worry about me then, I will just drop down dead somewhere (emotional blackmail).
- I don't know what I might do if ... does not happen (hinting at suicide ideation) (emotional blackmail).
- Someone who phones and asks for your name in order to complain before you have said anything (looking for trouble).
- You have different priorities to others you work with – (you think their standards are lower than yours).
- You don't like the way that others talk to you or how they write emails – (different communication styles that upset you/others).

Some passive aggressive or verbally aggressive behaviour is difficult to address. Communications by email and in written forms can be misinterpreted and can be very aggressive or not valuing of others. I am often shocked by communications I am copied into, and some of the worst offenders are senior management. These can range from top-down mandates that are communicated in a very terse style, with no pleasantries, to highly critical communications to individuals and teams. When we communicate in writing we need to make doubly sure that we do not alienate others or create unintentional or unwarranted distress. If there needs to be communication about a person's performance this needs to be carried out carefully to ensure that the person truly understands the importance of what is being said and can genuinely address the issues. Emotional blackmail and individuals who are looking for trouble are difficult to manage, but high emotional intelligence will always help us to communicate more effectively and compassionately.

Stone et al (1999) says that a difficult conversation is anything we find hard to talk about. We need to stop thinking about who is right and listen to each other. We all have different interpretations and perceptions, and we need to move from being sure to questioning. We need to avoid blame and express our feelings without blaming, attributing or judging. We might have responded badly because of past experiences or conflict inside ourselves. We need to accept our part in what has happened and take the lead in problem solving. We can then encourage others to do the same. To do this we need to understand different sorts of conflict.

DIFFERENT TYPES AND LEVELS OF CONFLICT

- Competitive conflict – individuals compete for goals which are incompatible
- Disruptive conflict – not about winning – the emphasis is on defeating, harming or driving away another person (Rungapadiachy 1999)
- Fights – force is involved and the prime object is to incapacitate or eliminate the opponent
- Games – the purpose is to win without eliminating the opponent
- Debates – the objective is to change the opinion of the opponent (Rapoport, 1960)

The Thomas-Kilmann Conflict Mode Instrument (Kilmann, and Thomas 1974) highlights different ways of approaching conflict:

- The vertical axis refers to the degree of **assertiveness** – which attempts to satisfy our own concerns
- The horizontal axis refers to the degree of **cooperativeness** – which attempts to satisfy the concerns of others
- **Avoidance** – withdrawal (low assertiveness, low cooperation)
- **Competition** – forcing and resisting (high assertiveness, low cooperation)
- **Accommodation** – smoothing over (low assertiveness, high cooperation)
- **Collaboration** – win-win and problem solving (high assertiveness and high cooperation)
- **Compromise** – mutually acceptable solution finding.

So, it is clear that we need to work on our compromising, but particularly our collaboration skills. Compromise or negotiation takes skill, as does integration and collaboration. We need to avoid suppression, denial or avoidance of conflict because it will cause problems further down the line. If there is compromise conflict can be averted but if there is no compromise conflict usually escalates. Conflict and cooperation are not necessarily symmetrical, in that both parties do not necessarily feel that they are both in conflict. We can cause upset without meaning to, and sometimes without being aware of what we have done to cause distress. So, we need to think about different perceptions of the situation, and what is actually true and an accurate view of what has taken place. It is possible in some cases that if the people involved are unaware of the situation conflict can be avoided.

Rungapadiachy (1999) says that there are different aspects of conflict:

- ***Affective experience*** – what do the people involved feel. If the nature of the interaction is personalised and one party is blamed, then conflict will arise. If things are depersonalised and the behaviour, rather than the person, is blamed then conflict can be avoided.

- **Behaviour manifestation** – there is a question of intent. If the behaviour is perceived as being intentional then prevention of achievement of goals and conflict will arise. If this is seen as accidental, conflict can be avoided.
- **Conflict resolution or suppression** – conflict is resolved or put on hold. Resolution will only take place if both parties are prepared to collaborate. Unresolved conflicts exist in life and attempts to resolve them can sometimes do more harm than good.
- **Resolution aftermath** – if there is one winner then the other could feel a sense of loss which could fuel further conflict. If the resolution has been amicable good feelings can result.

Rungapadiachy (1999) goes on to say that in managing conflict there are several outcomes:

Win-lose scenario: one winner and one loser but…

- One person does not have to lose for another to win
- Honesty and openness are key
- As is self-awareness
- It is essential to listen to the other's point of view
- We need to avoid blame and criticism, and creating a "tit for tat" stance
- Recognising each other's strengths is crucial.

Lose-lose scenario – there are no winners and nobody compromises

Win-win scenario – this involves a problem-solving approach where both parties are satisfied. Positive strategies are:

- Empathetic listening
- Allowing everyone to express their thoughts and feelings
- Communication skills and self-awareness can prevent or resolve conflict. One person does not need to lose for another to win.

Labrague and McEnroe-Petitte (2017) in their study say that nurses prefer using constructive and positive conflict management styles and that the students in the study benefitted from teaching programmes focusing on conflict management and simulation scenarios, role playing and reflective exercises. So, more input on how to resolve conflict would be helpful for nursing students and part of CPD for qualified nurses and MDT development with other health care professionals.

Weeks (1992) says that there are eight essential steps to conflict resolution:

- Creating an effective atmosphere – timing, place, and opening comments.
- Clarify perceptions – what are the real issues, and what are red herrings or less important, what are the perceptions of all those involved, what questions need to be asked, what communication strategies would be helpful.
- Individual and shared needs, needs of the relationship and of conflict resolution.
- Building shared positive power – negative and positive.
- Look to the future and learn from the past – and recognise the impact that the past has but focus on the present and the future
- Generate options – from both party's perspective.
- Stepping stones – what is doable and most likely to convert to action and success.
- Make mutual benefit agreements – and keep the conflict partnership resolution alive.

Weinstein (2018) believes that there are seven principles of conflict resolution:

- Acknowledging the fact that there is a conflict – are you irritated by someone, talking about someone behind their back, are you avoiding someone or do you feel uncomfortable around someone? Are you worried about something that has happened? Is there conflict within yourself or with others?
- Take control of your response – we need to behave like an adult and take responsibility for our part in the situation.
- Apply the resolution framework for difficult conversations (Part 1) – prepare for the conversation and think about your fears, wants and needs and then look at the bigger picture, get your facts straight, think about possible outcomes and options, what is the least and most that you would agree to, clarify your agenda and practice empathy and start to take back some control and set up a conversation.
- Apply the resolution framework for difficult conversations (Part 2) – have the conversation through active listening, summarising, paraphrasing and reframing to include listening for what is behind what is being said, ask questions and negotiate – think about accommodating, compromising, avoiding competing, collaborating.
- Manage the resolution – through ongoing discussion.
- Build a culture of early conflict resolution.
- Use conflict resolution in daily life.
- Know what to do when conflict resolution does not work.

I have put together the following strategies in relation to communication, self awareness and problem solving which could be helpful (Table 4.6).

Conflict usually involves having difficult conversations and there are various do's and don'ts to think about:

- Choose a suitable time and place – no interruptions, privacy, sufficient time, not just before a holiday or before another important meeting, think about the time of day and give advanced notice.
- State your intention upfront – explain what you want to talk about, why the conversation is necessary, what outcome you would like to see. Plan in advance and this plan should structure the conversation and get it back on track. Maybe go through your plan with a trusted colleague or mentor.
- Gather evidence and stick to the facts and direct observations and back up what you are saying whenever possible. Have examples ready but don't get sucked in and let one example dominate the discussion. Give examples of what made you come to the conclusions that you have.
- Don't wait until you are so cross that you boil over and react emotionally and overcritically and personally.
- Keep lines of communication open – you might need to follow HR policies but talk to the person first so they can give their explanation and their side of the story. Try not to make snap judgements or decisions before hearing their perspective. There could be circumstances which you know nothing about.
- Be clear about what needs to happen next including timescales, who else needs to be involved, and potential consequences.
- Don't procrastinate – the situation will probably continue and a lack of action could make things worse. You could also lose the respect and trust of your team if you do not deal with issues which affect them.

Table 4.6 Conflict management strategies

Communication	**Communication skills** • Create a welcoming and relaxed environment where they feel valued and cared about. They might forget what you said but not how you made them feel • Be honest and open • Ensure that there is privacy and confidentiality • Make it as difficult as possible for them to be antagonistic towards you • Try to get them to feel better about those involved than they did before the discussion. Feelings are emotions and you want them to be as positive as possible • Avoid defensive body language and use positive body language e.g smiling and eye contact • Active and empathetic listening – listen to what is being said and not said and do not multitask • Keep your voice low, calm and friendly even if they are not • Ask probing questions about what happened and clarify perceptions and develop a curiosity in difficult situations • Summarise, paraphrase and reframe and look for what is behind what is being said • Understand individual and shared needs, look for common interests • Listen actively and do not try to rush them – they need to tell their story. Do not rush to reassure, explain or suggest • Think before reacting – we need to think what might work best • Use direct less threatening communication and 'I' messages for example: • *I need feedback on x (not you have not told me x)* • *I am concerned about x (not I don't think you care about x)* • *I want to be part of the team (not you don't want to be)* • *I need more information (not you have not told me x)* • *I am feeling x (not you make me feel x)* • Look for common interests • Focus on the future • (Caspersen (2015) • Build shared positive power and problem solving **Differentiate between difficult people and difficult behaviour** (Boynton, 2019) • Someone might have a valid reason for complaining and saying that they are not happy helps • This helps to reveal underlying issues • It also helps you to develop ownership and this involves assertiveness and you being accountable for problem solving • Questioning them gives you more information about the problem which can be useful – so develop a curiosity about this • It helps you to think about new ways forward • It promotes healthy conversations and collaborative problem solving • Assume that useful dialogue is possible even if it is unlikely • Acknowledge the conflict and that they are very unhappy/angry • If you are making it worse…Stop and escalate it to someone else. **Change the conversation** • Create a relaxed and confidential environment • Ask how their role is going: are there any challenges that they are aware of • Say what they are good at and how much they are valued • Maybe say what you might find difficult – gain some ground and build bridges and similarities between you

(Continued)

Table 4.6 (Continued) Conflict management strategies

	• Start by explaining what you are aware of (external view) • Explain what you have seen/heard • How this might have made you feel if you had been on the receiving end? • Ask how do you think that the other person felt as a result • What were they feeling at the time? • How could this have been perceived by others? • Acknowledge that they did not intend this • Give them plenty of time to have their say • Admit what other issues can be challenging. **Facilitate listening and speaking** • Do not hear the attack – listen for what is behind the words • Figure out what is happening and not whose fault it is. • Resist the urge to attack, change the conversation from your position • Talk to the person's best self • Differentiate between needs, interests and strategies • Acknowledge their emotions – do not shy away from these and see them as signs • Differentiate between acknowledgement and agreement when listening and making suggestions • Differentiate between evaluation and observation • Test your assumptions, relinquish them if they turn out to be false • Escalate concerns to someone who has the power to solve the problem. If that is you, it might be best to ask them to come to see you or say that you will phone back, because their concern is too important to rush and you want to focus on what they are saying but you cannot do that right now • Ask them what they would like you to do "how can we sort this out together" • Think before reacting and consider what they are saying, and possible responses and solutions open to you both.
Self-awareness	• High self-awareness • Self-knowledge • Avoid blaming others • Do not make the situation about your feelings, your self-image and self-esteem • Attack the problem not each other • Emotions run very high when there is conflict – what is the problem underlying the emotion? • Think about how they may be feeling as a result of what happened • Give generous attention to the person who you are struggling with • Carry on working together and do not give up on each other • Accept responsibility – attempting to put blame on someone else creates anger and resentment. In order to resolve a conflict, we need to accept our share of the responsibility and stop blaming the other person. • Do not hide behind zero tolerance and what you/they will not tolerate • Keep your emotions at bay – conflict is very emotional and we are sometimes defensive or attack back – focus on the problem not the person. **Your behaviour** • Brusque care – you are competent but cold and insensitive • Polite care – briskly efficient, you smile but not with your eyes • Kindly care – interact with them as an individual, anticipate their needs, come back with a response, they felt cared for and it was clear that you enjoy your job • Compassionate care – when people are vulnerable, anxious, scared or in pain, you help them to feel better, comfortable, cared for and grateful

(Continued)

Table 4.6 (Continued) Conflict management strategies

	• People can tell the difference within seconds and the kindly and compassionate members of staff are therapeutic in their own right and people feel better as a result • A kind and compassionate approach also protects you from burnout • Think about what made you want to work in your role in the first place and be true to that • Think about people as if they were a friend or close member of your family • It does not take any longer to be kind and communicate well – it is your choice whether to be like this or more brusque and uncaring (Youngson, 2018).
Problem solving	• Prepare for the conversation • Look at the bigger picture • Recognise their strengths and concerns • Look for strategies and common ground • What would they suggest might be helpful • What does the person need from you right now • Work out what the problem is, not whose fault it is • Consider third party intervention if necessary • What would help in the future. ***Look for ways forward***: • Acknowledge that there is conflict – talk to the right people about real problems • Assume undiscovered options exist – seek solutions people will willingly support • Be explicit about arguments – be explicit when they change • Expect and plan for future conflict • Look to the future and learn from the past • What is the least and most you would agree to, and take back control and behave like an adult • Think about options and stepping stones for what is possible • Make mutual benefit agreements and keep conflict resolution alive through ongoing discussions • Build a culture of early conflict resolution and use this in everyday life • It is the little things that people notice, and that can create feelings. We need to measure positives and the rationale behind issues but also emotionally measurable issues. • Try to get them to a point where they want to promote the team in a positive light. After seeing you, would they recommend this as a good place to work. • What would you want them to say about how they felt after the encounter with you – that you were helpful, friendly, professional and that they thought that the meeting was helpful. • Avoid conflict developing and deescalate as fast as possible • Expect and plan for future conflict. • Allow them time to have their say • Accept responsibility for what is happening. They might need to accept some too, but blaming others leads to resentment and anger • Look for common ground • Focus on strategies for moving forward together • Do not force them into a corner in terms of what they are saying, this causes extreme and polarised views • When something has gone wrong it is an opportunity to change their views for the better.

(Continued)

Table 4.6 (Continued) Conflict management strategies

Individual and team conflict – Strategies for moving on....
• Maybe say "let's work on why you said this in the way that you did".
• Think about strategies for the future now that they are aware of the potential conflict
• What are the obstacles in moving forward, and how can you overcome this?
• How can we work together on ways to give (and receive) feedback respectfully?
• SMART action plan: Specific, Measurable, Achievable, Realistic, Time-orientated
• Tips.... Do not describe someone in terms of their behaviour – i.e. bullying
• A bully cannot exist without a victim or in an organisational culture which will not tolerate it
• Separate intention from impact
• Focus on how someone might feel and how this could be perceived by others.

- Don't start the conversation with "you". This sounds like an attack and will create defensiveness. Focus on the behaviour not the person, so how certain actions damage reputations etc and maybe also think about using "we" in terms of what needs to be discussed, resolved etc.
- Don't make assumptions – there could be mitigating circumstances, so use active listening to draw these out. Be respectful at all times.
- Don't let your emotions get in the way – sensitive subjects create emotional reactions. Try to keep your own emotions in check and stay focused and objective. Avoid hearsay or personal opinions and focus on facts. Maybe take a break, if you can, to give both of you space so you can both return with a clear head.
- Don't be afraid to move things on if your conversations are not having the desired effect. Escalate your concerns to your manager to take advice from HR if necessary and possible.
- People become defensive not about the facts, but the intention behind the facts, and the way that the message is delivered. We need to create a feeling of safety and use our emotional intelligence.
- Don't become defensive yourself. Combat defensiveness with curiosity about why a rational decent person would think or behave the way they have. Persuading them is about listening to them, understanding them and not being judgemental. Think about "what went before".

Some people can come across as being difficult but try to think about difficult situations, rather than thinking that the person is difficult, where you can. Try to stay calm and do not react or take it personally, listen and if appropriate apologise. Be assertive if you are not being allowed to respond and problem solve where you can. Support other team members when there has been conflict with a challenging situation, and someone has been rude; debrief from the situation and try to think about any changes that might be necessary to improve the service you offer. Open University (2021) https://app.goodpractice.net/#/open-university/s/snx1x8b74i.

I have tried to give some practical solutions to help you deal with conflict at an early stage. Unresolved previous conflict casts long shadows and these will not always go away. It is always best to predict conflict and deescalate it fast. Try to ensure that issues are resolved and that positive ways are found to ensure that feelings of distress and anger do not persist. I have now discussed conflict in detail, and what we can do to manage situations as positively as possible. However, it is impossible to take away all negative stressors from our lives so it is important to think about how we can care for ourselves as well as possible to maximise our resilience.

Why is it so important to care for ourselves in order to keep our stress levels manageable?

This section will discuss the importance of caring for ourselves, something we usually do much less well than caring for others. Kanner et al (1981) say that it is the small things that go well, or badly, every day that make us more, or less, able to cope with life's challenges. How we cope with everyday hassles, and focus on the uplifts, can be a better predictor of our level of psychological stress and resilience than big events that make us happy, or cause us distress. Therefore, the following self-assessment tool has been designed to help us to identify the small hassles, and the small counteracting positives, that can make a real difference in our lives. You might have other ideas for what these could be for you personally. Try to think creatively about the things that cause you irritation and enjoyment, and then try to identify what you can do to reduce or increase these on a day-to-day basis.

QUESTIONNAIRE 4.1 Hassles and uplifts assessment

(based on research by Kanner et al, 1981)

Assess the hassles and uplifts that have affected you in the past month and score these in terms of how much you feel they have affected your positivity and negativity:

Score 0 if these have not happened in the last month
Score 1 if the impact has been **somewhat** severe
Score 2 if the impact has been **moderately** severe
Score 3 if the impact has been **extremely** severe

Hassles	Score	Uplifts	Score
Misplacing or losing things		Getting enough sleep and rest	
Difficult relationships with others – neighbours, colleagues, friends, family		Having time for your hobbies and interests, learning something new, seeing friends and having time to talk etc	
Troubling thoughts and concerns about death, the future, meaning of life etc		Feeling as if things are going well	
Health worries about yourself, friends, family, pet etc		Having enough money for what you want to do	
Financial ongoing worries or tasks		Liking people you mix with	
Smoking, alcohol, use of drugs		Having time off, holidays etc	
Too many responsibilities		Giving back to others, giving your time, love, advice etc	
Work worries and insecurity or not enjoying your job		Feeling well or recovering from an illness or being physically active	

Worries about the future, pension – retirement etc	Finding something that you thought that you had lost
Too many interruptions and too much to do	Being with people whose company you enjoy
Having to wait or having too much time on your hands	Getting on well with people, partner, children, parents, colleagues, friends etc
Feeling lonely or isolated	Feeling that you have done something well
Making silly mistakes	Cutting down on alcohol, smoking, drugs, food etc
Worries about your appearance and body image	Receiving compliments
Sexual problems	Solving problems or conflicts and meeting a challenge
Fear of rejection	Doing things you enjoy – reading, shopping, music, laughing with friends, kissing, hugging, flirting
Not getting enough sleep or rest	Good news – locally or nationally
Too many administrative tasks	People you care about feeling better
Problems with ageing parents or children	Enjoying your job and feeling that you are doing it well
Worries about news events, crime, traffic, pollution	Feeling accepted, loved and appreciated and giving love to others
Work to do on your home	Meditating, praying, feeling at one with the world

Hassle overall assessment

Which hassles affect
you most

Positive actions to
reduce these hassles

Uplift overall assessment

Which uplifts affect you
most

Positive actions to
increase these uplifts

This assessment tool might help you with the minor things that go wrong in life, and maximise the moments of pleasure, and it would be really helpful to think about ways you can decrease and increase these, as appropriate. However, our lives can be full of ongoing demands which are incredibly difficult to balance and incredibly stressful to deal with. Our professional demands alone can be all consuming and create immense distress.

Radcliffe (2021b) refers to "guerrilla nursing" where we nurse in perpetual crisis which fundamentally changes our psychological state. This was true before the COVID-19 pandemic, but it has been even more true during this, and in the period since. Clinical supervision has largely disappeared, and when it is planned it is often deprioritised due to poor staffing levels. Even when it does take place the focus is usually on work outcomes, rather on our wellbeing or our professional development. Radcliffe (2020b) goes on to say that nursing has often prided itself on the challenges it can cope with, how much it can absorb, and its ability to endure, rather than on its resilience. Nursing often takes pride in its ability to suffer for the cause. Radcliffe (2020b) goes on to say that this culture is of course outdated, unprofessional, lacking in reflection and lacking in ongoing patient focus. "A failure to self-care is a failure to make nursing sustainable" (Radcliffe, 2020b, p15). So, we need to focus on protecting ourselves, and our employers need to focus on protection of their employees. Providing supervision, which actually happens, and focuses on the whole person, and not just our work, would be a good start.

The American Holistic Nurses Association (2013) identified six different components of self-care focusing on physical, mental, emotional, relational, choices and spiritual parts of our lives. However, it is very rare that we think of ourselves as holistically as this. Patwell (2021) also discusses the importance of caring for ourselves and working in an environment which promotes caring of others. The CARE model stands for Connect, Adapt, Routinize and Exercise and is a framework for building resilience, which enables us to be our best selves (Patwell, 2021). She says that the pandemic caused a state of grieving, due to the rapid pace of change, loss of loved ones, and the loss of what we normally enjoy and our normal connections with friends and families. So, the CARE framework focuses on:

- Connect – how are we really doing personally and professionally, how are we caring for ourselves and others, what has changed for us, what do we need and how are we communicating those needs? This involves managers checking in on employees regularly, providing opportunities for discussion, and helping them to make sense of changes, and in providing resources to enable people to cope with the changes.
- Adapt – what are our guiding principles, what values, behaviours and mindsets do we need, how can we take a lead on this, what resources do we need to use and how will we manage our success? This involves talking with employees to find out what changes mean for them, their mindsets and helping them to develop a plan to help them change.
- Routinise – what rituals and routines do we need, what can we capitalise on in our organisational culture, what processes do we need to use to adapt? This involves employers setting boundaries between work and play, realistic priority setting and problem solving, celebrating success, and putting in new routines and rituals which promote collaboration and learning from each other.
- Exercise – what are we doing to stay fit and well physically, mentally, emotionally and spiritually, are we getting what we need, how do we need to adapt to care for ourselves, our team, our family and friends, and others? This involves us all focusing on taking care of ourselves and taking time to reenergise, recharge and have fun.

Mojza (2010) in her longitudinal research study found that a lack of psychological detachment from work in off-time predicted an increase in emotional exhaustion a year later. This increases the chances of psychosomatic complaints and decreases work engagement over time. However, she also says that a lack of psychological detachment might not always be detrimental because reflecting on work issues can enhance problem solving, and talking about job related topics can enable employees to access support from family and friends (Halbesleben, 2006).

Hofmeyer et al (2020a) says that self-compassion involves:

- Protecting – we need to feel safe from harm and feel able to say no to people and factors that could harm us
- Providing – we need to know and provide ourselves with what we need to be well
- Motivating – we need to encourage ourselves to act with kindness and support.

The authors say that it is important to reconnect with what drew us to nursing in the first place and draw on this compassion. Knowledge and competence are important, but so are kindness and compassion, and we need resilience and kindness to deal with the distress inherent in our roles. Ken Schwartz an American lawyer who died in his 40s of lung cancer said that "Small acts of kindness can make the unbearable bearable" (Abbasi, 2012) and Schwartz rounds came from his belief that health care staff should support each other in the stressful roles they carried out through monthly meetings focusing on sharing their feelings about the care of particular patients.

Figley (2002) writes about what causes compassion fatigue in psychotherapists and the variables and what could alleviate this:

- Empathic ability – how much we notice the pain of others?
- Empathic concern – how motivated are we to respond to this distress?
- Exposure to the client – how much high exposure is there to this distress?
- Empathic response – to what extent do we respond to the distress?
- Compassion stress – how much emotional energy do we have left after an experience of patient distress and how much ongoing demand is there for support?
- Sense of achievement – how satisfied are we with how we responded to the need?
- Disengagement – to what extent could we "let go" of the distress of others afterwards?
- Prolonged exposure – do we have enough time to recover from the demands of patient distress – gaps in the day, between shifts, days off and holidays?
- Traumatic recollections – do we experience memories which trigger distress following exposure to the distress of others?
- Life disruption – how much do traumatic memories or unexpected changes in our responsibilities impact on the rest of our life?

So, we need to have sufficient empathic ability, concern and exposure to a patient's distress to elicit an empathic response. However, we need to reduce our compassion stress and limit prolonged exposure without time to recover, and let go of the stress caused by experiencing the stress of others. A strong sense of having helped, and a lack of flashbacks of feelings caused by others' distress and minimal disruption of our lives will also counter compassion fatigue.

Higher levels of self-compassion are associated with lower levels of burnout and lower barriers to compassion. Self-compassion prevents us from being overconscientious and striving for perfection, which can lead to higher levels of burnout. We can see ourselves as rescuers which can prevent us seeing when we are less effective at work, and we can justify our behaviour as being necessary for the benefit of patients (Dev et al, 2018). Mindful self-care and focusing on strategies to prevent burnout, like purposely shedding the role we have at work when we get home, as well as incorporating moments of self-care into our working day, can be really helpful when stress levels are high. An example of this could be focusing on the sensation of water on our skin, and sinking into this experience and focusing on our breathing as we are washing our hands for 20 seconds (Kearney et al, 2009). Another useful example is using time driving to and from work to focus on home for the first part of the journey into work and then focus on planning for the day for the rest of the journey. In the same way coming home from work, reflect on the day in the first part of the drive home, then think of home, social and family issues before reaching home.

A workplace culture needs to be safe and effective for patients, but also kind and caring for the patients in our care. Staff need to feel valued and enjoy working there, and they need to feel part of the team and engaged which all contributes to staff wellbeing. Positive and supportive workplaces understand what it feels like to work there, by acting on staff feedback, having well structured appraisals, mentorship, clinical supervision, ongoing learning and development opportunities. Staff need to work in well-defined teams where there are opportunities to get to know each other and there is time to reflect on shared goals, effectiveness, patient care, teamworking, challenges and innovations. Exploring values, beliefs and attitudes which influence our behaviour is an important part of this (Sanders and Shaw, 2019).

Sanchez- Reilly et al (2013) focus on the stress of caring for patients at the end of their lives, and the importance of clinicians using self-care and self-awareness strategies, so that their patient care is enhanced. They highlight the importance of medical training including an emphasis on communication skills, self-care, mindfulness, reflection and professional boundaries. There also needs to be education focusing on grief and bereavement, coping skills and counselling. Self-care strategies include focusing on close personal relationships, maintaining healthy lifestyles such as physical activity, a healthy diet, adequate sleep, time for holidays and time for self-development. Nursing curricula need to do the same, but there is so much to fit into professional training that this is less of a priority than it should be. Vanderbilt University's (Vanderbilt University, 2012, in Sanchez-Reilly et al, 2013) Wellness Wheel refers to six types of wellness – physical, intellectual, emotional, spiritual, social and occupational – all of which help individuals to reflect on life balance and self-care. Self-awareness can lead to greater job engagement and satisfaction and enhanced self-care and compassion (Sanchez-Reilly et al, 2013). Mindfulness strategies can be key to enhanced wellbeing and empathetic engagement and reduced anxiety in practitioners. Sanchez-Reilly et al (2013) also highlight the importance of team self-care and support, including an emphasis on interprofessional education and a focus on developing empathetic approaches and sharing personal and professional learning within a team environment.

Part of self-caring is not treating ourselves badly, and blaming ourselves for everything we do that is not perfect. We would not criticise others in this way, but we think it is acceptable to criticise ourselves. If we insult ourselves this will activate our flight or fight responses which increases our stress hormones and causes psychological and physiological damage. So, self-care is also related to self-compassion and being kind to ourselves. We need to show humanity to ourselves and believe that failing in things is a shared human experience. We need to notice when we are finding fault with ourselves and talk calmly, kindly and positively to ourselves and do this in a mindful focused way.

Neff (2020) has developed seven exercises to help develop self-compassion:

- How would I treat a friend in this situation?
- Take a self-compassion break to help you to overcome negative emotions.
- Explore self-compassion through writing – write a kind letter to yourself.
- Seek a supportive touch – get a massage or a hug to help you feel cared for.
- Change your critical self-talk – reframe to a kinder approach.
- Start a self-compassion journal – write compassionately to yourself about stressful events in your life.
- Identify what you really want – rather than what you do not want.

Barratt (2017) has developed five pathways to self-compassion:

- Physical – through our bodies by practising relaxation, exercising, eating nutritious food, avoiding substances that harm the body, receiving soothing touch.
- Mental – or allowing our thoughts to develop through meditation, mantra, visualisation and kind self-talk.
- Emotional – by befriending our feelings through developing acceptance of our emotions, engaging in enjoyable activities, practising loving kindness mediation, practicing forgiveness.
- Relational – by connecting with others and practising generosity and expressing kindness and love to them and deepening friendships.
- Spiritual – by nourishing our spirit through spending time in nature or with loved ones and seeing the beauty in our lives and identifying our values.

Orellana-Rios et al (2018) carried out research into the extent to which palliative care interdisciplinary team members benefitted from a mindfulness and compassion orientated meditation programme. Although they could not prove a link between the course and increased compassionate practice, practitioners reported benefits in relation to self-care, emotional regulation skills, work related distress, mindfulness at work and interpersonal connection skills. In addition, course members addressed areas that they felt would help them sustain their compassionate behaviour at work. So, compassion and wellbeing links appeared to be significant.

The problem with promoting self-care of individuals is that it can be perceived that staff who are stressed do not have sufficient resiliency strategies and this can be a victim blaming approach. There needs to be a commitment from organisations to understand that stress is inevitable in most care situations, and always when resources are limited and there is understaffing and over working. Organisations have a duty of care, and they need to understand that practitioners are doing a remarkable job in very challenging circumstances and that their physical and psychological mental health can be at risk. Employers need to take responsibility for this and develop organisational strategies to help their employees. Debriefing opportunities need to be the norm when there are traumatic situations in practice so that they do not go home distressed and unable to discuss events with someone.

Maben et al (2021) analysed four studies carried out following the Francis inquiry (2013) which focused on practitioner wellbeing and the links to compassionate care in acute hospital settings, which were seen as particularly relevant during the pandemic. Attending Schwartz rounds to provide a safe space to discuss positive and difficult work experiences was useful. Hearing other practitioners' stories improved teamworking, reduced isolation and encouraged attendees to show empathy and compassion for colleagues, patients and themselves (Maben et al, 2018). Creating Learning Environments for Compassionate Care (CLECC) involved workplace learning and support through a study day focusing on team building and patient experiences (Bridges et al, 2018). This was followed by team manager learning sets, peer observations of practice, classroom learning and strategies for creating spaces in busy shifts. Intentional Rounding (Harris et al, 2019) promoted better handovers of information, improved communication between staff and taking more responsibility for patient care, and this inevitably created safer care for patients. Older People's Shoes (Arthur et al, 2017) used old-age simulation suits to help health care assistants to experience care delivery; this enhanced care and empathy and helped them to build better relationships with patients. All these initiatives enhanced support for practitioners, improved patient care and staff wellbeing and compassionate care delivery. Maben et al (2021) stress the importance of initiatives like this, especially when care is even more stressful, for example during the pandemic.

Duffy (2018) emphasises how hard it is working in health care and says that less than half of physicians would choose a career in medicine if they were able to start over again, and 73% would not recommend that their children become doctors. She also says that 54% of all doctors are suffering from burnout. More organisational strategies need to be in place to help medics and other health care practitioners focus on their wellbeing. These strategies need to help practitioners to deliver care with compassion and empathy, without creating too much burden on themselves.

Physical, inner and social self-care is important, involving exercise, spirituality and meditation. Being in control of our own inner world, and relationships with family and friends and colleagues, is crucial (Galiana et al, 2015). Fairhall (2020) says that in her community trust during the pandemic the message was that "it is OK not to be OK" and that mechanisms were put in place to increase the level of emotional support for all working in health care. This included helping colleagues to stay up to date with changing COVID protocols, and treating others with care and compassion and ensuring that team members were taking breaks when they were struggling. Smith (2020) stresses the importance of employers helping staff to care for their colleagues and ensure that they stay hydrated, take breaks and discuss their mental wellbeing openly. This includes feeling sure that their needs will be prioritised and supported. Radcliffe (2020b) also says how important it is to address the stigma that there can be when nurses say that they are finding it difficult to cope. He differentiates between resilience and endurance and says that organisations need to understand this difference. We feel that resilience can be taken as the norm, and this can be used as a stick to beat individuals with who are struggling to cope. This victim blaming approach increases the stress that we feel when it all gets too much.

Williams (2021) says that during the pandemic self-care has been even more important than usual because it has not been possible to see family and friends, or to do the things that maintain our emotional stability. He says it is important to self-care and not just carry on doing tasks. We need to focus explicitly on our emotional wellbeing, and monitor our levels of stress, engage in physical activity, give ourselves space, go outside at times, learn to say no and practice mindfulness.

Neff (2003) has identified areas of self-compassion and questions that we need to ask ourselves. She says that self-compassion is positively associated with positive mental health and reduced anxiety and depression as well as higher levels of life satisfaction. Self-kindness is associated with higher levels of wellbeing and in one study carried out by Friis et al (2016) it also lowered HbA1c levels, depression and mood difficulties in patients with diabetes. Positive psychological strategies also link to higher self-esteem. Neff (2013) in her TED talk highlights the importance of self-kindness, understanding our common humanity and being mindful and focusing on self-compassion www.youtube.com/watch?v=lvtZBUSpir4.

Brown (2017 https://www.youtube.com/watch?v=DVD8YRgA-ck) makes the distinction between guilt and shame. Regretting something about our behaviour creates feelings of guilt. However, feelings of shame happen when we internalise this into feeling that we are always lacking in this way which makes us self-critical. An example she gave is that a child might have made a mess, but they might not be messy. We can feel guilt for something that we have done and regret this and apologise. However, if we internalise natural mistakes that are part of being human, with self-loathing and shame this can lead to poor mental health and even addiction issues. Shame is about secrecy, silence and judgement, and the antidote to this is empathy. Shame cannot survive when we experience empathy because we know that we are not alone. We need to use our listening skills to ask about how people are feeling, and not just go straight to reassurance, which is an empathic failure. We can help people to gain perspective and not feel alone. We also need to challenge negative or hateful things, and ask about what pain underlies this. We should not be hateful to ourselves or others, it makes us feel vulnerable. If we feel vulnerable because we have experienced emotional trauma then we need courage to counteract this. Brown (2017) says that students are "turtles without shells" and when people put on those shells they are in protection mode and cannot learn. A hoodie is an invisibility cloak, like in Harry Potter. Shame is the fear of not being lovable, and it cannot survive being spoken, if we share our feelings, we are no longer alone. We need to experience joy and to do this we need to feel gratitude. Brown's (2017) highly insightful points are worth reflecting on so that we can act on these in our lives. When we are in protection mode none of us can learn anything, so we need to stop feeling defensive and vulnerable and make changes.

Radcliffe (2021c) says that new students need to avoid health care assistants who say that what they are being taught is unrealistic and impossible in the "real world". If we need to compromise then we need to understand what that means, and the inherent risks and benefits. We should not lower our standards without understanding this. Students should also avoid lecturers who do not smile, avoid eye contact and appear unapproachable. This lack of social skills and negativity should not be role modelled, enhanced positivity should be modelled instead. We need to avoid negativity and not buy into this. This is another important point to reflect on. Do we know people whose social skills we would not wish to emulate, and how should we address this if one of our colleagues acts in this way?

Many studies have demonstrated that higher stress levels lead to higher levels of burnout and lower quality of life in health care practitioners. Self-compassion appears to correlate with lower stress and burnout and higher quality of life in physicians, nurses and medical students (Dev et al, 2020). Woods (2021) reinforces the message that self-compassion reduces stress, anxiety, depression, compassion fatigue and burnout, and says that self-compassion is something that we can learn and be taught. If we are compassionate towards ourselves, we have higher levels of compassion satisfaction and personal accomplishment, and can feel more empowered in stressful situations. We can also feel more motivated and make more positive steps towards our own wellbeing if we feel valued and supported by our organisation. Therefore, organisational strategies need to be put in place to focus on self-compassion, wellbeing and mindfulness. A compassionate culture will help to increase employee wellbeing and reduce the impact of stress in health care practitioner roles.

Mathieu (2012) says that it is imperative to maintain self-care in the following areas:

- Physical self-care – eating, exercising, taking time off sick when necessary, accessing medical care, sleeping, being sexual, taking holidays and days off.
- Psychological self-care – self-reflection, reading which is unrelated to work, using our other intelligences – for example going to theatre, museums, concerts.

- Emotional self-care – making opportunities to laugh and cry and spend time with others whose company we enjoy and doing things we enjoy.
- Spiritual self-care – meditation, singing, praying, reflecting.
- Workplace or professional self-care – taking breaks when possible, accessing peer support, chatting to colleagues, accessing supervision.

Much of self-care depends on our level of self-knowledge and self-awareness. We need to:

- Remember why we do what we do.
- Know what unwinds us and then make sure we do this.
- Take a moment to think and recover at times.
- Focus on the good things that happen, the silver linings and write down good experiences.
- Sometimes we won't be totally successful but those experiences can teach us something, so look for what we have learnt.
- Sometimes "good enough" is just that. We can not always be perfect.
- Notice the kindness of others.
- Walk and move more and go outside at times.

All the points in the literature discussed here are important for our wellbeing, and focusing on self-compassion is crucial. These are summed up in the following questions to reflect on, and actions that could be helpful. It can be helpful to think about the areas where we might not be so focused, and how we can maintain physical, psychological and workplace self-care. The final points relate to our leadership role and how we can take a lead on creating and maintaining a positive workplace environment where self-care is prioritised.

Questions to ask yourself

How compassionate am I to myself?

Self-kindness:

- Am I forgiving of the parts of my personality I am less happy about?
- How kind am I to myself when I am suffering in some way?
- Am I caring towards myself when life is difficult?
- Am I forgiving of my inadequacies and flaws?

Self-judgement;

- Do I criticise myself when I see parts of me that I do not like?
- Am I sometimes too hard on myself?
- Am I cold-hearted, disapproving, judgemental, intolerant or impatient in relation to my own flaws?

Common Humanity:

- Do I recognise that my feelings of inadequacy are shared by others too?
- Do I see having flaws as part of being human?
- Can I see that others also feel the way that I am when I feel down?
- Do I see that experiencing difficulties is part of life?

Isolation:

- Do I feel I need to be alone when I have failed at something?
- Do my inadequacies make me feel more separate from the world?
- Do I think that most people are happier, or having an easier time, than I am when I feel down or I am struggling?

Mindfulness:

- Do I make an effort to keep my emotions in balance?
- Am I curious and open about why I am feeling down?
- Do I try to take a balanced view of situations and do I try to keep things in perspective when I fail at something?

Over identification:

- Do I get carried away with my feelings when something goes wrong?
- Do I obsess, fixate and blow things out of proportion when things go wrong?
- When I fail at something do I become consumed by feelings of inadequacy?

(adapted from Neff, 2003)

Shame versus guilt:

- Do I differentiate between my behaviour and who I am when things go wrong?
- Do I feel a sense of guilt when something I have done has not gone well?
- Does this turn into feeling of shame that is about who I am?Brené Brown (2017) Daring Classrooms https://www.youtube.com/watch?v=DVD8Y-RgA-ck (accessed 15/10/21)

Actions to ensure we are caring for ourselves

Physical self-care:

- Plan regular exercise when possible – dancing, swimming, walking, running, sports, singing and other fun physical activities.
- Think about whether you need to control the use of alcohol, smoking, caffeine and over the counter medications in your life.
- Eat healthily and get enough sleep.
- Seek medical help if necessary.
- Take holidays, mini breaks, day trips when possible.
- Take time to be sexually active.

Psychological and emotional and social self-care:

- Create opportunities for time with friends and family and having a satisfying social life.
- Try to relax when possible.

- Do not expect too much of ourselves.
- Find workable strategies that promote our wellbeing and practice these regularly.
- Maintain a balance between physical, intellectual, emotional and social activities in our lives.
- Increase realistic optimism approaches.
- Create opportunities to increase connections and empathy with others.
- Increase our emotional intelligence and self and relationship awareness and management.
- Try to feel in charge of our own destiny and have an internal locus of control.
- Focus on resilience and self-efficacy as much as possible.
- Focus on wellbeing, rather than illness and stress.
- Increase feelings of gratitude for what we have.
- Maintain our sense of humour and maximise opportunities for this.
- Revisit favourite books and films.

Workplace and professional self-care:

- Increase our opportunities to feel worthwhile and valued at work.
- Try to encourage good team dynamics at work and find time to chat with colleagues.
- Take regular time off.
- Ask for employer support if needed.
- Tell others when we are feeling under pressure.
- Be kind to ourselves and others when they are showing signs of stress.
- Have a balance between our work and home lives.
- Identify what our organisation provides in relation to professional development, peer support and stress reduction, and access these as appropriate.

Actions to encourage healthy workplaces

- Prioritise wellbeing of employees.
- Provide supervision opportunities and prioritise time for this.
- Encourage healthy ways to resolve conflicts.
- Encourage staff have opportunities to learn and develop.
- Ensure that those in our care are respected and that there is sufficient respect from managers and colleagues.
- Encourage team support, positive attitudes and high morale.
- Try to ensure that strategies encourage a stable workforce with reasonable turnover levels, high attendance and good time keeping.
- Focus on wellbeing, self-care and access to counselling if necessary.
- Encourage teamworking and connections between colleagues.
- Look for ways to build diversity and job enrichment into work.
- Help staff to understand why decisions are made, and include them in decision making when possible.
- Express concern for staff wellbeing and not merely focus on the work they are doing.
- Try to remain positive, give positive and constructive feedback and praise staff and acknowledge effort and results when possible.

We need to take action when we see colleagues communicating in a way that is not acceptable to us. If we do not do this, others might feel that this is acceptable, and emulate this communication. So, we need to use our assertiveness skills to challenge unacceptable communication, whether this is with patients, loved ones, ourselves or other members of our team. We need to focus on not letting occasional feelings of guilt about something that could have been done better to become feelings of shame which means that we become too critical of ourselves. It is important to think about caring for ourselves and asking whether we are merely enduring the stresses in our lives, rather than developing resilience strategies. This chapter is about identifying positive ways forward, and maximising our resilience, and which is discussed next.

What strategies could I use to manage my stress and increase my resilience to maximise my ability to be compassionate?

This chapter has focused a great deal on the effect of the pandemic. Palmer (2021) discusses long COVID and the impact that this has had on mental health. Anxiety, depression and even confusion and dementia allied symptoms can arise from COVID symptoms lasting over 12 weeks. This could be linked with a cytokine storm caused by the immune response to the infection which affects the blood brain barrier. Palmer (2021) says that psychological, self-help, coping and self-care strategies, alongside appropriate medication can be helpful.

Pascoe and Edvardsson (2013) discuss the importance of benefit finding. Positively orientated coping strategies influence psychological and physical health outcomes. For example, finding some benefits in relation to cancer diagnosis and other illnesses can help survivors to deal with the stresses of negative health. Adverse health issues, such as COVID-19, can bring about positive behaviour change and better relationships with family members which can mitigate against the negative experiences and bring about a more positive quality of life. As health care practitioners we can help individuals to think about possible positive aspects of recent illness and adversity where appropriate. This could apply to ourselves and our friends and colleagues too.

Maxted (2021) highlights different resilience strategies for helping us to address stress in our lives. When we are chronically stressed our fight-or-flight reactions stay turned on with a surge of hormones such as adrenaline and cortisol and this takes its toll on us. These constantly raised hormone levels make us feel jittery and tired, and we can become angry and irritable. We can also misinterpret situations and our sense of reality can become skewed. Suggested strategies are:

- Running and physical activity – to release endorphins which calm us.
- More sleep – which can help us cope better and process information more helpfully.
- Deep breathing – to stimulate the vagus nerve which calms us.
- Interacting with a pet – this boosts feel-good oxytocin levels and reduces stress related cortisol levels.
- Meditation – also reduces cortisol levels.
- Knitting – can lower our heart rate.
- Listening to music or listening to podcasts or audiobooks – helps us relax.
- Writing by hand – helps us to organise our thoughts and feel more in control.
- Cold water swimming – stimulates our parasympathetic nervous system which calms us.

Kearney et al (2009) stress the importance of:

- **Work engagement** which is characterised by energy, involvement, efficiency, competence, pleasure and a perception of control.
- **Compassion satisfaction** – feeling that you have done the best you could for the patient in your care which reduces the potential for vicarious trauma and compassion fatigue due to this.
- **Post-traumatic growth and Vicarious Post-traumatic Growth** which is characterised by positive changes in interpersonal relationships, a sense of self and a focus on life rather than death. Vicarious post-traumatic growth relates to clinician growth which results in recognising the positive sequelae of other's experiences of trauma. So, for example, this can result in an increased meaning and peacefulness which enriches the lives of all involved.
- **Exquisite empathy** which is focusing on the present, within clear boundaries, and empathetic engagement which is of reciprocal benefit to patients and caregivers.
- **Meaning-centred team interventions** which focus on spirituality and finding meaning in life.
- **Self-awareness** which helps us to access a broader range of choices than the often restricted range we tend to utilise when we are highly stressed. This can be helped by mindfulness meditation and reflective writing.
- **Self-awareness to enhance self-care** which allows care givers to be aware of the patient in their care as well as their own needs, so they do not lose perspective and empathy and do not experience such high levels of stress.

It is useful to focus on our coping strategies and how helpful these are:

Questions to ask yourself

Your coping strategies

To what extent do you:

- deal well with changing circumstances
- believe that coping with stress makes you stronger
- stay focused under pressure
- see yourself as a strong personality
- ask advice when you need to
- search for resources when you are unsure about what to do
- Use alcohol, medication, smoking or eating in the belief they will make you feel better (negative coping strategies).
- Use your spiritual beliefs to make you feel better
- use your sense of humour to help situations
- use work and other substitute activities to distract yourself
- access emotional support from friends and relatives.

Based on Carver et al (1989) *Coping Behaviour Questionnaire*

Many people have more Type A personality traits; it might be helpful if we tried to adopt more Type B behaviour patterns, rather than Type A, because these patterns can moderate the influences between stressors and strain. Type A individuals are more likely to display high levels of concentration, ambition, competitiveness, aggression and impatience. Whereas Type B individuals demonstrate an absence of these characteristics. Friedman and Rosenman in their seminal text (Rosenman et al, 1964) identified Type A characteristics as being associated with more signs of coronary heart disease, and Type B characteristics have therefore been perceived as a moderating influence in relation to how we cope with stressors.

So, Type A individuals tend to be-competitive, hardworking, impatient with themselves and others, inflexible in their approach, generally aggressive achievers who set themselves unrealistic deadlines and push themselves hard. Often described as workaholics, they like deadlines and pressure. They can also be intolerant of weakness in themselves and others, like to be in control and hate having to wait or queue. Any provocation can result in angry and hostile outbursts, and they can try to multitask often inappropriately (Hartley, 1995, Cooper et al, 2001). Their personal causes of stress can include being obsessional, over identification with their jobs, blaming themselves, low risk taking and low sensation seeking. Sexual stereotyping can also be unhelpful with men being perceived as being more likely to get angry and aggressive (fight responses) and women being perceived as more likely to go off sick or start to cry (flight responses). Therefore, women becoming more aggressive and having angry outbursts, or men becoming depressed and withdrawn, can be perceived very negatively which can add to the stress on individuals who are acting out of line with gender stereotypical perceptions.

Adopting more Type B characteristics include:

- Using humour and laughter
- Widening our horizons beyond our immediate "to do" lists
- Developing a better understanding of others
- Creating a better balance in life
- Delegating more where we can
- Having more relaxed time schedules where possible
- Being more patient with ourselves and others
- Being more optimistic
- Feeling more in control
- Feeling valued
- Achieving our life objectives
- Achieving more than we thought possible
- Valuing ourselves
- Accessing more social and emotional support
- Thinking about our level of boredom
- Having sufficient time for ourselves and what we need to achieve.

People who feel that the locus of control (Rotter, 1966) is with them, and that they are the masters of their own destiny, still feel stressed and anxious like other people do, but they respond to this differently. Bradberry (2015) says that "since the empowered believe that they have control over the outcomes in their lives, their anxiety fuels passion instead of pity, drive in lieu of despair, and tenacity over trepidation". So, they redouble their efforts and follow the maxim, "when the going gets tough, the tough get going". People who perform best in life tend to manage their emotions better at times of stress. We are conditioned to not take any action until we feel some sort of anxiety, or stress, and that heightens our performance. So, we are at our best when we are experiencing moderate levels of anxiety. If we generally feel empowered and able to take control of our lives we anticipate change, and plan for it. We also revisit situations that have not gone as well as we would have hoped, and think about what we could have done differently, and focus on thinking about strategies, and not our feelings about how we could have done better. We also focus on the positive and do not let ourselves become weighed down by negative thinking. All these strategies help us to remain in control of our destiny, and feel more able to cope with stress, and treat this anxiety as a way to act at the peak of our performance. At times our stress can tip into distress and we need to know how to cope with this too. Pascoe (2014) talks about the importance of breaking down what is making us feel distressed into more manageable tasks. Because these tasks are more achievable this can help us to feel more in control again, in addition to focusing on our strengths, rather than our perceived deficits. In essence we need to treat distress seriously and work out ways to manage this in ways that are helpful to us on a personal level.

Another factor that can be protective in relation to stress is what Kobasa (1979) refers to as the "hardy personality" where there is a high degree of *commitment* to solving problems, as well as a strong internal locus of *control* (Rotter, 1954). There is also a degree of self-efficacy to see change as a *challenge* not a threat (Bandura, 1977 cited in Maes et al, 1987) and a sense of *coherence* (Antonovsky, 1979 cited in Maes et al, 1987). So, we need to adopt that sense of control and self-efficacy that allows us to perceive change as a challenge. This relates strongly to resilience, which is key to developing helpful coping strategies to deal with stressors in our lives.

Using our different intelligences (Furnham, 2008) can be helpful in reducing our stress. We know that using our intellectual intelligence (IQ) as well as our technical/ operational (TQ), motivational (MQ), experience (XQ), people (PQ), learning (LQ) and cultural (CQ) intelligences can make us more effective, and this can have a positive impact on our stress levels. However, our greatest tool is perhaps our emotional intelligence (EI) which focuses on our self and relationship awareness and our self and relationship management, which will be discussed in greater detail in Chapter 5.

Other strategies that can be helpful in dealing with stressful periods in our lives can be to adopt a different mindset in relation to the aspects of our lives that are causing us stress. A very relevant motto in life is:

> God grant me the serenity to accept the things that I cannot change, the courage to change the things I can and the wisdom to know the difference.
>
> (Reinhold Niebuhr).

Yet, we spend so much time worrying about things that we cannot change, and being less effective than we might be about what we can influence, which is a waste of time, energy and emotion. If we just focused our minds on fighting battles that we can win, we would feel much more in control and empowered. So, it is crucial that we can tell the difference between those aspects of our life that we can change, and those that we cannot.

Other helpful strategies centre around achieving a total health balance, as discussed earlier. For example, making sure that our physical health is as good as it could be by taking regular exercise, trying to make sure that we get as much sleep as we need, using meditation and relaxation techniques as appropriate, and trying to focus on eating as healthily as we can. Our emotional, social and intellectual health are also key to maximising our health potential, and managing our stress levels. Sometimes we are very busy, but under stimulated either intellectually or socially, which does not allow us to have the balance in life that we all need. So those of us who focus more exclusively on our work and exercise regimes can become very socially isolated, less cerebrally stimulated and less emotionally involved than is ideal for our total health. Taking the time to think about issues that are bigger than ourselves, or to do something that engages our brain, whether it is a crossword, Sudoku or other puzzle, or other activity that engages our brain, can be really helpful and help us to concentrate on something other than our day to day worries. In addition, spending time with others in a shared interest, sharing views and having a healthy debate, or giving ourselves the opportunity to have a laugh and relax with people whose company we enjoy can also help us to relax. We need to take time to enjoy music, art, theatre, or whatever interests we enjoy, and make emotional connections with others and have loving and sexual relationships with those who are most important to us.

We need to understand what stress is, and how it can influence how we feel. We need to identify our major causes of stress, anticipate stressful periods and plan for them, and practice a variety of stress management techniques developing a repertoire which works for us. Having an awareness of when our stress levels are reaching unmanageable levels is key to being able to adopt helpful strategies at times of greater stress.

We need to stop worrying about what might not happen, and enjoy each moment for what it is, and be able to learn from past mistakes. Sometimes we need to make a place of peace in our busy environments so that we can truly relax. That could be spending time in the garden, going for a walk, sitting on the balcony of your flat or just taking a long leisurely bath or shower without interruption. There are times when we might need to release pent up frustration by shouting, singing, doing physical exercise or just taking the time to have a laugh or a cry if we need to. We need to delegate as much as possible and try to master time and reward ourselves when we have done particularly well. We need to cope more successfully with waiting and have activities with us that could help us use empty time more productively for enjoyment or managing other parts of our lives. So, when we are waiting in a queue, we could spend the time making a shopping list, sorting out our "to do" lists, read or just consciously "people watch" or chat to others in the queue. We might not feel so much that our time has been wasted and we start to feel more in control and more positive as a result.

Other strategies could be discussing our stress with others, or writing down our thoughts or thinking about worst case scenarios and imagining that we have lived through this experience. We could even imagine that it has all happened in the past, or think about exaggerating the situation even further in our minds, or take active steps to address the problem and imagine that these steps have been successful. All these ways of thinking through the situation can help to put it into perspective, so that we can perhaps minimise its impact, or maximise our ability to deal with it, or just find a way to forget about it for a while. Sometimes thinking through the reasons why a situation is less worrying than we think, can help us to keep everything in proportion. Thinking the situation through can take some time though, and this can involve time that we do not have. So, one idea could be postponing our worry until a certain time of the day, or only once per hour, which can be a way for us to delay the worry but still keep in control, knowing that we will need to think about it. Sometimes also writing on a piece of paper why the situation is manageable can be a way of keeping our stress under control. If we have the piece of paper about our person, simply having it there can be a source of comfort, even if we do not have the opportunity to actually read it. We can always read it later when we have the time to do so, but we might not need to do this if our stress has been managed effectively earlier.

If absolutely necessary, and we are really worried about our stress levels, then the only strategy that is open to us could be to put our life on hold, go to bed and sleep for a couple of days. Then when we do start to return to life we can start by reading light and funny articles and then books or watch similar television programmes or films. When we do return to work we need to make greater efforts to relax in the evenings and have a better work life balance. However, these strategies would only be required in worst case scenarios when stress symptoms have become completely unmanageable. Being aware of causes and symptoms of stress, and taking steps to avoid or alleviate stress, are much more helpful and productive strategies. Being proactive in managing our stress is much healthier and more empowering and this enables us to maintain control of our lives.

Reflective practice can be used to reflect on a traumatic critical incident so that the enormity of what has just happened, and the trauma of witnessing it, can be diffused by identifying how the incident has made us feel and what impact this has had on us. If reflection is carried out in a facilitated reflective group setting in the work environment then emotions that are discussed at the session can be "held" by others there, which can make it easier to cope with feelings and to think about them (Winnicott, 1945). It is important that formal supervision, reflection, mentorship and peer support are part of everyday practice so that the emotional labour of nursing can be managed in a proactive manner. Difficult emotions can be acknowledged, and the impact of emotional work can be recognised and normalised and this can play a big part in reducing burnout and emotional exhaustion. The RCN report (2013) on wellbeing and stress advocates this, as well as support for staff with mental health issues. The report (RCN, 2013) also highlights the risks of people being present at work when they are not well enough to be. This presenteeism creates risks to the individual and patients or clients and creates health and safety issues and risks to productivity. However, it also puts a burden on colleagues through needing to support them, as well as in providing cover for the parts of their role that they are unable to perform. So, I have put together the following questions to ask yourself which might help you to focus on aspects of how you respond to stress, and increasing your self help strategies.

Questions to ask yourself

- Do you sometimes let life's challenges overwhelm you? Could you find ways to recognise issues but think that things will work out in the end and work on finding ways to start to address inevitable challenges at work and home?

- Do you accept who you are, with your strengths and limitations, and grasp opportunities for personal growth and positive relationships with others? If not, what could you do to make this happen to a greater extent at work and in your personal life?

- Do you feel able to cope with life's problems, and do you feel satisfied with your life? It is rare that we always feel that this is the case so try to think about when you feel challenged in these areas, and what you could do to increase your problem solving and feelings of satisfaction with life.

- Which positive coping strategies do you find most effective? Could you start to increase the repertoire of strategies that you could use?

- How empowered do you feel? Are you in control of your day to day life and your work situation? Could you think of ways in which you could feel more in control?
- Can you recognise signs of having a hardy personality? Are you committed to problem solving, do you have an internal locus of control and do you see change as a challenge? Do you generally feel as if there is a sense of coherence in what happens in your life? If any of these answers are no, can you think of any ways that you could increase your "hardiness", and encourage others to do the same?
- Do you have sufficient levels of stress to stimulate you, or are you over stimulated? What level of stimulation would you think is ideal for you, and what changes would you need to make in order to maintain that level of simulation?
- How is your physical, emotional, social and intellectual health? Are there any areas where you need to become healthier, and do you have sufficient balance in your life between these areas of health?
- Are you more of a Type A personality, and if so, how could you become more Type B in your outlook? Could you be more optimistic and introduce more fun and laughter into your life?
- Are you sometimes guilty of stereotyping people by gender? Could you be more supportive of people who exhibit signs of stress which are more suited to the opposite gender? If so, what could you do differently?
- Do you sometimes fight battles that you can not win? Could you take steps to focus primarily on situations which you can influence?
- Could you do more to anticipate or recognise stress in its early stages? If so, how could you do this?
- Could you make your anxieties more manageable? Could you deal with waiting more effectively? Think about strategies that could help you here.
- Could you do more to reduce the amount of change in your life at times? What strategies could you use to identify times when the amount of change becomes too high and causes undue stress?
- Could you take a lead in ensuring that there are sufficient opportunities in your workplace for reflection, supervision, mentorship and peer support? Are there any opportunities to acknowledge difficult emotions? How could you enhance the support available for yourself and colleagues within your work area?

I have carried an extensive search of the literature to try to collate ideas around areas of stress, resilience strategies and the benefits of these (seeTable 4.7 below).

Hopefully the table above will help you to see the evidence base behind resilience strategies you might want to adopt within your life. Some of these strategies are actions you can take yourself and encourage your colleagues to do as well. Others are actions you can use as a team, or they could be adopted across your organisation, so you could perhaps consider how great your sphere of influence could be and take a lead in making changes where possible. The next section focuses on strategies for ourselves as individuals and leaders and organisational strategies to enhance resilience in our home and work lives and across our practice areas.

Table 4.7 Stress management and resilience strategies

Stress / resilience issue	Resilience strategy	Benefits	Literature source
Not having the opportunity to debrief after traumatic situations	Schwartz rounds to share trauma and sadness, and time out of practice to reflect. Using emotional touchpoints to discuss negative emotions at work. Debriefing, staff support and personal reflection (Turner et al, 2011)	MDT increased shared knowledge and better collaborative relationships. Emotional touchpoint discussions help to recognise and discuss feelings, receive feedback and see more positive aspects of care. This approach also helps to develop relationships, recognise and reinforce good practice and helps people to shape future services (Brodie, 2021)	Hargreaves (2015) Maben and Bridges (2020) and Bridges et al (2020) Brodie (2021) Turner et al (2011)
Not having the opportunity to rest and reenergise	Six types of rest: • Mental rest • Sensory rest • Creative rest • Emotional rest • Social rest • Spiritual rest	• Break from thinking • Break from stimulation • Hobbies to inspire • Processing of emotions • Spending time with those who support and bring out the best in us • Activities which give us a sense of purpose • Less medical errors and enhanced patient care	Dalton-Smith (2021) Maben and Bridges (2020)
Thinking negatively and assuming the worst	• See compassion as a priority • Be respectful, inclusive and non judgemental • Encourage self-care and self-awareness • Appreciative feedback	Increased positivity and a focus on self-care and compassion. Appreciative inquiry focuses on what motivates us and what we care about because that increases shared knowledge and team motivation (Sharp and Dewar (2017)	Bregman (2020) Sharp and Dewar (2017) Griffiths (2022)
Not feeling as if you belong in your work environment, and feeling excluded leads to team and self sabotage	Social belonging is a fundamental human need, so focusing on feeling part of the team is essential. Understanding why people feel excluded and empowering team leaders to restructure team experience to be more inclusive and enjoyable	Belonging leads to increased job performance (56% increase) and lower staff turnover (50% reduction) and fewer sick days (75% reduction). In a 10,000 person company this would equate to a £40 million saving. A focus on collegiate relationship and getting to know colleagues is important. A focus on teamworking increases engagement and practitioner wellbeing (Montgomery et al, 2015 and Malliarou et al, 2008)	Carr et al (2019) Montgomery et al (2015) Malliarou et al (2008) Maben and Bridges (2020) Woodford et al (2020) Hofmeyer et al (2020b)
Too much emphasis on acquiring knowledge and skills, and on outcomes, rather than on caring with compassion	More emphasis on the patient, and less on checklists. More inclusion of the nature of compassion in nursing curricula.	A focus on compassion speeds up the recovery of older people's recovery and the quality of their care, and creates a deeper understanding of their needs. This also can result in reduced practitioner stress.	Nathoo et al (2016) de Zulueta (2013)

(Continued)

Table 4.7 (Continued) Stress management and resilience strategies

Stress / resilience issue	Resilience strategy	Benefits	Literature source
A lack of focus on practitioner wellbeing and stress reduction strategies	Mindfulness, meditation, effective communication, stress reduction strategies. Personal, family and professional support and self-care strategies. Access to restorative supervision. Resilience training programmes to focus on shared experiences of trauma and connecting with colleagues	Sustained engagement and resilience and more effective coping strategies and greater emotional intelligence. Self-care strategies and support networks help you to cope with the demands of your role. Focusing on coping mechanisms, cognitive flexibility, the importance of a supportive network, exercising and having a sense of humour enhances a more balanced lifestyle and greater coping mechanisms	Penberthy et al (2018) Woodford et al (2020) Mealer et al (2014) Hylton Rushton et al (2009) Carrieri et al (2020)
Resilience being seen as an individual responsibility, not a collective one	Resilience seen as a collective and organisational responsibility, with team and management support. Enhanced occupational health services and support.	Organisational responsibility to support staff enables individuals not to feel alone, and blamed if they are not coping, especially through the pandemic. Assessment, treatment and counselling being available which help practitioners to cope with challenges of their role. A focus on reducing emotional exhaustion through education on resilience strategies and creating healthy and harmonious environments.	Maben and Bridges (2020) Mitchell (2021) Hofmeyer et al (2020b) Marine et al (2006) Zhang et al (2021)
Lack of awareness of own psychological needs	Greater self-awareness about own needs and ability to ask for support. Peer support and looking after each other.	Greater understanding of shared needs for support in times of high challenge, including during the pandemic	Maben and Bridges (2020)
Lack of compassionate leadership	Compassionate, inclusive and collective leadership – attending, understanding, empathising and helping. Primary interventions – reducing time pressures and increasing control over work. Secondary interventions – supporting those under stress e.g. resilience training, mindfulness etc. Tertiary interventions – remedial support, counselling etc (West al 2020)	Leaders listening with fascination and taking thoughtful and intelligent action to help health care practitioners which is compassionate leadership. Inclusive leadership promotes equality and positive diversity. Collective leadership shares leadership to where expertise, capability and motivation sits in the organisation. Command and control management demoralises and causes suffering.	West, Bailey and Williams (2020) de Zulueta(2013) Woodford et al (2020) Moore (2020) West et al (2020) Marine et al (2006)

A lack of control over own life and being able to act within own values. Also feeling a sense of belonging and effective at work and deliver valued outcomes	Feeling **autonomous**, a sense of **belonging** and **contribution** (ABC framework of nurses' and midwives core needs, West, Bailey and Williams, 2020). Focus on values based actions and what matters most to you and increase opportunities to express your values in actions, notice when actions move away from your values and focus on value consistent actions.	Increases wellbeing and motivation at work where people can flourish and thrive. Focus on values-based actions in a team environment increases staff support and helps staff to self-refer to psychological therapy as appropriate. Personal and professional invigoration and enhanced resilience and more proactive approaches to dealing with stressful events resulted from a focus on this approach	West, Bailey and Williams (2020) Jennings et al (2017)
Not focusing on what we can influence and control but using energy to focus on issues outside our control.	Focusing on concerns we have, but can not influence, can take valuable energy. We then feel victimised and focus on blame, and our circle of influence decreases and we are seen as negative and critical.	Proactive people focus on what they can do whereas reactive people focus on things outside their control. Focusing on what we can influence allows us to make effective changes. We are then perceived as effective people and this increases our power and influence. Self-efficacy helps us with our feelings, thoughts and actions and helps us to cope with more challenging tasks and traumatic patient situations, set higher goals, achieve better outcomes and have better coping strategies.	Covey (1989) Zhang et al (2021)
Stress especially during COVID-19 causing anxiety, loss of control and sense of professional worth with a negative impact on wellbeing and reduced capacity to cope with health visiting role	Emotional wellbeing at work programme to support health visitors based on person-centred and group processes and reflective, restorative and strengths based approaches. Restorative supervision and group supervision able to be accessed by staff Reduced job demands and increased job resources and increased meaning in the work carried out (Jourdain and Chenevert, 2010)	Emotional wellbeing at work programme resulted in improved staff wellbeing, reduced stress and anxiety, improved sense of control and self-worth, greater capacity to cope with job demands and higher quality care and greater job satisfaction, staff retention and better outcomes for clients, children and families. Restorative supervision increases resilience in relation to the negative impacts of work, reduces burnout, enhances physical and mental health, empathy and compassion and increases the quality of patient care. Group clinical supervision can increase resilience through increasing confidence, regulating emotions, enhanced coping strategies, managing expectations and developing self-awareness as individuals and as a team.	Baldwin et al (2020a and b) Baldwin and Kelly (2020) Jourdain and Chenevert (2010) Francis and Bulman (2019) Capito et al (2022) Griffiths (2022)

(Continued)

Table 4.7 (Continued) Stress management and resilience strategies

Stress / resilience issue	Resilience strategy	Benefits	Literature source
Use self-help strategies	Acknowledge sadness, understand emotions, disrupt negative thoughts, resolve inner conflict, learn to say no, be kind and pretend to feel more positive until you do. Self-awareness and self-compassion help us to develop greater resilience.	All these strategies are powerful self-help strategies that help us feel more in control and help us to be more positive and resilient. Resilience, self-efficacy and self-regulation mediates the relationship between job demands, exhaustion and task performance and subsequent risk of burnout. Mindfulness, emotional self-regulation, retaining core values and boundaries, being receptive to change, having compassion for others and shared learning increases our resilience.	Slater (2015) Ceschi et al (2017) Stephen and Pettit (2015) Jennings et al (2017)
Taking on too much and "hurry sickness"	Action orientated strategies – question why something is necessary, be more assertive about what you can take on, stop multitasking and spreading yourself too thinly, prioritise and time manage to focus on effectiveness rather than activities. Acceptance orientated strategies – accept that you have no power to change some situations, slow down, take breaks and seek support. Emotion orientated strategies – stay positive, improve your self-regulation and use EI	Acknowledging your limits, and what is and is not possible for you to manage, enables us to say no sometimes and switch off and relax. If we do not do this we become less able to stop and think and see the bigger picture and are likely to make more mistakes. Our personal relationships can be affected too, and we can develop severe health problems due to high stress levels	Friedman and Rosenman (1964) and Burke and Deszca (1982) Open University (2021)
Not understanding the nature or importance of resilience	Greater awareness of the four components of resilience – confidence, purposefulness, adaptability and social support.	Carrying out an assessment of our own resilience, and what helps and hinders our resilience, could increase our awareness and help us develop strategies to enhance our resilience www.robertsoncooper.com/iresilience/	Robertson Cooper (accessed 2022)

Strategies raised in Chapter 3 focusing on stress management

COVID related

- More available PPE and equipment
- Redeploying staff to less stressful areas
- Taking turns in high pressure roles and reducing repetitive exposure
- Shift patterns that allow staff to rest between shifts
- More available mental health support
- Strategies to help with insomnia and stress management
- Encourage use of humour
- Self-esteem boosting
- Debriefing after stressful shifts
- Preparing and supporting students
- Specialist support when suffering from long COVID.

Other strategies

- Reducing amount of change where possible
- Symptoms of stress physically, emotionally, behaviourally, cognitively
- Balance of life – physical, emotional, social, intellectual
- Supervision and positive reappraisal
- Access to CPD
- Conflict de-escalation and anti bullying strategies
- Minimisation of errors
- Peer and psychological support
- Management awareness of burnout
- Training in self-care and compassion
- Staff wellbeing and positive impact of role and feeling valued
- Focus on stress management, resilience, positivity, self-care, mindfulness, reflective practice, problem solving, communication, end of life care and unexpected death, relaxation
- Focusing on vicarious trauma and coping with grief and loss
- Control over work environment, annual leave and shifts where possible
- Management of working hours
- Culture of support and respect
- Restorative supervision
- Courageous conversations to challenge dysfunctional organisational systems and processes
- Leadership development programmes
- More social contact with colleagues
- Collaborative approach with MDT and a focus on teamworking
- Emotional distancing when at home
- More appreciation from management
- Support in stressful patient situation care
- Not encouraging suppression of negative emotions
- Reducing role ambiguity and role conflict
- More focus on recovery activities and low effort activities
- Recognising burnout and emotional exhaustion
- Running and physical activity
- More sleep

- Deep breathing, meditation and mindfulness
- Interacting with a pet
- Knitting and crafts
- Listening to music or listening to podcasts or audiobooks
- Writing by hand
- Cold water swimming.

RECOMMENDATIONS FOR LEADERSHIP AS INDIVIDUAL PRACTITIONERS, LEADERS AND ORGANISATIONS

The NMC's survey on nurses leaving the profession (2020) found that 18% had left because of toxic workplaces where there were blame cultures, bullying and unsupportive management. As Benison (2021, p 421)) says "staff as well as patients need better care". The HSCC report (2021) on the pandemic's impact on staff burnout highlights understaffing as a significant factor. Benison (2021) says that staff were overstretched and under supported even before the pandemic and have been working with extraordinary commitment in circumstances that have been even more challenging. A blame culture, and victim blaming, is unhelpful and more investment is certainly needed to ensure that nurses have sufficient resources to provide the care that they want, and need, to give.

Radcliffe (2021b) discusses the Francis report's (Francis, 2013) "guerrilla nursing" where nurses focus on merely getting through the shift, rather than on helping patients to get well. Burnout, a lack of support and supervision, reduced staffing and a lack of clinical leadership increases the chances of unsafe care and a lack of ability to maintain safe standards, and certainly not best practice. Radcliffe (2021b) says that:

> to not speak about (poor practice) is to normalise it and that is not an option…… poor nursing care may be a consequence of bad politics, weak leadership, COVID-19 and austerity, but it is the responsibility of nursing and nurses. Is that necessarily fair? Maybe not, is it true, yes?
>
> (Radcliffe, 2021b, p 15)

So, burnout might seem to be inevitable during the pandemic, but if the nursing profession does not seize its leadership role to address its manifestations in their practice areas, then nobody else will. Therefore, the following section highlights the role that nurses can play in addressing stress and burnout, and increasing resilience, before going on to discuss wellbeing and the role of positivity in Chapter 5.

Focusing on resilience and compassionate care as individual practitioners and leaders

Robson (2018) highlights the importance of looking out for each other and recognising when things are getting too much. He writes about a time when he was a junior doctor and he made clear plans to commit suicide and how colleagues knocked on his door and interrupted his plans. He said that this was probably just good luck that they did this. However, another colleague of his from that time responded to his blog and said that they were aware and had staged an intervention. However, in those days they were unable to help more and were unskilled and untrained and unable to discuss how he might have been feeling. Robson (2018) encourages people to speak out and seek help and treatment and not collude with the code of silence around mental health.

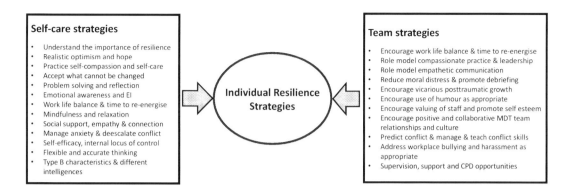

Figure 4.1 Individual and team resilience strategies

Compson (2015) cites the CARE heuristic of Compassion, Awareness, Resilient Responding and Empowerment which helps us to develop strategies to help treat or protect against burnout. So, we need to be compassionate towards ourselves and others, and be aware of the risk of burnout and strategies to mediate against this. Also increasing our resilience and feelings of empowerment and having an internal locus of control and self-efficacy.is important.

Thompson and Thompson (2008) discuss the Control Influence Accept model where we use our skills and abilities to **control** the aspects of situations that we can control, and **influence** the elements that we cannot control where we can make a difference. Finally, we need to **accept** situations that we cannot control or influence, and adapt as necessary. If we use the influence that we do have then we can feel less overwhelmed by situations. It is exhausting to keep fighting things that we cannot change and it can be healthier to adapt to situations and re-evaluate our goals, priorities and strategies. An example has been the pandemic which has caused major disruptions to our lives, on top of the worries, health issues and distress that is discussed so much in Chapter 3. We have not been able to control or influence the disruptions, and we have lost major celebrations and holidays and time with family and friends. However, we have changed how we have been doing things and how we have kept our connections with others and managed to find some new ways to enjoy life. We need to think about the self-care strategies that we could use in everyday life and how we can take a lead in encouraging these within our teams (Figure 4.1)

Focusing on resilience and compassionate care as organisations

Employers need to focus on minimising stress and maximising resilience in their employees. Sallon et al 2017 studied 97 nurses, technicians, dieticians, administrators and doctors in Israel. They participated in an eight-month programme of weekly sessions and workshops. These focused on cognitive practices such as mindfulness, meditation and relaxation. Somatic body awareness strategies focused on balance, posture and the muscular skeletal system to help alleviate symptoms caused by long hours of sitting, standing and activity. Energising strategies were also used to help release muscle tension, express emotions and focus on connectiveness, joy and laughter and medium impact cardiovascular exercises. Participants were encouraged to be open, expressive and empathetic and actively listen to each other. Hands on strategies such as acupressure and palm massage were also part of the programme. As a result, participants reported less upper respiratory infections and family doctor visits. They also were more energetic, able to relax and cope with stress at work and at home, and they also felt they had an improved mental state and felt happier and more at peace.

Graham and van Witteloostuijn (2010) highlight the importance of high quality relationships between employers and their managers, along with frequent interactions, in nurturing employee wellbeing and preventing emotional exhaustion. I have adapted the organisational strategies in relation to stress in Chapter 3 to include those in relation to resilience. These cultural and educational strategies are fairly similar because reducing stress and increasing resilience are so closely related (Figure 4.2). Skovholt and Trotter-Mathison (2016) pp. xx–xxi say that it is imperative that we maintain some kind of professional and personal vitality and address our personal and professional stressors. This involves:

- Professional vitality – finding work meaningful, using self-care strategies, maintaining some level of control and avoiding excessive demands from others.
- Personal vitality – being loved by those we are intimate with, having fun, being financially secure, doing things we enjoy, having sufficient restorative sleep, eating healthily.
- Professional stress – having high but not unreachable or unrealistic standards, keeping work conflict low, positive relationships with colleagues and supervisors, experiencing learning opportunities, being generous within reasonable boundaries.
- Personal stress – being cared for as well as caring for others, satisfying family relationships and relationships with others, coping with losses in life, adhering to our own personal values and beliefs, taking time for reflection.

This management of personal and professional stressors and maintaining personal and professional vitality is essential to our resilience. It is also important to acknowledge that we need to nurture our different selves Skovholt and Trotter Mathison (2016) pp161–75 says that we need to nurture the following:

- Our emotional selves
- Our financial selves
- Our humorous selves
- Our loving selves
- Our nutritious selves
- Our physical selves
- Our playful selves
- Our priority setting selves

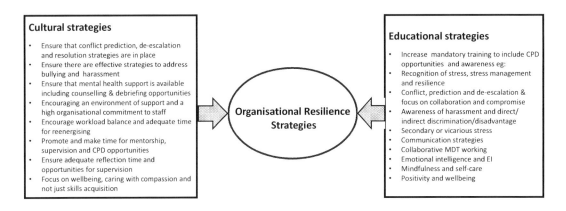

Figure 4.2 Organisational resilience strategies

- Our recreational selves
- Our relaxation/stress reduction selves.

Finally, generosity of ourselves sustains us and this is put very clearly in the following poem:

> Do all the good you can
> By all the means you can
> In all the ways you can
> In all the places you can
> At all the times you can
> To all the people you can
> As long as ever you can.
>
> (Although attributed to John Wesley, the author is unknown
> (according to John Wesley expert R. Thompson, Director
> Wesley Centre, personal communication July 21, 2015,
> cited in Skovholt and Trotter-Mathison, 2016, p136)

This chapter has built on Chapter 3 and the discussion of stress and the importance of managing this and developing stress management strategies in our everyday lives. This chapter focused on resilience strategies which we need to make specific to our lives. We can then encourage others to do the same and take a lead in trying to create organisational change where possible. This is very difficult to make happen because health and social care organisations are very large and like ocean going ships they cannot stop or change quickly. Changes that do happen tend to be following criticism, adverse incidents and "never events" when the services have been found wanting and full investigations have been put in place. The Francis inquiry (2013) is one such event. The Ockenden review of Shrewsbury maternity failings resulting in many child deaths and also maternal deaths (Ockenden, 2022) is another example. Individual child deaths such as Maria Colwell, in 1973, Jasmine Beckford in 2003 and Arthur Labinjo Hughes in 2021 are other examples where changes have been made or are in the process of being made. We could ask why there need to be tragedies and deaths for change to be implemented, and many would argue that changes are not radical enough and are difficult to sustain. We would all like to see more protection of the wellbeing of staff, and for acknowledgement and change to take place following the distress caused by caring for patients through the pandemic to result in more wellbeing measures being put in place. So, the next chapter will focus on positivity and wellbeing.

REFERENCES

Abbasi K. (2012) Making the Unbearable Bearable. *Journal of the Royal Society of Medicine*, 105(3): 93.

Adamson C, Beddoe L, Davys A. (2014) Building Resilient Practitioners: Definitions and Practitioner Understandings. *British Journal of Social Work*, 44(3): 522–41.

Alladin A. (2015) *Integrative CBT for Anxiety Disorders: An Evidence-Based Approach to Enhancing Cognitive Behavioural Therapy with Mindfulness and Hypnotherapy.* Oxford: Wiley-Blackwell.

Aloufi M, Jarden R, Gerdtz M, Kapp S. (2021) Reducing Stress Anxiety and Depression in Undergraduate Nursing Students: Systematic Review. *Nurse Education Today*, 102: 104877 https://doi.org/10.1016/j.nedt.2021.104877.

American Psychological Association (2014) *The Road to Resilience.* Washington DC: American Psychological Association.

Antonovsky A. (1979) *Health, Stress and Coping*. In: Maes S, Vingerhoets A, Van Heck G. (1987) The Study of Stress and Disease: Some Developments and Requirements. *Social Science and Medicine,* 25(6): 567–78.

Arthur A, Aldus C, Sarre S, Maben J, Wharrad H, Schneider J, Barton G, Argyle E, Clark A, Nouri F, Nicholson C. (2017) Can Health-care Assistant Training Improve the Relational Care of Older People? (CHAT): A Development and Feasibility Study of a Complex Intervention. *Health Services and Delivery Research*, 5(10).

Atkinson P, Martin C, Rankin J. (2009) Resilience Revisited. *Journal of Psychiatric Mental Health Nursing*, 16(2): 137–45.

Baldwin S, Stephen R, Bishop P, Kelly P. (2020a) Development of the Emotional Wellbeing at Work Virtual Programme to Support UK Health Visiting Teams. *Journal of Health Visiting*, 8(12): 516–22.

Baldwin S, Dowdican-McAndrew G, Clark-Maxwell A, Ellis T, Foley C, Hynes C, Kelly P, Lalljee F, Naick F, Schafer R, Ward C. (2020b) The Role of the Clinical Education Team in the Response to COVID-19. *Nursing Times*, 116(12): 53–56.

Baldwin S, Kelly P. (2020) A Flexible Multi-faceted Profession: Supporting Frontline Practitioners in the Fight Against COVID-19. *Journal of Health Visiting*, 8(5): 204–06.

Bandura A. (1977) *Social Learning Theory*. In: Maes S, Vingerhoets A, Van Heck G. (1987) The Study of Stress and Disease: Some Developments and Requirements. *Social Science and Medicine*, 25(6): 567–78.

Barratt C. (2017) Exploring How Mindfulness and Self-compassion Can Enhance Compassionate Care. *Nursing Standard*, 31(21): 55–63.

Beddoe L, Davys A, Adamson C. (2013) Educating Resilient Practitioners. *Social Work Education*, 32(1): 100–17.

Benison L. (2021) Shifting the Blame Will Not Help. *British Journal of Community Nursing*, 26(9): 421.

Boynton B. (2019) *5 Reasons to Distinguish Between Difficult People and Difficult Behaviour*. https://www.healthecareers.com/career-resources/on-the-job/5-reasons-to-distinguish-between-difficult-people-and-difficult-behavior (Accessed 13/9/23).

Bradberry T. (2015) *How Successful People Handle Stress*. https://www.forbes.com/sites/travis-bradberry/2015/05/26/how-successful-people-turn-stress-and-anxiety-into-top-performance/?sh=154083903867 (Accessed 13/9/2023).

Bradshaw J. (2009) *Reclaiming Virtue*. London: Hatchette.

Bregman R. (2020) *Humankind: A Hopeful History*. London: Bloomsbury Publishing.

Breslin H. (2023) *Reframing Resilience: "Bouncing Back" as a Problematic Paradigm*. http://blog.heprofessional.co.uk/edition/reframing-resilience-bouncing-back-as-a-problematic-paradigm#:~:text=The%20language%20of%20resilience&text=It%20is%20frequently%20described%20as, an%20appropriate%20orientation%20and%20trajectory (Accessed 13/09/2023).

Bridges J, Pickering R, Barker H, Chable R, Fuller A, Gould L, Libberton P, Mesa-Eguiagaray I, Raftery J, Sayer A, Westwood G, Wigley W, Yao G, Zhu S, Griffiths P. (2018) Implementing the Creating Learning Environments for Compassionate Care (CLECC) Programme in Acute Hospital Settings: A Pilot RCT and Feasibility Study. *Health Services and Delivery Research*. **6**(33): 1–166.

Bridges J, Harris R, Maben J, Arthur A. (2020) Research that Supports Nursing Teams Part 1 of 4: How Research Can Improve Patient Care and Nurse Wellbeing. *Nursing Times*, 116(10): 23–25.

Brodie J. (2021) Using "Emotional Touchpoints" to Support Staff During COVID-19. *Nursing Times*, 117(12): 23–25.

Burke R, Deszca E. (1982) Career Success and Personal Failure Experiences and Type A Behaviour. *Journal of Organizational Behavior*, 3(2): 161–70.

Calhoun L, Tedeschi R (2014) *Handbook of Posttraumatic Growth: Research and Practice*. New York: Psychology Press.

Capito C, Keegan C, Lachanudis L, Tyler J, McKellow C. (2022) Professional Midwifery Advocates: Delivering Restorative Clinical Supervision. *Nursing Times*, 118(2): 26–28.

Caouette J, Price C. (2018) *The Moral Psychology of Compassion*. London: Rowman and Littlefield International.

Carr E, Reece A, Rosen-Kellerman G, Robichaux A. (2019) *The Value of Belonging at Work.* https://hbr.org/2019/12/the-value-of-belonging-at-work (Accessed 13/9/23).

Carrieri D, Pearson M, Mattick K, Papoutsi C, Briscoe S, Wong G, Jackson M. (2020) Interventions to Minimise Doctors' Mental Ill-health and its Impact on the Workforce and Patient Care: The Care Under Pressure Realist Review. *Health Services and Delivery Research,* 8(19): April 2020.

Carver C, Scheier M, Weintraub J. (1989) Assessing Coping Strategies: A Theoretically Based Approach. *Journal of Personality and Social Psychology,* 56(2): 267–83.

Caspersen D. (2015) *Changing the conversation: The 17 Principles of Conflict Resolution.* London: Profile Books Ltd.

Ceschi A, Fraccaroli F, Constantini A, Sartori R. (2017) Turning Bad into Good: How Resilience Resources Protect Organizations from Demanding Work Environments. *Journal of Workplace Behavioral Health,* 32(4): 267–89.

Charney D. (2004) Psychobiological Mechanisms of Resilience and Vulnerability: Implications for Successful Adaptation to Extreme Stress. *American Journal of Psychiatry,* 161(2): 195–216.

Compson J. (2015) The CARE Heuristic for Addressing Burnout in Nurses. *Journal of Nursing Education and Practice,* 5(7): 63–74.

Connor K, Davidson J. (2003) Development of a New Resilience Scale: The Connor-Davidson Resilience Scale (CD-RISC). *Depression & Anxiety,* 18(2): 76–82.

Cooper C, Dewe P, O'Driscoll M. (2001) *Organizational Stress: A Review and Critique of Theory, Research, and Applications.* London: Sage Publications.

Covey S. (1989) *The 7 Habits of Highly Effective People.* Salt Lake City: Franklin Covey Co.

Dalton-Smith S. (2021) *Burnout: The 7 types of Rest Everyone Needs – and How to Get Them.* https://ideas.ted.com/the-7-types-of-rest-that-every-person-needs/ (Accessed 13/9/23).

De Zulueta P. (2013) Compassion in 21st Century Medicine: Is it Sustainable? *Clinical Ethics,* 8(4): 119–28.

Dev V, Fernando A, Lim A, Consedine N. (2018) Does Self-compassion Mitigate the Relationship Between Burnout and Barriers to Compassion? A Cross-sectional Quantitative Study of 799 Nurses. *International Journal of Nursing Studies,* 81: 81–88.

Dev V, Fernando A, Consedine N. (2020) Self-compassion as a Stress Moderator: A Cross-sectional Study of 1700 Doctors, Nurses, and Medical Students. *Mindfulness,* 11(5): 1170–81.

Duffy B. (2018) *Ending Physician Burnout: It's Time for Physicians to Take Back Control of Their Environment and How They Deliver Care.* https://www.linkedin.com/pulse/ending-physician-burnout-its-time-physicians-take-back-duffy-md (Accessed 13/9/23).

Ewen H, Kinney J. (2014) Application of the Model of Allostasis to Older Women's Relocation to Senior Housing. *Biological Research for Nursing,* 16(2): 197–208.

Fairhall J. (2020) Support for Nurses During the Pandemic. *British Journal of Community Nursing,* 25(8): 369.

Fan L, Blumenthal J, Watkins L, Sherwood A. (2015) Work and Home Stress: Associations with Anxiety and Depression Symptoms. *Occupational Medicine,* 65(2): 110–16.

Figley C. (2002) Compassion Fatigue: Psychotherapists' Chronic Lack of Self Care. *Journal of Clinical Psychology,* 58(11): 1433–41.

Fineberg N, Haddad P, Carpenter L, Gannon B, Sharpe R, Young A, Joyce E, Rowe J, Wellsted D, Nutt D, Sahakian B. (2013) The Size, Burden and Cost of Disorders of the Brain in the UK. *Journal of Psychopharmacology,* 27(9): 761–70.

Francis A, Bulman C. (2019) In What Ways Might Group Clinical Supervision Affect the Development of Resilience in Hospice Nurses? *International Journal of Palliative Nursing,* 25(8): 387–96.

Francis R. (2013) *Report of the Mid Staffordshire NHS Foundation Trust Public Inquiry.* London: The Stationery Office

Friedman M, Rosenman R. (1964) *Hurry Sickness: 10 Ways to Overcome Constant Panic and Rush.* https://www.mindtools.com/pages/article/how-to-beat-hurry-sickness.htm (Accessed 13/9/23).

Friis A, Johnson M, Cutfield R, Consedine N. (2016) Kindness Matters: A Randomised Controlled Trial of a Mindful Self-Compassion Intervention Improves Depression, Distress, and HbA$_{1C}$ Among Patients with Diabetes. *Diabetes Care,* 39(11): 1963–71.

Furnham A. (2008) *Management Intelligence: Sense and Nonsense for the Successful Manager.* Hampshire: Palgrave Macmillan.

Galiana L, Oliver A, Sanso N, Benito E. (2015) Validation of a New Instrument for Self-care in Spanish Palliative Care Professionals Nationwide. *The Spanish Journal of Psychology*, 18(E67): 1–9.

Graham L, van Witteloostuijn A. (2010) *Leader-Member Exchange, Communication Frequency and Burnout.* Working Papers 10–08, Utrecht School of Economics.

Grant L, Kinman G. (2013) *The Importance of Emotional Resilience for Staff and Students in the 'Helping' Professions: Developing an Emotional Curriculum.* York: The Higher Education Academy.

Grant L, Kinman G. (2014) Emotional Resilience in the Helping Professions and how it can be Enhanced. *Health and Social Care Education*, 3(1): 23–34.

Grant L, Kinman G. (2020) *Developing Emotional Resilience and Wellbeing: A Practical Guide for Social Workers.* London: Community Care Inform.

Griffiths, K. (2022) Using Restorative Supervision to Help Nurses During the COVID-19 Pandemic. *Nursing Times*, 118(3): 33–36.

Halbesleben J. (2006) Sources of Social Support and Burnout: A Meta-analytic Test of the Conservation of Resources Model. *Journal of Applied Psychology*, 91(5): 1134–45.

Hargreaves R. (2015) The Value of Schwartz Rounds Should not be Underestimated. *Nursing Times*, 111(14): 11

Harris R, Sims S, Leamy M, Levenson R, Davies N, Brearley S, Grant R, Gourlay S, Favato G, Ross F. (2019) Intentional Rounding in Hospital Wards to Improve Regular Interaction and Engagement Between Nurses and Patients: A Realist Evaluation. *Health Services and Delivery Research*, 7(35).

Hartley M. (1995) *The Good Stress Guide.* London: Sheldon Press.

Health Education England (HEE). (2016) *Values Based Recruitment Framework.* NHS Health Education England.

Health and Social Care Committee (HSCC). (2021) *Workforce Burnout and Resilience in the NHS and Social Care.* https://committees.parliament.uk/publications/6158/documents/68766/default/ (Accessed 13/9/23).

Hofmeyer A, Taylor R, Kennedy K. (2020a) Knowledge for Nurses to Better Care for Themselves So They Can Better Care for Others During the COVID-19 Pandemic and Beyond. *Nurse Education Today*, 94(104503) doi:10.1016/j.nedt.2020.104503.

Hofmeyer A, Taylor R, Kennedy K. (2020b) Fostering Compassion and Reducing Burnout: How Can Health System Leaders Respond in the COVID-19 Pandemic and Beyond? *Nurse Education Today*, 94: 104502 https://doi.org/10.1016/j.nedt.2020.104502.

Hoge E, Ivkovic A, Fricchione G. (2012) Generalized Anxiety Disorder: Diagnosis and Treatment. BMJ. 2012:345 doi: https://doi.org/10.1136/bmj.e7500.

Hunter B, Warren L. (2014) Midwives' Experiences of Workplace Resilience. *Journal of Midwifery*, 30(8): 926–34.

Hylton Rushton C, Sellers D, Heller K, Spring B, Dossey B, Halifax J. (2009) Impact of a Contemplative End-of-life Training Program: Being with Dying. *Palliative and Supportive Care*, 7(4): 405–14.

Jarvis P. (1996) *Commentary on a Case Study of a Patient-Centred Nurse.* In: Fulford K.W M, Ersser S, Hope T. (1996) *Essential Practice in Patient-centred Care.* Oxford: Blackwell Science.

Jennings P, Flaxman P, Egdell K, Pestell S, Whipday E, Herbert A. (2017) A Resilience Training Programme to Improve Nurses' Mental Health. *Nursing Times*, 113(10): 22–26.

Jourdain G, Chênevert D. (2010) Job Demands – Resources, Burnout and Intention to Leave the Nursing Profession: A Questionnaire Survey. *International Journal of Nursing Studies*, 47(6): 709–22.

Kanner A, Coyne J, Schaefer C, Lazarus R. (1981) Comparison of Two Modes of Stress Measurement: Daily Hassles and Uplifts versus Major Life Events. *Journal of Behavioral Medicine*, 4(1): 1–39.

Karatsoreos I, McEwen B. (2013) Resilience and Vulnerability: A Neurobiological Perspective. *F1000 Prime Reports* 5,13. doi:10.12703/P5–13.

Kearney M, Weininger R, Vachon M, Harrison R, Mount B (2009) Self-care of Physicians Caring for Patients at the End of Life: "Being Connected…A Key to My Survival". *JAMA*, 301(11): 1155–64.

Kilmann R, Thomas K. (1974) *The Thomas-Kilmann Conflict Mode Instrument*. Tuxedo, NY: XICOM

Knollman-Porter K, Burshni V, (2020). Optimizing Effective Communication While Wearing a Mask During the COVID-19 Pandemic. *Journal of Gerontological Nursing*, 46(11): pp.7–11.

Kobasa S. (1979) Stressful Life Events, Personality, Health: An Enquiry into Hardiness. *Journal of Personality and Social Psychology*, 37(1): 1–11.

Kristjansson K, Arthur J, Moller F. Ferkanym M. (2017) *Virtuous Practice in Nursing: Research Report*. University of Birmingham: The Jubilee Centre for Character & Virtues.

Labrague L, McEnroe-Petitte D. (2017) An Integrative Review on Conflict Management Styles Among Nursing Students: Implications for Nurse Education. *Nurse Education Today*, 59: 45é52.

Leiter M, Gascon S, Martinez-Jarreta B. (2010) Making Sense of Work Life: A Structural Model of Burnout. *Journal of Applied Social Psychology*, 40(1): 57–75.

Lintern S. (2014) Test for Nursing Values Unveiled. *Nursing Times*, 110(43): 2.

Maben J, Harris R, Arthur A, Bridges J. (2021) Nursing Interventions that Provide Team Members' Psychological Wellbeing. *Nursing Times*, 117(1): 44–47.

Maben J, Bridges J. (2020) COVID-19: Supporting Nurses' Psychological and Mental Health. *Journal of Clinical Nursing*, 29(15–16): 2742–50.

Maben J, Taylor C, Dawson J, Leamy M, McCarthy I, Reynolds E, Ross S, Shuldham C, Bennett L, Foot C. (2018) A Realist Informed Mixed-methods Evaluation of Schwartz Center Rounds in England. *Health Services and Delivery Research*, 6(37).

Malliarou M, Moustaka E, Konstantinidis T. (2008) Burnout of Nursing Personnel in a Regional University Hospital. *Health Service Journal*, 2(3): 140–52.

Marine A, Ruotsalainen j, Serra C, Verbeek J. (2006) Preventing Occupational Stress in Health care Workers. *Cochrane Database Systematic Review*, 18(4): CD002892 doi:10.1002/14651858.

Mathieu F. (2012) *The Compassion Fatigue Workbook*. East Sussex: Taylor & Francis Group.

Maxted A. (2021) Under Pressure – Should You be Worried About Your Stress Levels. *The Times*. Sept 11th 2021. p2/3.

Mealer M, Conrad D, Evans J, Jooste K, Salyntjes J, Rothbaum B, Moss M. (2014) Feasibility and Acceptability of a Resilience Training Program for Intensive Care Unit Nurses. American Journal of Critical Care. 23(6) e97-e105 doi: http://dx.doi.org/10.4037/ajcc2014747.

Mealer M, Jones J, Newman J, McFann K, Rothbaum B, Moss M. (2012) The Presence of Resilience is Associated with a Healthier Psychological Profile in Intensive Care Unit (ICU) Nurses: Results of a National Survey. *International Journal of Nursing Studies*, 49(3): 292–99.

Milne M, Munro M. (2020) Symptoms and Causes of Anxiety and its Diagnosis and Management. *Nursing Times*, 116(10): 18–22.

Mitchell G. (2021) Pioneering Service Supporting Nurse Mental Health Across Five Trusts. *Nursing Times*, 117(4): 19.

Mojza E. (2010) Staying Well and Engaged When Demands Are High: The Role of Psychological Detachment. *Journal of Applied Psychology*, 95(5): 965–76.

Montgomery A, Spann F, Baban A, Panagopoulou E. (2015) Job Demands, Burnout, and Engagement Among Nurses: A Multi-level Analysis of ORCAB Data Investigating the Moderating Effect of Teamwork. *Burnout Research*, 2(2–3): 71–79.

Moore C. (2020) Nurse Leadership During a Crisis: Ideas to Support You and Your Team. *Nursing Times*, 116(12): 34–37.

Nathoo S, Shaw D, Sandy P. (2016) Determinants of Compassion in Providing Care to Older People: Educational Implications *Nurse Education Today*, 101: 104878. https://doi.org/10.1016/j.nedt.2021.104878.

Neff K. (2003) The Development and Validation of a Scale to Measure Self-Compassion. *Self and Identity*, 2(3): 223–50.

Neff K. (2013) *Self Compassion: The Proven Power of Being Kind to Yourself.* Lousiville, Co: Sounds True.

Neff K. (2020) *Self compassion – Guided Meditation and Exercises.* Center for Mindful Self-Compassion. https://centerformsc.org/practice-msc/guided-meditations-and-exercises (Accessed 13/9/23).

Niebuhr R. (c1937) *The Serenity Prayer* https://www.aa.org/sites/default/files/literature/assets/smf-129_en.pdf.

Nolan S. (2020) No Health care Worker Should Have to Cry Alone. *Nursing Times.* https://www.nursingtimes.net/opinion/no-healthcare-worker-should-have-to-cry-alone-03-07-2020/ (Accessed 13/9/23).

Nursing and Midwifery Council (2018) *The Code.* London: NMC.

Nursing and Midwifery Council Leavers Survey (2020) Why do People Leave the NMC Register? https://tinyurl.com/r4y3chs (Accessed 9/8/21).

Nyatanga B (2020) Enhancing Spiritual Harmony in Palliative Care. *British Journal of Community Nursing*, 25(8): 411.

Ockenden D. (2022) *Ockenden Review: Summary of Findings, Conclusions and Essential Actions.* London: Crown Copyright

Open University (2021) *OU KnowHow How to handle rude customers* https://app.goodpractice.net/#/open-university/s/snx1x8b74i (Accessed 13/9/23).

Orellana-Rios C, Radbruch L, Kern M, Regel Y, Anton A, Sinclair S, Schmidt S. (2018) Mindfulness and Compassion – Oriented Pactices at Work Reduce Distress and Enhance Self-care of Palliative Care Teams: A Mixed-method Evaluation of an "on the Job" Program. *BMC Palliative Care*, 17(3): 1–15.

Palmer S. (2021) Long COVID and Mental Health. *British Journal of Community Nursing*, 26(8): 406–09.

Pascoe L, Edvardson D. (2013) Benefit Finding in Cancer: A Review of Influencing Factors and Outcomes. *European Journal of Oncology Nursing*, 17(6): 760–66.

Pascoe S. (2014) Learn How to Cope with Distress. *Nursing Times*, 110(11): 33.

Patwell B. (2021) Reflecting on Leading Meaningful Change Through COVID. *Academic Letters Article.* https://doi.org/10.20935/AL480 (Accessed 05.05.2021).

Penberthy J, Chhabra D, Ducar D, Avitabile N, Lynch M, Khanna S, Xu Y, Ait-Daoud N, Schorling J. (2018) Impact of Coping and Communication Skills Program on Physician Burnout, Quality of Life and Emotional Flooding. *Safety and Health at Work*, 9(4): 381–87.

Radcliffe M. (2020a) Being Brilliant at Nursing is Transcendent and Life Affirming. *Nursing Times*, 116(4): 15.

Radcliffe M. (2020b) Not Addressing Mental Ill Health and its Stigma is a False Economy. *Nursing Times*, 116(11) 15.

Radcliffe M. (2021a) Covid is Highlighting the Value and Ubiquity of Human Kindness. *Nursing Times*, 117(2): 15.

Radcliffe M. (2021b) To Not Speak About Poor Care is to Normalise it. *Nursing Times*, 117(9): 15.

Radcliffe M. (2021c) There are Some People Who Students Would do Best to Avoid. *Nursing Times*, 117(10): 15.

Rahim M. (2011) *Managing Conflict in Organizations.* Abingdon: Routledge

Rapoport A. (1960) *Fights, Games, and Debates.* Michigan: University of Michigan Press.

Rhoads J, Murphy P. (2015) *Anxiety Disorders.* In: Rhoads, J, Murphy, P. (2015) *Clinical Consult to Psychiatric Nursing for Advanced Practice.* New York: Springer Publishing Co.

Robertsoncooper. *i-Resilience Report.* https://www.robertsoncooper.com/iresilience/ (Accessed 2022).

Robson S. (2018) *Learn From Me: Speak Out, Seek Help, Get Treatment.* https://practitionerhealth.ie/learn-from-me-speak-out-seek-help-get-treatment/ (Accessed 13/9/23).

Rosenman R, Friedman M, Straus R, Wurm M, Kositchek R, Hahn W, Werthessen N. (1964) A Predictive Study of Coronary Heart Disease: The Western Collaborative Group Study. *Journal of the American Medical Association*, 189: 15–22.

Rotter J. (1954) *Social Learning and Clinical Psychology.* New Jersey: Prentice-Hall.

Rotter J. (1966) Generalised Expectancies for Internal Versus External Control of Reinforcement. *Psychological Monographs*, 80(1): 1–28.

Royal College of Nursing (2013) *Beyond Breaking Point – A Survey Report of RCN Members on Health, Wellbeing and Stress.* https://www.iosh.co.uk/~/media/Documents/Networks/Group/Health%20and%20Social%20Care/Beyond%20Breaking%20Point.pdf?la=en (Accessed 13/9/23).

Rungapadiachy D.M. (1999) *Interpersonal Communication and Psychology: Theory and Practice.* Edinburgh: Butterworth-Heineman

Rungapadiachy D.M. (2008) *Self-awareness in Health Care: Engaging in Helping Relationships.* Basingstoke: Palgrave Macmillan

Sallon S, Katz-Eisner D, Yaffe H, Bdolah-Abram T. (2017) Caring for the Caregivers: Results of an Extended, Five-component Stress–reduction Intervention for Hospital Staff. *Behavioral Medicine*, 43(1) 47–60.

Sanchez-Reilly S, Morrison l, Carey E, Bernacki R, O'Neill L, Kapo J, Periyakoil V.S, Thomas J.de L. (2013) Caring for Oneself to Care for Others: Physicians and their Self-care. *Journal of Support Oncology*, 11(2): 75–81.

Sanders K, Shaw T. (2019) Creating Caring Cultures: Getting Started. *Foundation of Nursing Studies.* https://www.fons.org/resources/documents/Creating-Caring-Cultures/Creating-Caring-Cultures-2nd-Edition.pdf (Accessed 13/9/23).

Sharp C, Dewar B. (2017) Learning in Action: Extending our Understanding of Appreciative Inquiry. In: Zuber-Skerritt O (ed.) (2017) *Conferences as Sites of Learning and Development: Using Participatory Action Learning and Action Research Approaches.* Abingdon: Routledge

Skovholt T, Trotter-Mathison M. (2016) *The Resilient Practitioner.* Abingdon: Routledge.

Slater E. (2015) DIY Therapy – 10 key exercises. *The Times.* Nov 28th Body & Soul p5.

Smajdor A. (2013) Should Compassionate Practice be Incentivised. *Nursing Times*, 109(49/50): 18–19.

Smith B, Dalen J, Wiggins K, Tooley E, Christopher P, Bernard J. (2008) The Brief Resilience Scale: Assessing the Ability to Bounce Back. *International Journal of Behavioral Medicine*, 15(3): 194–200.

Smith R. (2020) Nurses And All Staff Must Be Cared For Just As They Care For Us. *Nursing Times*, 116(11): 13.

Snyder M. (2014) *Positive Health: Flourishing Lives, Well-Being in Doctors.* Bloomington, IN: Balboa Press.

Stephen R, Petit A. (2015) *Developing Resilience in Practice: A Health Visiting Framework.* London: Institute of Health Visiting.

Stone D, Patton B, Heen S. (1999) *Difficult Conversations: How to Discuss What Matters Most.* London: Penguin Books Ltd.

The American Holistic Nurses Association (AHNA), American Nurses Association (ANA) (2013) *Holistic Nursing: Scope and Standards of Practice.* 2nd ed. Silver Springs, MD: NurseBooks. org

Thompson S, Thompson N. (2008) *The Critically Reflective Practitioner.* Basingstoke: Palgrave Macmillan

Turner J, Kelly B, Girgis A. (2011) Supporting Oncology Health Professionals: A Review. *Psycho-Oncologie.* 5(2): 77–82.

Weeks D. (1992) *The Eight Essential Steps to Conflict Resolution: Preserving Relationships at Work, at Home and in the Community.* New York: Penguin Putnam Inc.

Weinstein L. (2018) *The 7 Principles of Conflict Resolution: How to Resolve Disputes, Defuse Difficult Situations and Reach Agreement.* Harlow: Pearson Education Limited.

West M, Bailey S, Williams E. (2020) *The Courage of Compassion: Supporting Nurses and Midwives to Deliver High-Quality Care.* London: The King's Fund.

Williams T. (2021) Nurses Need to Look After Their Emotional Wellbeing. *Nursing Times*, 117(1): 12–13.

Winnicott D. (1945) *Primitive Emotional Development.* In: *Through Paediatrics to Psychoanalyis: Collected Papers.* London: Tavistock.

Woodford H, Gunning H, Langdon S, Whelan J. (2020) Aiding Staff Wellbeing and Resilience During the Coronavirus Pandemic. *Nursing Times*, 116(9): 20–23.

Woods L. (2021) The Importance of Self-compassion for Health Visitors' Wellbeing. *Journal of Health Visiting*, 9(12): 501–15.

Youngson R. (2018) *Take the Test: Are You Kindly, Compassionate or Just Competent.* https:/tiapana.co.nz/take-the-test-are-you-kindly-compassionate-or-just-competent (Accessed 13/9/23).

Zhang J, Wang X, Xu T, Li J, Li H, Wu Y, Li Y, Chen Y, Zhang J. (2021) The Effect of Resilience and Self-efficacy on Nurses' Compassion Fatigue: A Cross-sectional Study. *Journal of Advanced Nursing*, 78(1): 1–12.

5

How can I reduce my negative thinking and increase my positivity?

- Introduction
- Discussion – main points and evidence with case studies, exercises, aide mémoires and questions

  - Why is emotional intelligence crucial for compassionate care?
  - The importance of different intelligences and cultural competence
  - Why is empathy important in increasing positivity?
  - Why is it so important to maximise our engagement and enthusiasm in our work?
  - How do positivity, happiness and wellbeing interact with each other?
  - Mindfulness and the window of tolerance.

- Recommendations for leadership as individual practitioners, leaders and organisations

  - Focusing on positivity and compassionate care as individual practitioners and leaders
  - Focusing on positivity and compassionate care as organisations.

INTRODUCTION

Previous chapters have focused on stress management and resilience, but this chapter will focus primarily on positivity because so often we can dwell on what is going wrong, and not on what is going well. We need to appreciate the positives in what we are managing to accomplish in difficult times, and what we are doing well in adverse situations, and then appreciate these for the positives that they are. This chapter will also focus on the importance of emotional intelligence as a tool for enhancing our communication with others. Self-awareness and self-management and relationship awareness and management are so important in ensuring that our relationships with our multiprofessional team colleagues, managers and of course patients and clients, can be as positive as possible. It will also focus on the importance of our other intelligences, and cultural intelligence and our empathy in order to stay positive. Finally, it will focus on maintaining engagement and enthusiasm within our work roles.

Again, the format will be:

- Case study
- Discussions

- Exercises and aide mémoires
- Recommendations for leadership as individual practitioners, team leaders and organisations

DISCUSSION

Case Study 5.1

Jen's focus on social stimulation

Whilst on student placement in a community hospital, I had got to know some of the longer stay patients and had begun to build a rapport with them. This made it easier for me to recognise when they needed assistance or were uncomfortable.

At the start of one of my shifts I could hear Mr X immediately as soon as I entered the ward. He has vascular dementia but is usually very settled and happy. He had constantly been trying to get out of bed and pressing his call bell for the last hour, according to colleagues. Due to his mobility issues, he is unable to walk at present and so was at risk of falls. The bay was generally quite busy but the majority of patients in his bay were now in the day room.

I sat with Mr X for a few minutes to try and ascertain what was causing him distress. I asked if he wanted to go to the day room, checked that he had eaten and had sufficient fluids and that he was comfortable. Mr X declined to go to the day room but still appeared unsettled. I thought about his social needs and reminded him about his radio and TV, which he normally enjoyed. Again, this was declined. I then recalled a conversation we had had previously, regarding his younger years as a Paratrooper for the RAF. I also recalled, having gone through the books for another patient, that there was an interesting book on World War II aircraft in the day room full of pictures and quick facts about the aircraft. I excused myself from Mr X and went to retrieve the book. On my return I showed him the book and his eyes lit up. I helped him to sit up, put the hospital table over his bed and ensured that he could access the book. I went through one or two of the pages and then left Mr X to look through the rest.

He settled for the next hour and a half and thoroughly enjoyed looking through this book. He remained settled through lunch, napped in the afternoon and appeared much happier and settled. I had naturally assumed that Mr X's distress was caused by a physical pain or perhaps hunger or thirst. However, on taking the time to assess him holistically, I realised that he was bored and lacking attention and stimulation. Most of his friends were in the day room and there was no one for him to chat to.

It is important to recognise that not all distress is caused by pain or infection but that someone can become distressed because of their environment, the lighting, too much noise or lack of interaction. It is essential to get to know a patient, we are then able to differentiate differences in behaviour and therefore resolve the cause of distress quicker. For Mr X, he was showing a difference in his usual behaviour pattern but was unable to communicate why he was distressed. By assessing his emotional needs, as well as his physical needs, I realised that he needed something to occupy him.

This incident reminded me that whilst we are health care professionals, not everything is due to an ailment or physical change. It was important to assess each patient as a whole and not jump to conclusions. By taking a few minutes to chat with Mr X I was able to de-escalate his distress and provide better care for him as an individual, ensuring person-centred care. I feel that my response to Mr X was an appropriate response to meet his needs. I feel that I was able to assess all of his needs and respond accordingly. I will continue to uphold this practice and remember to assess not only physical needs, but emotional needs too.

Case Study 5.2

Melissa's focus on enhancing self-esteem and psychological wellbeing

During my placement in cardiology I looked after a patient who was receiving palliative care due to congestive heart failure. He had been in hospital for four weeks waiting for a package of care. He was confined to bed due to his shortness of breath and he had been unable to use the commode due to his increased breathlessness which made this unsafe. He was struggling physically because his breathing was so compromised. However, he was better than when he first came in as he was able to talk to me without stopping to get his breath back and was able to discuss his views and needs.

One Sunday morning the night staff reported that the patient had been able to use the commode during the night and had his bowels open. That morning I walked past his side room and noticed that he was in his chair and looking out of the window. He seemed to have good posture in the chair and did not look distressed with his breathing.

His actions indicated new strengths and maybe I could help him do more. I asked how he was today and he told me that he felt really good about using the commode and he thought he would see how he was sitting out in the chair which he was managing really well. He was so happy with his achievements, and he had a smile on his face and was extremely proud of himself.

I then wondered about whether he could now have a shower. Other patients have said that a shower made them feel fresh and generally happier about themselves, and I would feel the same way. The patient was able to transfer as he did when he used the commode and into the chair. He was unable to walk to the shower, but I could get a wheelchair to take him, but could he manage sitting upright for a long period? He did not seem distressed breathing at the moment though. If I gathered all the equipment, I needed I would be able to reduce the time he was sitting. The aim was to minimise the amount of physical activity for the patient and I needed to have all the equipment ready, not leave him alone and reduce the time he was out of bed, and that would reduce the risk to him. Also, by carrying this out in the afternoon, which was usually quieter, nurses would be able to offer me support as needed because they would not be doing a drug round.

When I asked him if he would like to go for a shower his face lit up with a smile and he said that he would love that. I told him to rest now for the morning and in the afternoon after lunch I could help him with his shower. He was so excited and happy that he was going for a shower. I would monitor his condition for any deterioration and would stop, abort the plan or try something else. All went smoothly and there was only one time where I was concerned about the patient. He was in the shower at the time and had his eyes closed and was breathing deeply and not saying much. I asked him if he was alright and he said that he was just enjoying this moment. After the shower he thanked me and said that he felt fresh and energised. I thought about the patient's "bio-psycho-social" needs and how much this had contributed to his wellbeing and how positive he felt.

I have a flowchart in my head where I see people at different stages of their ability while in hospital. When they are dressed in a hospital gown and tend to have a strip wash in bed these tend to be poorly patients. The next stage is where they can help and have pyjamas or a nightdress on. At the next stage they are feeling better and can go for a shower and start to wear their own clothes. So, when I work on a Sunday, I will use that day to see if can make a difference to patients' bio-psycho-social wellbeing. I will also think about the weekday routine as patients generally get washed in the mornings, but some of them get worried about missing the doctors. It would be better in some cases to have a wash in the afternoon when it is quieter and more support is available. There is also more time to assess a patient's abilities, rather than thinking about the next patient to be washed.

Case Study 5.3

Jen's focus on enhancing self-esteem and patients feeling valued

During one of my ward placements, a patient was showing signs and symptoms of Clostridium Difficile. The night staff had spoken to him, explained all the precautions that they would need to take, and the rationale for these, and had then placed him in a separate bay for isolation. Mr X had capacity to absorb all this information and had given full consent for this to happen. During the day, Mr X repeatedly pressed his buzzer for small requests, such as fresh water, a newspaper or in needing assistance with something he had previously been able to do independently.

When I returned the next day, Mr X was showing signs of distress. He was standing in the doorway to his room and was shouting out to other patients, asking them to come to him. At handover, it was also mentioned that he had been awake a lot during the night and was requiring assistance more than usual. After donning PPE, I chatted with him and it became very apparent that he was lonely. He became quite tearful and stated that although he had agreed with all of the precautions, understood them and did not object to them in any way, he felt isolated from his fellow in-patients and was finding the isolation really difficult.

I sat and talked to him about what we could do to resolve this and how we could make the situation easier for him. Mr X stated that he just wanted to feel part of the ward again and to be able to join in the activities. I explained to Mr X that once his results were back, we would have a better understanding of the time scale for the isolation, but that for now, he needed to stay in the bay if he wishes to continue with the precautions. After some discussion, I suggested that maybe he could make something for the Easter display. I explained that if the C-Diff test came back positive, we may not be able to display it outside the room, but that we could display it in his room and make the room a bit more colourful for him. We discussed what he would like to do, and with what materials. I then collected some card (to make egg baskets), the instructions on how to make them and some shredding paper for the nests. The ward sister was making bonnets for eggs and I explained that I was sure she would have some spare. I left Mr X making these and he seemed much more settled. I notified the staff nurse of our conversation and she said she would check on him later.

Mr X was quite an active patient and regularly sat in the lounge interacting with other patients and so the separation was really difficult for him, even though he knew the rationale and wanted to protect others. Mr X had the choice whether to agree with the isolation or not, but he found the isolation harder to deal with than he thought. I learnt a lot by taking the time to get to the root of the problem and reacting accordingly. By sitting with him and finding the cause of his anxiety and recognising the signs of his distress I could respond to this, whilst respecting him as an individual and treating him with compassion. My local trust isolation policy states that we must consider both the physical and psychological safety of patients. By explaining the procedure to Mr X and involving him, we included him in his care whilst protecting others from potential harm. He was risk assessed prior to the isolation and was at low risk of any harm. He did feel short term effects of isolation, but this did not affect him long term.

We received the results for Mr X later that day and he did not have C-Difficile and so we were able to allow him back into the main ward and he took his Easter baskets and added them to the display. This made him feel better and allowed him to feel as if he had contributed. He later thanked me for taking the time to chat with him. Even though Mr X was at low risk in relation to his isolation, he showed some clinical signs of depression due to the lack of stimulation, social interaction and less one to one contact. He felt low in mood, was agitated and had altered behaviour.

This experience has reiterated to me that I need to take all aspects of a person's wellbeing into my assessment of that person. I need to be more aware of the implications of changes within somebody's routine or care and how that can impact on that person. I will take some extra time in the future to check on the psychological changes with individuals in similar situations.

Case Study 5.4

Philippa's focus on working in partnership

Whilst working in an Intermediate Care Team, I was asked to see a gentleman who had had multiple falls at his home. He did not sustain any major injuries and was assessed as safe; however, the GP was concerned about his ability to manage so asked for him to be monitored in his home environment. The cause of the falls was put down to frailty and a shuffling gait causing him to trip. When I went to see this gentleman, his house was very run down and only had an electric heater in his lounge despite it being autumn and cold. In himself he was very depressed at his loss of independence and was not happy about receiving help. He struggled with hearing, particularly due to the PPE and wearing of masks meaning he was unable to lip read.

When I went in, I introduced myself and knelt at his feet due to him having a stoop which meant sitting up to look at me would have caused him discomfort. My name was not easy for him to hear through the mask so I showed him my name badge which he could read. I tried to maintain eye contact so he could see I was open and concerned for him but that he was in control. I was trying to enable him to be independent rather than deprive him of his freedom. This was a difficult balance as during the COVID pandemic we were supposed to maintain distance from patients; however, this had to be disregarded due to the need to be understood and listen.

At first, he was very closed off and did not want to discuss his needs or his condition. He maintained he did not need support and there was nothing wrong. To try to make him more comfortable I looked around his home and noticed he had lots of artefacts from Native Americans. I asked what his connection was and he appeared to enjoy telling me about his trips there. Once the conversation was flowing, I offered him a cup of tea. He admitted he has not been eating as he has no appetite. He then commented that he hadn't had his bowels opened for a long time, he was unsure how long. He also confided that he wasn't able to get to the toilet in time and often wet himself. I started to suspect a urine infection and constipation and upon examining him he had swollen legs which would have contributed to his decline in mobility. It emerged that he is sleeping in his chair because it was too cold. I explained the importance of laying down to sleep if possible and the advantages this would have for his bladder, bowels and swollen legs. I offered, and he accepted, me finding another electric heater and placing this in his bedroom. As it was late evening, he agreed I could assist him to bed later on.

Whilst trying to persuade him to eat he declined and said he couldn't see the point if he didn't want to. As much as it would have been polite and easy to accept his choice, I knew this would not improve his situation, he would further decline and possibly fall again and do damage this time. I gently explained to him that if he chose not to eat or drink, he would not get better or get his independence back. This felt like I was pushing him to do something he really didn't want to do but I hoped I could make him see that it wasn't a choice between eating now or not, it was a bigger choice of continuing to decline or taking actions to intervene and attempt to get better. He started with a quarter of a sandwich and a glass of coke, which although not ideal, was a start and I did not want him to lose his trust in me.

He allowed me to wash him and find a change of clothes. He was a private man, so I encouraged him to wash independently where possible. I made a conscious effort to avert my gaze or busy myself elsewhere whilst he washed in order for him to remain comfortable. I explained that I would need to check pressure areas such as his sacrum and he was happy for me to do that. We continued having a discussion about his experiences of being a war evacuee and he enjoyed telling me stories and I made sure I was attentive and interested to put him at ease. Prior to leaving I arranged for him to have a commode delivered so he was able to get to the toilet more easily, a urine bottle so he didn't have to mobilise when unaccompanied and left him plenty of fluids and food to hand. He agreed to going to bed with my assistance, and to having a wheeled Zimmer frame I had bought from our stores so that he could get to bed safely. I advised him on ways of walking that would reduce his risk of falls such as having his feet slightly further apart and lifting his feet rather than shuffling.

Communication was extremely important throughout this assessment. Had I not taken the time for him to understand I was not in a hurry and was not going to force any services upon him he would have become far less welcoming. He even seemed to enjoy the interaction. I do not feel that he would have responded as well had I attempted a far stricter stance. I think that by taking the softer approach as I did, he was able to retain control of the situation and not see this as a threat to his independence. I feel his satisfaction with the approach was evidenced by him being agreeable to my suggestions. It would have been good for me to assess him at greater length, perhaps by obtaining blood tests, but they happened later, as did witnessing him attempt activities of daily living. This assessment was purely an opportunity to build a rapport and ensure he was safe and comfortable and enable me to identify problems and gather information.

Again, with their permission, I have used my students' reflections on their practice. In the first case study Jen has thought about the social needs of her patient and how he needed more stimulation, but that this needed to be in a way that he could relate to. His interest in planes guided Jen to get a book for him to look at which captivated his interest. In the next case study Melissa took a strategic problem-solving approach to this challenging situation, and made such a difference to the patient's quality of life. She has not just accepted the status quo but has thought about how she could do more for this patient. She applied her theoretical learning and developed new strategies for other situations in the future. Her sensitivity and compassion shines out in helping this patient to increase his independence and have a much wanted shower. This same approach is demonstrated, again by Jen's reflection in relation to the importance of social stimulation and self-esteem. Jen again used a creative person-centred approach to enable him to feel included and valued by taking part in making Easter decorations. Philippa used her extremely high communication skills to gently work with a man who was intensely private and did not think he needed help. He accepted the many interventions that she put in place, and this was possible only through her unhurried and interactive approach. These reflections are excellent, and demonstrate the students' exemplary practice, and they use their practice experiences to demonstrate their proactive problem solving and person-centred care. It is also so easy to see their positivity and love of their nursing role, which I find humbling and inspiring to see.

Case Study 5.5

Olivia's reflection on why she wanted to become a nurse

Someone once asked me why I wanted to become a nurse. My answer consisted of: "I enjoy and want to help people, I am a people person, I like caring for those in their time of need". Yes, those are still relevant to me today, but since embarking on my nurse training I have truly seen and learnt what nurses experience day to day and what the job role entails on the front line.

One day nurses are there to be a shoulder to cry on for either a patient, a relative or a colleague. Other days they are there to be shouted at, bitten, or scratched by a distressed patient (the sad reality of the effects of dementia and brain metastases). They may be shouted at by an upset relative who doesn't want to accept the devastating prognosis of their loved one, the diagnosis nurses have to break to patients and the news that changes people's lives for the worst. Nurses have to endure heartache, but then still carry on the rest of their shift putting on a brave face and trying to tell themselves; "this is my job".

But nurses are also there when patients' relatives cannot be, to hold their hand and comfort them in those final moments in the world. Nurses are often there through a patient's entire cancer journey, from the start when the terrible news is given, through the plan of treatment, through the chemotherapy, through the sickness and hair loss, through the tears and through relatives' fear that their loved one may not make it through. Nurses need to be the person that provides reassurance even when they are not sure of what the outcome is going to be. The silver lining is that the nurse is able to be there when the patient and their family finally receive the all clear, and have come out of the other side.

Nurses can change someone's day; they can make the most terrifying situation not seem so frightening. They have the power to truly make a difference for the better.

Nurses have the opportunity to have a huge impact on someone, to mean so much to someone that they say: "I could not have done this without you". Words so powerful that an individual feels that they appreciated having you there – to have a positive impact on someone and make a difference, when it is "ust my job".

Well, that is some job, and that is why I want to be a nurse.

Olivia has said in these few eloquent words why she chose to be a nurse and what nursing means to her. This degree of positivity would give her a great deal of resilience to buffer her against the most stressful of days. This piece of very moving writing says so much about what nursing can and should be. I am not sure that she knows how insightful her words are, or how inspiring they would be to those who are thinking of making a career in nursing, or those who are already in practice.

These case studies all focus on positive and creative approaches to patient centred care, and all these students were only in their first year when they wrote these reflections. However, they are now qualified nurses. And their role modelling is so important for others in their teams, and they will be taking a lead in promoting positivity and exemplary care.

Why is emotional intelligence crucial for compassionate care?

Case Study 5.6

Lisa's use of emotional intelligence to be an advocate and escalate her concerns

A patient was admitted with a head injury for observation and it was suspected that he had been under the influence of alcohol. The patient was an outlier, therefore under a consultant from a different ward, but had not been seen by any consultant. He was supposed to be having four-hourly observations; the nurse and health care assistant had not been monitoring him as they thought that he was drunk and could sleep it off. I noticed that the patient was becoming increasingly unwell, and repeatedly escalated this to the nurse in charge. When no action was taken, I took the patient's observations hourly and I escalated my concerns to the consultant on the ward, who reviewed the patient. He was assessed and was diagnosed with a subdural haematoma and transferred to intensive care and was subsequently in hospital a long time.

In the episode of care, I switched between different leadership styles and became more directive because I needed to be an advocate for my patient and seek assistance on his behalf. My leadership in this situation was underpinned by emotional intelligence. Goleman et al (2002) state that emotional intelligence is having confidence, being self-aware, empathetic, and being able to adapt your leadership style and self-management. Firstly, I demonstrated my emotional intelligence by having the confidence in my own skills. I recognised the importance of soft signs and utilised this by having the confidence to escalate above the nurse. Secondly, by being self-aware and self-managing my emotions, due to the lack of response to my concerns, I kept my emotions under control rather than becoming angry and frustrated, and escalated my concerns to the doctor. Thirdly,

I used my empathy and recognised that my concerns were not being acted upon and the patient's deteriorating health status was not being taken seriously.

The Health care Leadership model (NHS Leadership Academy, 2014) states the importance of emotional intelligence, and cites having personal qualities such as confidence, knowledge, self-awareness and control of emotions creates a foundation for how we act. Both the health care leadership model (NHS Leadership Academy, 2014) and emotional intelligence (Goleman et al, 2002) demonstrate how we manage our emotional self is fundamental to being a successful leader.

The episode of care demonstrated autonomous practice and I demonstrated this by drawing upon my own knowledge of physical signs of deterioration. However, I holistically assessed the patient by not solely relying on figures from the National Early Warning Score (Royal College of Physicians, 2017), in this episode of care the patient was not scoring a worrying NEWS score, but I recognised the importance of soft signs, such as periods of incoherence and sensitivity to light, I carried out hourly observations rather than the four-hourly observations in the plan of the patient.

The challenges to leadership and autonomous practice from reflecting upon this episode of care are having the courage to escalate and challenge behaviour. I demonstrated courage by seeking assistance for the patient's care and recognised negative stereotyping from the nurse and health care assistant who referred to the patient as a drunk and letting them sleep it off. This stereotyping had a direct impact on the patient care, regardless of whether the patient had been drinking or had alcohol dependency issues we have a duty to provide care and not provide less care because of one's opinion. Unconscious bias was being displayed by the nurse and the health care assistant which can lead to poor decision making, forming the wrong conclusion and result in misdiagnosis. In this episode of care, this unconscious bias of the nurse and health care assistant, showed a lack of cultural competence, and if not for my intervention could have had devastating consequences for the patient.

In future practice I intend to demonstrate compassionate practice and will create a culture of speaking up and ensuring that others' opinions and values are listened to. Leading by example would have a knock-on effect on other staff, challenging unconscious bias supported by using emotional intelligence and utilising leadership styles. When I am a registered nurse I will utilise the coaching method, as this allows you to explore and rationalise thinking and empower others into discussion, helping team working with different views. Leadership takes courage and compassion and strengthens autonomous practice, and this is something I will continue to advocate from student nurse to a registered nurse.

Lisa's emotional intelligence was clearly evident in how she escalated her concerns to senior colleagues. She did not just accept the status quo and could see the judgmental approach that others were taking to the patient in her care. It would have been so easy for her frustration and concern to affect how she communicated with others, and this would not have helped her patient. By staying calm and evidence-based and using her excellent communication skills she was able to explain her concerns, and these were taken seriously by the consultant and action was taken. This takes courage and emotional brilliance, and Lisa should be very proud of all that she achieved.

PPE

These dry hands
Gloved, cocooned in plastic
Separate our skin
I hope you feel my touch
To let you know I am here.

These fatigued smiles
Masked, concealed in fabric
Separate our view.
I hope you see my kindness
To let you know I care.

These exhausted bodies
Gowned, wrapped in scrub
Separate our souls.
I hope you value my dedication
To let you know behind all this I am me.

By Sarah Quinn

Compassion, the life blood of the NHS

We are here for you 24/7, in your darkest, most vulnerable and weakest moments

We are the holding of a hand to show you we are here through it all.
We are people who make porridge at 4am for that eight-year-old boy whose beloved granddad just died and was in need of distraction.
We are the first people you see when you wake up after surgery and tell you it all went well
We are the ears who listen to that 90-year-old lady recite from memory her favourite poem perfectly because no family come to visit.
We are the eyes you show your wounds to which we dress without batting an eyelid.
We are the assistants who help you learn to walk again, and who motivate you to try again after falling.
We are the people who make you a cup of tea after you find out the child you were carrying will never be born alive.
We are the carers who shave you when you can't, so you look smart for your wife even in your hospital bed.
We are the staff who learn to sign their name so they can communicate in a way you understand.
We are the staff that turn up every day and see so much. In this never ending battle we still try. A little compassion goes further than you may ever know.
We are the NHS.

by Sarah Quinn

Sarah Quinn was a Masters nursing student at Oxford Brookes University when she wrote these insightful poems, and they clearly articulate the challenges of communicating when wearing PPE, and the importance of small but so very important acts of compassionate practice. They also demonstrate emotional intelligence, which is also the focus for Lisa's excellent practice and advocacy in the previous case study where she challenged the status quo and escalated her concerns. Lisa did this in an emotionally intelligent manner, thereby minimising the possibility of conflict and creating the right environment for her concerns to be taken seriously.

Emotional intelligence (EI) is crucial for us to develop as people, and to help us to cope with our own emotions, but also with the emotions and behaviour of others. Salovey and Mayer (1990) describe emotional intelligence as the ability to assess the feelings and emotions in ourselves and others, so that we can discriminate between them and use this information to guide how we think and what we do. This involves us perceiving emotions and understanding them, as well as reasoning with emotion and managing the emotions which drive us. This is far from easy, especially when we are not prepared for the situations which can arise in our lives. Goleman et al (2002) describes the four domains of emotional intelligence as being **self-awareness**, **self-management**, **social awareness** and **relationship management**. These are inextricably linked because if we are not aware of our own emotions, we cannot understand the impact that these could have on others. Therefore we cannot manage these same emotions and our relationships with others will suffer. If we are self-aware we are aware of how our feelings affect us in the situations we are in, and in the relationships we have with other people, and this is the bedrock of emotional intelligence. This self-awareness also plays a part in being **empathetic** because we understand the feelings of others better and can control how we express our emotions. We are then more socially aware and can develop resonance and maintain relationships with others.

The emotional and social intelligence leadership competency model Goleman and Boyatzis https://www.keystepmedia.com/shop/12-leadership-competency-primers/#.YiH7ay2l1R0 (accessed 04/03/22) highlights EI competencies as:

- Self-awareness – emotional self-awareness, accurate self-assessment, self-confidence.
- Self-management – emotional self-control, transparency and adaptability, achievement orientation and positive outlook, trustworthiness, conscientiousness, drive to meet internal excellence, taking the initiative.
- Social awareness – empathy and organizational awareness, ability to recognise the needs of others.
- Relationship management – influencing, coaching, mentorship and developing others, communication, being a change catalyst, conflict management, building bonds, teamwork and collaboration and inspirational and visionary leadership.

(Goleman et al 2002)

Furnham (2008) agrees with this and discusses emotional intelligences at work in the form of personal competencies:

- Self-awareness – emotional self-awareness, accurate self-assessment, self-confidence.
- Self-regulation – self-control, trustworthiness, conscientiousness, adaptability, innovation.
- Motivation – achievement drive, commitment, initiative, optimism.
- Empathy – understanding and developing others, service orientation, cultivating opportunities through different kinds of people, political awareness.
- Social skills – influence, communication, conflict management, leadership, being a change catalyst, building relationships, collaboration and cooperation, team capabilities.

It is worth thinking about what comes naturally to us in relation to these competencies. Also, what we struggle with, because then we can plan goals to address the challenges we face. If we do not have sufficient awareness about what we find difficult, we cannot work out what might be helpful. Also, if we cannot be honest about our own failings, we cannot help others to develop strategies to deal with their challenging areas. As leaders and managers we need to display EI ourselves to be effective leaders. We need to be motivated and self-aware and demonstrate empathy and social skills in order to accept responsibility and be accountable for our actions (Clancy, 2014).

We need to be aware of our own emotions to understand their effect on our behaviour and relationships. We then need to be able to self-manage and cope with our disruptive emotions so that we can be effective in challenging situations. Emotional brilliance is a term that Goleman (1996) used to describe very high levels of emotional intelligence, which is needed when we are feeling particularly threatened. So, when someone is angry with us about something that is really not our fault, we need to use our emotional brilliance to try to pacify them and de-escalate the conflict. We can also use our emotional brilliance to try to predict when conflict might start to occur. In order to do that we need to understand the stress of others and use our positivity to think the best of them, even though their behaviour is not showing themselves in the best light. We can also use our empathy and understanding of their feelings to bring their emotions out into the open, and try to seek common ground, so that we can seek solutions that are acceptable to all. As resonant and sensitive leaders (Goleman et al, 2002) we can coach others, and influence, inspire and motivate ourselves and others. This allows us to develop others' emotional intelligence too. We also need to create and sustain teams that can work towards shared goals through positive relationships and be able to be flexible and adapt to change. In order to do this, we need to have some organisational awareness so we can sense emotional undercurrents and influencing factors and dynamics which affect decision making.

Not everybody exhibits emotional intelligence though, and it can be hard working with someone who is not self-aware and does not manage their own emotions, or their stress. People who experience alexithymia have feelings but cannot put them into words, they lack self-awareness and insight and are "emotionally tone deaf" (Chambers and Ryder, 2012, p. 109). People like this can rise to the top of an organisation, and this can be true in health and social care too. They often interview very well and have a lot of evidence of having met targets, made major progress with projects and they excel in outcome measurable objective measures. However, this can be at the expense of collaborative team working, and they can cause a great deal of stress and distress within the work environment. You might want to think about who you might know who behaves in this way. They might, or might not, manage their own stress or understand yours, and sometimes their behaviour can be unreasonable in the workplace and they do not always manage their own emotions well. This can manifest itself in the person shouting, bursting into tears, precipitously leaving meetings, slamming doors etc, and definitely not demonstrating that they can manage their own emotions. This is incredibly stressful within any environment, and it is counterproductive in every way in a care environment. An example of a person who interacts in an alexithymic manner could be the Consultant Surgeon Sir Lancelot Spratt in the *Doctor in the House* (Gordon, 1952) book. He had no understanding of the emotions or sensitivities of patients in his care and caused great stress and distress to nursing and medical colleagues on his ward rounds. If you work with someone who operates in this manner in your work environment you need to find ways to manage situations that arise because of the inappropriate management of their emotions. You also need to find ways to engage with someone so that they understand the rationale for some action that you are recommending. For example, if you explained the need for an action based on the fact that members of staff were unhappy about a new initiative, this would be unlikely to be of interest to a manager who has an alexithymic approach. They would be much more likely to be concerned about how targets could be at risk because staff might leave. It might be necessary to address the problems that are being caused by someone with little emotional intelligence. However, if this person is creating a good impression to their managers because targets are being met to a high standard, then senior managers might be more concerned if there were starting to be complaints about harassment from members of staff, which could create additional work and concerns which might start to affect working relationships and practice. These are difficult issues to address and we need to have some political awareness and astuteness to identify the best ways to move forward. If these issues are left unaddressed then members of staff can feel demotivated, suffer low morale and be apathetic. Sparrow and Knight (2006) say that "where there is a sense of apathy within an organisation, staff morale will be very low and customer satisfaction poor" (p184). This is clearly crucial to patient satisfaction too, however, whether apathy leads to low morale, or whether low morale leads to apathy is open to debate and the cause and affect links can be unclear.

At the other end of the continuum from alexithymia is emotional brilliance where somebody is able to maintain their emotional intelligence, with all its empathy, self-awareness and management of emotion when there is a high level of stress within a situation. Goleman (1996) gives the example of emotional brilliance as being when dealing with someone at the peak of rage. However, another example could be when somebody is very unwell and is suffering distressing symptoms. Some managers, however, do not recognise the challenging situations that their staff experience on a day to day basis. In addition, they do not treat the people they manage with respect. They could express inappropriate emotions, and do not understand the emotions of others. They do not understand emotions and do not respond appropriately to them, and they are unable to problem solve or predict or deal with conflict. This is the antithesis of emotional intelligence and managers who lack self-awareness and cannot deal with their own stress or understand their emotional needs, or those of others, will cause additional stress to those they work with. In our last book there was a focus on stress within the workplace and we said that "leaders can be so stressed that they cannot identify unhealthy stress levels in their colleagues or understand that another change would be a step too far at the moment" (Chambers and Ryder, 2012, p17). This level of stress within the workplace is endemic within today's health and social care environment. However, if managers are this stressed they will act in a detrimental way to all those they work with. As Marques (2007) says, without emotional intelligence a leader cannot relate to the hidden messages behind what someone is saying, or the things that are not being said. Marques goes on to say that in terms of leadership, emotional intelligence and passion are interlinked. A leader needs to have a passion for their role and to identify the needs of the patients and the service they lead. Integral to leadership is the need to have charisma and love for our work, and the progress to be made, the people and the environment. It is clear that in Lisa's case study (5.6) she combined a passion for compassionate nursing care with advocacy for the patient in her care. She was then able to challenge the judgmental attitudes of her colleagues and escalate her concerns so that the fact that her patient was deteriorating could be recognised and treated.

So, what would a compassionate care environment feel like to those who work there? This would be when we feel supported by our team, where we feel able to ask for help and say when we have less knowledge or skills. We would also feel able to express feelings of under confidence and distress at the experiences that we have. That helps us to ask for support, and to receive it. Some practitioners and students can feel unsupported and leave, or feel very stressed and unsupported. So, a compassionate work environment is key to safe care for patients, and to health care practitioners being able to develop new skills and cope with the emotional demands of their roles.

Brand (2007) says that understanding our own emotions, and those of others, helps to reduce conflict in the workplace, and in the home environment. Focusing on the development of effective interpersonal relationships, combined with training on EI, helps us to manage our positive and negative emotions and control extreme negative emotions such as anger, stress and anxiety. This then has a positive impact on our relationships inside and outside work.

In a study at Edinburgh Napier University, EI was measured in nursing students throughout their programme. Although their EI scores did not appear to be related to their performance on the course as such, students whose EI levels fell sharply were more likely to leave. So, this could be helpful in relation to understanding recruitment and retention issues (Snowden and Stenhouse (2016). There needs be ongoing research about the impact of EI on patients and health care teams. However, rather like compassion we know what it is not sometimes more than what it is. When people lack EI we can see the problems this causes. We also know that EI adds to the art of nursing, and when combined with evidence-based practice we can be both effective and compassionate practitioners.

The Boston EI questionnaire (https//geminicapital.ie/wp-content/uploads/2021/12/The-Boston-EI-Questionnaire.pdf) is often used as a tool to measure EI and there are four possible responses to each of the 25 questions. The questions focus on self-awareness and self-perception, management of emotions, resilience and also the extent you can resolve conflict, demonstrate empathy and energise others. I have put together our own EI tool to help you to assess your own emotional intelligence, drawing on my reading and the perspectives of key leaders in this field.

QUESTIONNAIRE 5.1 Emotional intelligence

Think about the following statements in relation to yourself and score them according to the key listed below. Add strategies you might want to adopt and add a time frame for when you would like this to happen. If you are feeling brave you could also ask others to assess you on these statements and give you feedback.

Key	1 *Never*	2 *Rarely*	3 *Sometimes*	4 *Usually*	5 *Always*

1. Self-awareness

Statement	Score	What could I do about this and how soon do I need to do it
I know when I am happy and what makes me happy		
I am aware of when: • I am being unreasonable and why • I am getting annoyed or angry and why • My emotions are activated, and when I am being emotional, and why		

- Someone has upset me and why
- I am stressed and why
- I am anxious and why
- When I am avoiding tasks and why
- When my actions might have upset someone and why
- When someone is unhappy with me and why

| I tend to see the bigger picture and why people are acting as they are |
| I am aware of my weaknesses as well as my strengths |
| I am able to laugh at myself and see having a sense of humour as important. |
| I ask others for constructive criticism and feedback, and I tend to respond positively to this. |
| I like meeting other people, getting to know them and how they think, and I like communicating with others |
| I find people interesting and I ask questions and I like the differences there are between people |
| I try to see people as not being difficult but that they just think differently to me. I see them as a challenge in how I can communicate with them positively and win them over |

2. Self-management

Statement	Score	Comments/Suggestions
I can stay calm in stressful situations and can let go of stress/anger quite quickly once I have left the situation		
Others are often not aware of what sort of mood I am in and I can supress my feelings if I need to		
I can focus on changing my frame of mind and can often change my perspective on what is happening if I need to		
I am good at managing my time, multitasking, meeting deadlines and prioritising		
I think that motivating myself is important, especially if I am feeling low		
I can persuade myself to do tasks I do not want to do, and might do the difficult task first or might focus on doing one difficult task a day		
I am generally open and honest		

Statement	Score	Comments/Suggestions
I am generally able to adapt to new challenges and work out new strategies.		
I tend not to worry overmuch and am optimistic about life		
I like to focus on making the most of opportunities and taking the initiative when I can		
I try not to interrupt others and want to hear their views		

3. Relationship/social awareness

Statement	Score	Comments/Suggestions
I can sense the mood of a person, or a group, and can tell if people are not getting on with each other		
I am tactful and considerate when dealing with sensitive situations		
I enjoy relating to people from a range of different backgrounds and cultures		
I can understand the perspectives of others and can empathise with them		
I have got a good idea of what patients think is important, and what they need		
I can motivate others to deliver excellent patient care		

4. Relationship/social management

Statement	Score	Comments/Suggestions
I can inspire and encourage others and have a vision of what is important		
I believe that it is important to build good relationships		
I am a good listener and can empathise with others		
I can be a skilful negotiator and can understand others' perspectives		
I can predict and work towards de-escalating conflict		
I am passionate about what is important to me and can influence others		
I like to help others to succeed and develop		
I can be an effective change agent and can work towards overcoming resistance to change		
I am a team player and like to encourage others to work as a team		

Bradberry (2016) says that signs that we lack EI are that:

- We get stressed easily.
- We have difficulty being assertive.
- We have a limited emotional vocabulary and use few words to describe feelings.
- We make assumptions quickly and defend them vehemently.
- We hold grudges.
- We do not let go of our mistakes and dwell on them.
- We often feel misunderstood.
- We do not know our triggers.
- We do not get angry but emotions simmer inside.
- We blame others for how they make us feel.
- We are easily offended.

We need to train ourselves to think in more EI focused ways and then these negative and destructive emotions will be overridden by more positive emotions. Bradberry (2017) says that "emotional intelligence is a balance between the rational and emotional brain". He also says that EI is the foundation for critical skills such as stress tolerance, time management, decision making, change tolerance, empathy, teamwork, communication, presentation skills, anger management, trust, assertiveness, accountability, flexibility, social skills and customer service (Bradberry, 2017). In order to care for others and treat them with compassion we need to be able to show compassion to ourselves. This is a crucial part of EI (Heffernan et al, 2010).

Conversely, habits of emotionally intelligent people are seen to be:

- Labelling our feelings, rather than labelling people or situations
- Distinguishing between thoughts and feelings
- Taking responsibility for our feelings
- Using our emotions to help make decisions
- Showing respect for others' feelings
- Feeling energised not angry
- Validating others' feelings
- Practising getting a positive value from our negative emotions
- Not advising, commanding, controlling, criticising, blaming or judging others
- Avoiding people who invalidate us or do not respect our feelings.

(Chapman 2001 p88: summarised Hein's (1996) work.

Emotional intelligence allows us to use ourselves therapeutically to help others. We need to be aware of our own emotions, and those who we are caring for, to bring about positive outcomes for patients in our care. We also need to be emotionally intelligent leaders who can help colleagues through the inevitable changes that take place in the care environment. Hurley and Linsley (2012) highlight the importance of "resonant" or relational leaders who can reduce the emotional impact that change has on staff. Emotionally intelligent practice supervisors and assessors can also help students to cope with the many demands in new placements and in their professional development in their journey to become newly qualified nurses. Health care students need to anticipate and manage change on an ongoing basis, and they need to manage their emotions and their relationships with others through increasing their self-awareness, empathy and communication skills. Bar-On (2000) say that high emotional intelligence involves the following:

- Intrapersonal EI – self-awareness and self-expression which involves positive self-regard, understanding our emotions, being assertive and independent and maximising our potential through self-actualisation.
- Interpersonal EI – social awareness and interaction through empathy, social responsibility and mutually satisfying relationships.
- Adaptability EI – change management through validating our feelings in relation to external reality, coping with and adapting to change and problem solving.
- Stress management EI – emotional management and control through tolerating stress and controlling our impulses by constructively managing our emotions.
- General mood EI – self-motivation through a positive outlook, optimism, feeling content and happiness.

Sparrow and Knight (2006) also highlight the importance of self-awareness and self-knowledge as well as awareness of others. However, they also say that in order to manage ourselves we need to have the emotional resilience to bounce back, feel that we have some personal power, have goals but have some flexibility, be open and feel connected to others and be able to be trusted by others. In terms of managing our relationships we have to be able to trust others appropriately, have a balanced sense of optimism, or realistic optimism and be able to express our emotions but also control them. We also need to handle conflict and be assertive, be independent but also a team player. So, it is clear that if we are emotionally intelligent we have an innate sense of balance between:

- Being trusting and being able to trust
- Being independent but also part of a team
- Expressing emotions but also containing them
- Being optimistic but also realistic.

It is worth thinking about to what extent this balance is in our feelings and evident in our personal and professional lives. Emotional intelligence is crucial for compassionate communication and patient care, and for compassionate communication and leadership with colleagues. However, emotional intelligence is not the only intelligence that we use in our relationships with others. This will be discussed in the next section, but firstly it is important to sum up what we can do as individuals and leaders to maximise emotional intelligence.

The importance of different intelligences and cultural competence

In Chapter 2 the importance of using our different intelligences was discussed in relation to being compassionate. Furnham (2008) has identified these as being:

- Intelligence quotient (IQ) which involves processing information, a good memory and the ability to learn.
- Technical/Operational quotient (TQ) which involves our ability to manage ideas and projects, understand relevant technology and generally get things done.
- Motivational quotient (MQ) where we want to achieve, lead and succeed.

Table 5.1 Emotional intelligence as individuals and team leaders

Area of EI	What we can do ourselves	What we can do as leaders
Self-awareness	Accurate self-assessment Self-confidence	Understand the emotional needs of self and others Take responsibility for our own feelings Have positive values and take these from our negative emotions Treat others with compassion and provide support
Self-management	Self-control Adaptability Transparency Positive outlook Striving for excellence Be proactive	Treat everyone with respect Do not blame, criticise or control Be energised, have a love for our work and passion for compassionate care Use our charisma to make a positive difference
Social awareness	Organisational awareness Understand the needs of others	Be a visionary leader Be an effective leader Be a resonant and relationship orientated leader Political awareness and astuteness
Relationship management	Coaching and mentorship Be a catalyst for change Focus on communication Conflict management Emotional brilliance	Bring out the emotions of others and seek common ground Focus on stress management and recognise stress in individuals and situations Look for hidden messages behind words and actions Understand the rationale for actions and behaviour Predict and de-escalate conflict
Empathy	Understand the needs of others Cultivate opportunities to maximise potential	Develop others Create teams with diverse skills Be an advocate for others
Motivation	Drive for achievement Commitment to compassionate care Be proactive Be optimistic	Influence, inspire and motivate team members Create and sustain teams which are flexible and can adapt to change Enhance decision making Appropriate recruitment and staff retention Create compassionate teams and encourage teamworking and supportive relationships

- Experience quotient (XQ) which relates the quality and quantity of our experience.
- People quotient (PQ) which relates to our self-awareness and self-management of our motives, emotions, actions and the impact of these on others.
- Learning quotient (LQ) which involves our ability to think, manage and solve problems in different ways (Furnham, 2008, pp9–10).

We would also add another intelligence (Chambers and Ryder, 2012, p112):

- Cultural intelligence (CQ) which involves the ability to adapt to new cultural contexts and acquire new ways to deal with new situations (Gudykunst and Hammer 1983, cited in Berry et al, 2011).

Walsh (2019) discusses the importance of moving beyond self-awareness (how we are doing) to social awareness (how others are doing) to self-leadership (managing ourselves) and social leadership (influencing others). In order to do this we need to use all our different intelligences – this includes our evidence based (IQ) and technical knowledge (TQ), which builds on our past experiences (XQ) which allows us to maximise our learning and problem solving for this and other situations in the future (LQ). All these competencies are more around knowledge base and technical skills which we could say is more around the science of nursing; however, the softer skills are also crucial, and these are more based around the art of nursing. Our people skills (PQ), which incorporates self-awareness and EI and our cultural skills and experiences (CQ) allow us to adapt our compassionate communication to different people in a range of different situations. However, how we lead others in relation to all these areas depends on where our motivations lie (MQ), and what we believe is important to patients in our care, and the team we are part of.

Papadopoulos's model (2018) for culturally competent compassion in health care professionals highlights different components of cultural competence.

Cultural awareness	Self-compassion Universal elements of compassion Philosophies and religions
Cultural knowledge	Cultural compassion beliefs Cultural similarities and differences in understanding compassion
Cultural competence	Compassionate assessment Compassionate care giving Courage and compassion Barriers and challenges of compassion
Cultural sensitivity	Giving and receiving appropriate compassion Forming compassionate therapeutic relationships
Values	Human rights Citizenship
Principles	Intercultural education

Papadopoulos (2018) says that the following are essential prerequisites for culturally competent compassionate care:

- Understanding our own cultural values and beliefs and knowing how these impact on our understanding of compassion
- Believing that all humans should have equal value and respect
- Being motivated to learn about cultural health beliefs and behaviours
- Engaging with all patients through culturally sensitive and compassionate communication
- Having the humility to challenge our own assumptions and question our actions
- Providing all patients equal access to care and treatments
- Utilising all available resources – for example, interpreters to benefit the patients who need them.

This "takes time, education, good role models, a clinical environment that promotes and nurtures compassion and lots of practice" (Papadopoulos, 2018, p65). The importance of role modelling culturally competent compassionate care for colleagues and students cannot be underestimated and we also need leaders and managers who will demonstrate this in their attitude to patients and members of their teams, and inspire others to do the same.

It is useful to think about how we use our other intelligences in our practice, and our communication with others. Then we can try to develop our thinking further in relation to developing strategies focusing on sharing our thinking in order to help, inspire, motivate and lead others.

Why is empathy important in increasing positivity?

Morse et al (1992) explains their empathy model which differentiates between a patient or self-focused approach, which creates an engaged and connected approach, or alternatively an anti-engaged approach where the carer is protecting themselves from the sufferer's experience. It is important to differentiate between the extent to which an individual is giving learned responses, rather than spontaneous responses which might mean that they are pseudo engaged and professional, or not engaged at all and detached. The authors say that *pity* is an expression of someone else's plight, and *sympathy* is an expression of sorrow of that plight. *Consolation* moves on to trying to soothe distress but *compassion* shows recognition of that despair or pain, active listening and genuine understanding of their distress. Then we can go from *commiseration* and passive listening through to *reflexive reassurance* which is more active and tries to balance and counteract the sufferer's feelings.

Zaluski (2017) differentiates between the three types of empathy:

- *Perfect empathy* – which includes cognitive and affective empathy, and the tendency to take empathetic actions. Cognitively, it is important to truly understand from an ethical perspective the emotions of others. Affective empathy involves an ability to respond emotionally to the distress of others, and then empathetic action tendency means that we are likely to take actions to help or console others in an ethical way.
- *Truncated empathy* – lacks one component of the three areas (cognitive or affective empathy or empathetic actions), or one element exists in a very abbreviated form.
- *Contaminated empathy* – involves amoral or non-moral elements of perfect empathy where we might feel *relief* that we are not in the sufferer's position, *anxious* about whether this could happen to us, and feel pity which gives us a sense of *superiority* and *personal distress* at seeing the distress of others.

Zaluski (2017) says that if any of the four elements of contaminated empathy are present then the overriding feeling is *pseudo empathy*. Therefore, we need all elements of perfect empathy to genuinely care about others and to be compassionate. Minor (2018) says that doctors who are empathetic and build relationships with their patients train their emotional muscles better and become more emotionally evolved. They also treat themselves with greater compassion and are therefore more resilient for the future and can deal with challenges much better.

Brown https://www.youtube.com/watch?v=1Evwgu369Jw focuses on empathy and discusses the differences between sympathy and empathy. Sympathy is wanting to care for ourselves and at the same time being too critical of ourselves. We need to accept our differences and suspend judgement of ourselves and then forgive ourselves and realise that we all make mistakes. We can then be empathetic and can be in touch with how others feel which can lead to greater acceptance and learning about ourselves. Nyatanga (2019) also makes the distinction between *pity, sympathy and empathy*. If we are in a deep hole and someone comes along and says that I am sorry you are in that hole, that is pure *pity* which can be condescending and patronising. If someone gets into the hole with us they can experience the same feelings but can become stuck in the hole too, and that is *sympathy*. If a genuinely *empathetic* person comes along and actually tries to get us out of the hole, this is the most effective and compassionate response. This brings us closer to the patient and enhances their experience and helps their quality of life or end of life experience.

Denner et al (2019) talk about the importance of compassion and the different levels of communication in health care practice:

- Positively enriching communication means that patients express positivity about their care and there is a bond between the carer and the patient.
- Enriching communication where a carer shows genuine concern for the patient with good eye contact and warm communication, and the patient might or might not show appreciation for the care given.
- Neutral communication where there is no positive or negative impact, and the carer carries out care but in a mundane and functional way.
- Negatively controlling communication where no choice is given to the patient and the patient is excluded from the conversation and the carer appears reluctant, dismissive and possibly domineering and there is no eye contact and the patient can feel reprimanded or judged.
- Negatively restricting communication where the patient is ignored, told they are difficult, and the carer is rude or rough or leaves the call bell or table out of reach.

The differentiation in terms of communication can also be passive (you are ok, I am not), assertive (we are both ok) or aggressive (I am ok, and you are not). It is important to be assertive and this can be challenging when we are too busy and stressed. www.getselfhelp.co.uk/ccount/click.php?id=36 (Accessed 28/08/23).

Empathy is an important element of emotional intelligence and compassionate communication so try to think about the points that have been raised and maybe question whether you could adapt your approach to others and develop your empathy further.

Why is it so important to maximise our engagement and enthusiasm in our work?

There is a great deal of evidence saying being engaged and motivated at work makes us happier, and a positive work environment helps us, and others, to be happy. This in turn means that patients feel more positive, and that makes them more likely to maximise their own health potential and give us more positive responses and feedback. Again, this goes back to encouraging virtuous rather than vicious spirals (Campling 2013/2014) where negativity breeds more negativity, and positivity creates much better outcomes for us all.

A vicious spiral means that high job demands and low job and personal resources to deal with these can undermine any feelings of positivity. This leads to strain and work disengagement and low job performance and failure can easily follow.

However, the opposite can be true and in a virtuous spiral the job demands are also high but there are high job and personal resources to try to manage this. That can lead to high job crafting and greater motivation and work engagement which usually leads to higher job performance and achievement.

However, as has been said before it essential that a victim blaming approach is not taken, whereby the person suffering from burnout is criticised for their lack of stress management and resilience. The employer and those in a management and leadership position must take responsibility, and take action, when morale and motivation is poor. It is essential that a transformational leadership approach is taken in order to facilitate job engagement. Employees being over controlled and micromanaged is a barrier to job engagement and leaders need to promote a culture of social support and job-related feedback. Also, employees need to have space to be creative, skilled, learn new things and make decisions. Avolio et al (1999) says that leaders need to delegate responsibility and decision making, develop their employees, have a clear vision for the future and be optimistic, and communicate well with team members. Koppula (2008) talks about the importance of enthusiasm at work and feeling inspired, being immersed in work and persevering when things do not go well.

It is important that we can trust those in higher positions in our work environment. If there is a psychological breach in contract this links to altered "norms of reciprocity" and also to how supported and valued we feel. A breach in in the psychological contract will bring about a significant loss of resources in terms of how hard people want to work, and whether they want to stay in their role and organisation. This leads to even lower work engagement and job satisfaction. Unmet employee expectations will reduce employee engagement so managing an engaged workforce is crucial in ensuring positive employee attitudes and behaviour. Engaged employees have positive attitudes, are more likely to take the initiative, be more willing to develop their skills and abilities and feel more proud of their work. Therefore, considering the negative impact of a psychological breach in contract and the costs a disengaged workforce creates means that organisations should act quickly to restore broken promises when they happen Rayton and Yalabik (2014).

Low motivation is a significant predictor of burnout, and vice versa. However, feeling engaged at work has a positive impact on this and can mediate between emotional exhaustion, cynicism and turnover intention (Mangi and Jalbani, 2013)

Brummelhuis et al (2011) highlights the fact that increased job demands, for example work overload, and a decrease in job resources, for example social support and information, causes burnout. External regulation creates burnout and an accumulation of demands. Intrinsic motivation mitigates against burnout and resource loss, so it is an important factor in helping to break the negative cycle of burnout. Intrinsically motivated people are more likely to seek support and invest in collegiate relationships, cope more efficiently with tasks, participate in decision making and problem solve, and therefore make the most of resources available, and increase their part in these, whilst not decreasing their job demands.

A great deal has been written about workaholism, which is linked to emotional exhaustion, personal accomplishment and depersonalisation. This therefore is seen as negative and linked to "not working well" and to negative implications for co-workers and a need for professional assistance (Hamidizadeh et al 2014). Workaholics score high on perfectionism, non-delegation and job stress so it is important that individuals and organisations try to mitigate this. Too little engagement makes us more vulnerable to burnout whereas too much engagement, without being a workaholic, can lead to blocking of alert signals making us less likely to spot accumulating fatigue. However, there are different perspectives on workaholism.

The workaholism triad focuses on work involvement, feeling driven to work and work enjoyment. Workaholics score high on work involvement and feeling driven to work and low on work enjoyment. Whereas work enthusiasts score high on work involvement and enjoyment and low on being driven to work. Enthusiastic workaholics score high on all three area, work involvement and enjoyment and motivation to work. Having a positive view of workaholism is beneficial for individuals and organisations. A negative perception sees workaholism as an irrational commitment to excessive work and an addiction. The positive view is that workaholism is due to a love of work and the intrinsic desire to work long and hard because of this. (Spence and Robbins 1992).

Chirkowska-Smolak (2012) says that a high work demand may lead to emotional exhaustion, but we may retain our sense of vigour because we are achieving high standards in how we work. Exhaustion and vigour are not at opposite ends of the continuum. High levels of engagement might mitigate high demands. Therefore, organisations should aim to have high employee job fit and encourage role engagement, and also encourage an organisational culture which focuses on workload, recognition, values, control, fairness and a sense of community.

Engagement is the positive antithesis of burnout, and we need to focus on this as it will have a valuable contribution on our health and wellbeing (Maslach et al, 2001). Bakker et al (2011) says that:

> to achieve a genuine system of engagement we believe that employers and employees need jointly to craft a positive, trusting, civil, respectful, and mutually beneficial working relationship such that all parties genuinely believe there is the potential for equity, fairness, opportunity, and meaningful growth within the system. Just as at the level of the individual and the work team, we need systems, training, and supports to effectively work together and communicate with genuine openness, civility, and respect (Leiter et al, 2010 Leiter et al, 2011) — so too do organisations.
>
> (Bakker et al, 2011, p 85)

It is important to understand what motivates us. **Harmonising passion** is related to how employees perform. Enjoying the job and being willing to do what is necessary, rather than feeling obligated, reinforces individual identity, self-endorsement and volition. It is important that we do not just feel obliged to do more. If we are highly engaged we are able to also detach from work when necessary and enjoy other parts of our lives. **Obsessive passion** is an internal driver which helps maintain self-esteem, and feeling socially accepted and valued by others. Therefore, enjoying work gives an ego boost but if we are consumed by work to such an extent that we are unable to disconnect this leads to conflict in all domains of our lives. High job demands can cause obsessive passion, and increase obligation, and therefore increasing obsessive passion, to the detriment of harmonious passion, will make it less likely for us to enjoy our jobs. This can be because of constantly dealing with patient demands which can make it difficult to detach ourselves when doing admin tasks or relaxing at home (Trepanier et al, 2013).

Job resources contribute not only to work engagement but also to prevention of burnout via harmonious passion. It is important to take into account the type of passion employees have when assessing their psychological needs. It is not necessarily the amount of investment employees put into their work, but rather the quality of their investment, that predicts how they will function at work. People who are harmoniously passionate would be able to release themselves from work as they would have a higher sense of volition and flexibility. For example, if people are tired and cannot concentrate they are more likely to disengage from their work without feeling guilty or anxious, which prevents further energy depletion Harmonious passion creates higher work engagement, higher emotional energy and fulfilment and, because of increased flexibility, we are more likely to focus better, complete tasks and achieve positive outcomes. Whereas people with obsessive passion are too inclined to work hard but not enjoy their work and not achieve positive outcomes. People with harmonious passion are doubly beneficial in terms of psychological health at work because they are less exhausted and have more vigour. Obsessive passion creates psychological costs due to high exhaustion but they are less likely to seek social support or make best use of job resources to mitigate their exhaustion. From the organisational perspective employers need to:

1. Exercise some sort of control to either reduce job demands where possible or help employees' perceptions of demands, for example by focusing on self-efficacy.

2. Increase positive and stimulating job characteristics because this can buffer high job demands.
3. Promote harmonious passion at work by increasing autonomy and flexibility in relation to individuals' work.
4. Increase feelings of authenticity in individuals' roles which helps promote engagement.

Job demands and resources can influence whether somebody is harmoniously passionate or obsessively passionate which then has an important role in predicting psychological gain and costs at work. (Trepanier et al, 2013)

Workaholism tends to be viewed negatively and people who work hard can be perceived as being overly dependent on perfectionism and achievement. However, if we are work enthusiasts we would see work as a positive and something that motivates and inspires us. (Snir and Harpaz 2004) We are therefore more likely to feel fulfilled and fulfilment relates strongly to engagement and these both have a mitigating impact on burnout. Feeling engaged also has a positive impact on our work attitudes. Drivers such as high-level supervisor support, a sense of autonomy, use of skills as well as personal resources such as optimism, positivity, resilience and hope are all more likely to increase our role engagement. (Priyadarshi and Raina 2014)

Work engagement is a state that involves vigour, dedication and absorption. Job and personal resources are the main predictors of engagement and this becomes even more crucial when job demands are high. Engaged employees are more creative, more productive and more willing to go the extra mile. They also perform better, experience more positive emotions, including happiness, joy and enthusiasm. They are also more healthy and create their own job and personal resources and transfer their engagement to others (emotional contagion). So, it is essential that organisations work towards creating and sustaining work engagement. Individuals need to be given more choice and control and have the right skills and attitudes and engage in a constant programme of personal career development (Bakker and Demerouti, 2008).

Gutermann et al (2017) say that employee engagement is positively linked to performance, and negatively linked to turnover intention. Leaders who are engaged are more positive leaders and they are more likely to create an organisational culture of engagement. Organisational strategies for fostering engagement at a managerial level could include making engagement a focus of leadership development efforts and having this as a core organisational value. This could then cascade down through managerial levels in terms of promoting high quality leadership and development. Focusing on work engagement, relationship building and maintenance and having large scale work engagement surveys could also promote engagement in employees. Having this organisational emphasis could provide starting points for development workshops to help to foster a positive work engagement culture.

Cankir and Arikan (2019) say that job satisfaction seems to be a more powerful predictor of negative attitudes such as intention to quit, whilst work engagement may be more related to positive results like performance. The findings of their study were evaluated by considering the previous literature on job satisfaction and performance relationship, which have been debated since the1950s. In accordance with the current literature on work engagement they concluded that work engagement could be a better predictor of performance for education sector employees, but this applies to many work environments, including health care. I have summed up the findings of Blanch et al (2018) in the table below (Table 5.2).

Table 5.2 Characteristics of engaged workers (Blanch et al, 2018)

Personal attributes	Health attributes	Work attributes	Impact on the work environment
Active Autonomous Self-reliant Responsible Optimistic Flexible Adaptable Proactive Motivated Energetic Have a positive self-concept Self-evaluation skills Self-esteem Have social skills Do not undermine ourselves Self-efficacy Have realistic Expectations Be secure in self and abilities	High levels of physical and mental health High levels of well being Low levels of anxiety, depression and burnout Emotionally stability Low levels of exhaustion and malaise/illness	Quality of work life High performance Take the initiative Creative Achievement motivated Loyal and committed to the organisation Show minimal intention to leave job, organisation and profession Require less supervision Satisfied with their work Problem solve in relation to work demands Complain little Rarely conflictive and generates few tensions	Craft job to restructure job demands and job resources which acts as a buffer and helps to meet organisational goals Create a positive social climate and a great place to work where there is: Low turnover intention, absenteeism, accidents, injuries and conflict, errors, High levels of productivity, innovation and employee performance Help to create a more competitive and sustainable organisation

Bakker et al, 2011, say that engaged employees influence their colleagues and therefore they tend to work better as a team. They are not passive in their work environment, but act as change agents when required. Engaged employees have "greater psychological capital, seem to create their own resources, perform better, and have happier clients" (p 17). So, are there any downsides of being engaged? Having higher self-esteem can lead to an over confidence and an underestimation of the time needed to carry out work and can create unrealistic expectations and unrealistic optimism leading to inappropriate persistence. This can hinder subsequent performance and cause frustration and diminished productivity. Also, engaged employees can become workaholics and a lack of work life balance can lead to health problems. The authors also say that high arousal can be distracting for cognitive performance. So, it is worth bearing these points in mind.

In conclusion, the main drivers of work engagement are job and personal resources. Job resources reduce the impact of job demands on strain, are functional in achieving work goals, and stimulate personal growth, learning and development. In addition, job resources particularly have motivational potential in the face of high job demands. Also, engaged employees do seem to differ from other employees in terms of their personal characteristics. They score higher on extraversion and conscientiousness, and lower on neuroticism. Further research could take this thinking further. Finally, engaged workers possess more personal resources, including optimism, self-efficacy, self-esteem, resilience and an active coping style. These resources seem to help engaged workers to control and influence their work environment. Further research could examine whether engagement helps individuals to cope with their demands, mobilise their resources, stay healthy and perform well. More than just considering employees as a means to achieve the desired end of higher performance, positive organisational behaviour approaches must also include the pursuit of employee happiness, health and engagement as viable goals or ends in themselves (Bakker, 2009). I have tried to sum up the difference between high and low engagement on a personal and organisational level in the table below (Table 5.3).

The importance of fostering work engagement has been discussed, both in ourselves and our teams, but this relies heavily on being happy, positive and optimistic, which protects and enhances our wellbeing. So, this will be discussed in the next section.

Table 5.3 High and low personal and organisational engagement characteristics

High engagement – personal	Low engagement – personal
Happier and more optimistic staff Exercise high job crafting and create our own job role and use choice and control Are highly motivated and have high job satisfaction, job performance and achievement This leads to positive patients who give positive feedback Enthusiastic and have a sense of vigour Have high personal resources – extravert, optimistic, high self-efficacy, self-esteem, resilience and coping strategies Contribute to a positive work environment which creates virtuous spirals. This helps with emotional exhaustion, cynicism and low turnover intention Mitigate high job demands with high job and personal resources Are work enthusiasts who are highly involved with work and have a drive to work but also enjoy their work	Work strain and disengagement Low job performance and failure Too high self-esteem can cause overconfidence, underestimation of the time needed and unrealistic optimism High job demands and low job and personal resources and cause vicious downward spirals Too high levels of arousal can lead to reduced cognitive performance

High engagement – organisational	Low engagement – organisational
Take action when morale and motivation are low Create a positive and stimulating environment Use transformational and relationship focused leadership which promotes engagement Promote a culture of social support and constructive job feedback Understand the difference between work enthusiasts and workaholics Understand that inspired employees who are immersed in their work also persevere when things go less well Give space to allow people to be creative, learn and make decisions and act as change agents Delegate responsibility and create decision makers who take the initiative Ensure that there is a high job fit at recruitment Recognise work overload issues and take action as possible Focus on values, fairness, equity, openness and a sense of community Be optimistic and enthusiastic in communications and give clear information Give high support which creates optimism, autonomy, positivity and resilience Focus on employee health, happiness and engagement Create a culture where employees feel trusted, valued and supported Encourage harmonising passion which allows disengagement from work at times and prevents further energy depletion Foster feelings of choice, autonomy, authenticity and flexibility	Victim blame when people are suffering from burnout and blame poor stress management and resilience Overcontrol and micromanage. Too much regulation leads to high demands being made and increased burnout. Create unmet expectations and breaches in the psychological contract Are not aware that low motivation creates burnout and vice versa Do not help to avoid workaholism where there is high work involvement and drive to work but poor work enjoyment Do not discourage obsessive passion where there is a poor work life balance where staff are not able to switch off from work and are more susceptible to health problems Do not focus on work engagement and relationship building and maintenance Do not create career development opportunities Do not carry out engagement surveys and facilitate workshops on being engaged Are not engaged and do not role model this and facilitate more engaged staff.

How do positivity, happiness and wellbeing interact with each other?

Recognising when situations are becoming too much for us, and there is a shift in the negativity we feel, is crucial. Teater and Ludgate (2014) say that it is important to identify exactly what emotions we are experiencing, and how intense these are. We also need to identify which situations make us feel this way, and our thoughts and beliefs in relation to the distress we feel. So, our emotions, the trigger, and our automatic thoughts are important. If we can identify these we can then analyse the impact of these thoughts and beliefs.

We need to think about what makes us feel negative in order to understand what would make us feel more positive. Fredrickson (2009) says that we can choose to see many experiences in a positive or a negative light. If we let our negative side take over, we let our frustrations make inroads into our positive feelings, which creates more negative feelings.

If we choose to take the positive view it makes us more positive, and others too because emotions are contagious. We need to recognise that feelings of joy are rare and elusive so we need to actively seek and recognise when we are feeling happy and celebrate this. Sima (2022) refers to this as "joy snacking", where we recognise times when we are happy and content through each day and mindfully focus on these feelings. Savouring these small pieces of joy through the day can really increase our happiness and our feeling that our lives are meaningful. Positive emotions trigger upward spirals for ourselves and others and we need a 3:1 ratio of positive to negative thoughts to be able to be sensitive and give more to others

So, positivity stops us feeling negative and creates a tipping point where good things are more likely to happen.

However, we need to understand that being overly optimistic can lead to unmet expectations which can increase our negativity. We need to be realistically optimistic so that most of the time our expectations are met. We need to use our emotional intelligence to do this, and recognise that "being nice" does not mean that we let everyone trample over us. Assertiveness is part of being aware when we are not being treated fairly and well, and then doing something about it. Sometimes we have to make waves in order to protect ourselves, patients in our care, and colleagues. However, how we do this is crucial to our success and we need to use our communication skills, and how we manage ourselves, to keep calm and exercise our assertiveness so that conflict is not created.

David (2018) is concerned about the "tyranny of positivity", where we only strive for happiness and only perceive pleasant emotions as good. She says that this can mean being rigidly positive even in the face of obvious problems. This can lead to greater unhappiness and lower levels of resilience. David (2018) says that we need to build our lives around what we value, and happiness will be a by-product of this. For instance, if there is an ethical lapse, or someone voices racism, or a co-worker's rudeness harms another, the emotionally intelligent response would not be silence, but rather speaking up to call attention to the problem, even if that creates a ripple of hard feeling (Goleman, 2022).

Ballatt and Campling (2011) make the same point about kindness not being just warm and fuzzy sentimentality that does not fit in the challenging complex world of health care. They say kindness inspires a focus on the efforts of staff in their relationships with patients and each other. "Kindness is not a 'nice' side issue in the project of competitive progress. It is the 'glue' of cooperation required for such progress to be of the most benefit to most people" (Ballatt and Campling, 2011, p16). Fredrikson (2013) makes the same point that positivity is not just mindless optimism but about optimistic attitudes triggering positive emotions. Brain imaging studies found that pleasure centres in our brains light up when we act compassionately, in the same way as when we eat chocolate, or something similarly pleasurable (National Institute of Health (2014). Happiness is about the small things that go right every day, rather than the rarer bigger events in life. Health, happiness and success are generated also by our emotional intelligence (Sparrow and Knight, 2006).

Eudaemonic refers to what is conducive to happiness. Fredrikson (1998) refers to positive emotional states and Isen (2000) discusses how being positive can help us to make better decisions and think better (Fredrikson and Branigan, 2005). This links to psychoneuroimmunology which refers to how our psychology impacts on our brains and produces different chemistry that impacts on our immune systems. If we are happy our brains produce serotonin which stabilises our mood, endorphins which reduce pain, dopamine which is the reward chemical and oxytocin which is the love hormone. These are soothing system chemicals which we need to feel mentally well. So, our mood is more stable, we feel less pain and feel more rewarded and loved. Mental Health England has some excellent resources to help with our positivity and thought processes https://mhfaengland.org/mhfa-centre/resources/.

However, we can often undermine our own potential to be happy and we need to work out how we can do this. So, I have put together the questionnaire below so that we can work out ways that we can inadvertently do this (Questionnaire 5.2.).

QUESTIONNAIRE 5.2 Ways we undermine ourselves and increase our unhappiness

Adapted from Teater and Ludgate (2014) *Overcoming Compassion Fatigue: A Practical Resilience Workbook*

What messages do you give yourself?

We tend to be much more critical of ourselves than we would be of others. We can easily make ourselves feel bad and we do it without thinking. We genuinely believe that our perspective is accurate, but it could be just the way we are feeling, and not the whole picture. We can do this all the time, particularly when we are feeling at our lowest. We can alter how we think about things and catch our negative thoughts before they make us feel worse. Try to identify your negative messages in the following questionnaire. How much of the time do you give yourself these messages:

5 = All of the time, 4= Most of the time, 3= Sometimes
2= Occasionally, 1= Very occasionally, 0= Never

Seeing things in terms of extremes:

Everything is either a complete success or a complete disaster. For example, you make one small mistake and the whole occasion/day is ruined for you.

5	4	3	2	1	0

Examples and how it affects your life:

_____

_____

Making one negative thing an example of things always going wrong:

You feel like bad things are always happening to you. For example, you always feel like you are in the slowest lane in the car or the supermarket.

5	4	3	2	1	0

223

Examples and how it affects your life:

_____

_____

_____

Always seeing the negatives:

You always zone in on the negative side of situations and experiences. For example, you are given a lot of very positive feedback about how you handled a situation and you start worrying about the one aspect that someone said that you could have done differently.

5	4	3	2	1	0

Examples and how it affects your life:

_____

_____

_____

Predicting the worst outcome:

You hear about a bad situation that has happened to someone else and you immediately think that will happen to you too. For example, someone is being investigated for a possible brain tumour and you immediately think that is what it will be. Then you think that your occasional headaches might also be caused by a tumour.

5	4	3	2	1	0

Examples and how it affects your life:

_____

_____

_____

Trying to read other people's minds:

You start to think that you did not handle a situation well, and then assume everyone is thinking that too. For example, someone is busy and rushed and you assume that you have upset them in some way.

5	4	3	2	1	0

Examples and how it affects your life:

_____

_____

_____

Thinking that you can predict the future:

You assume that the only possible outcome of a situation is that you will fail in some way. For example, you are planning to discuss a change in how you need to carry out something at work and you automatically think that the other person will take this the wrong way and they will be upset with you.

5	4	3	2	1	0

Examples and how it affects your life:

_____

_____

_____

Making things bigger or smaller:

You either make things seem more important than they are if you receive some negative feedback. Or alternatively, you underplay the importance of something that someone says that puts you in a positive light. For example, you carry out something well and all but one comment praises you for how clearly you explained the situation. These positive comments you ignore as being what anyone would be able to do. However, you do keep returning to the one comment that says that they could not understand one small point about what you were saying.

5	4	3	2	1	0

Examples and how it affects your life:

_____

_____

_____

Viewing a situation from an emotional perspective:

You assume that how you feel about something that happened is an accurate representation of what actually took place. For example, you assume that because you are feeling anxious that something bad is going to happen.

5	4	3	2	1	0

Examples and how it affects your life:

_____

_____

_____

Thinking in terms of should or musts:

You think that you "should" always act in a certain way or that things "must" get done that way. For example, you think that you should have cleaned out the fridge by now, or that you must always do the washing on Saturdays.

5	4	3	2	1	0

Examples and how it affects your life:

_____

_____

_____

Describing yourself in a negative way:

You think of yourself as unattractive, unable to communicate well with others, or unsuccessful in certain situations. For example, you tell yourself that everyone will think that you are a failure, or that you always look a mess, rather than acknowledging that we all get things wrong at times, and we cannot look good all the time.

5	4	3	2	1	0

Examples and how it affects your life:

Blaming ourselves when it is not our fault:

You always assume that you were the one that should make things go well, and that it is your fault that it did not, even though the situation was not totally within your control. For example, you assume that if someone seems unhappy it is because you must have upset them in some way.

5	4	3	2	1	0

Examples and how it affects your life:

Focus on one of your negative thoughts:

- What was the negative thought?

- How much do you believe this as a percentage (0–100%)?

Evidence for thinking this way	Evidence against thinking this way

- How much do you believe this now (0–100%)?

- What do you intend to do to further test for this thought:

How can you deal with negative thoughts more effectively:

- What stressful situations are you dealing with?

- Which situations make you feel worse about yourself?

- How do you feel emotionally and physically when these situations arise?

- What are you thinking at these times?

- How do your feelings affect your behaviour?

- What do you believe about yourself that contribute to you feeling this way?

- What is the evidence for and against thinking this way?

- How could I think about this in a different way?

- What is the worst thing that could happen?

- What would I do if the worst did happen?

- What is the likelihood of things going this badly (0–100%)?

- What could I do to help me to deal more effectively with this situation?

- What can I do and how can I think that will help me to deal with this sort of situation in the future?

- What can I do in the future to help me to reduce my feelings of stress, distress or inadequacy?

- In what ways have I changed how I feel since I have started to think about this differently?

- Are my strategies working, if not what else could I try?

This last questionnaire has hopefully helped you to work out what sort of negative messages you give yourself, and how perceiving life experiences in terms of extremes, and what others think, and what we think we must do, all creates self-blame and this all has a negative impact on our happiness. Focusing on a negative thought and really thinking about how true this is, and how much we actually believe it, can help us to deal with these negative thoughts more effectively.

Pessimistic approaches are problematic because this leads to learned helplessness and is related to the inability to influence outcomes. Pessimism is strongly linked to depression and inertia, and this makes us feel bad and makes us less likely to succeed in the future and this leads to poor physical health. We can choose to be more optimistic but we have to reset our innate ability to be positive. We can learn to reprocess our thoughts and see stressors as a challenge not a threat. We also need to think about how we can practice random acts of kindness and be grateful for what we have in our lives (Achor, 2011a).

Fox (2012) makes a strong case for optimism. Optimism originates from 'optimum', or the best possible so this means accepting that there are inevitable challenges and limitations and then working through strategies to minimise these. Pessimism originates from 'pessimus', which is the worst possible, and every setback is seen as evidence that the world is against us. If we see things in this way, we will always find proof of this. Optimists, however, see problems as challenges to be overcome, whereas pessimists see problems as insurmountable and not within their power to overcome. Anhedonia is the inability to experience pleasure, which can be part of pessimism or depression. If we cannot enjoy positive experiences or sensations, for example tastes and smells, and focus on negative thoughts, both can have a negative impact on our ability to be happy, positive and optimistic. Rozanski et al (2019) says that greater optimism can lead to better problem solving and less depression, which in turn can lead to greater recovery after cardiovascular events, and mortality from many causes.

Being positive is not just the opposite of being negative and we can reduce our negative thoughts without increasing our positive thinking (Watson et al 1988). We can also increase our positive thinking without reducing our negative thoughts (Garamoni et al 1992). So, we need to work on both our negative and positive thinking. This involves being realistically optimistic because unrealistic optimism is not healthy because we are not prepared for the reality of situations as they occur. We need to think ahead, anticipate challenges and increase our problem solving. We also need to seek advice and support which helps us to enhance our coping strategies (Style 2011).

Lyubomirsky (2007) says that sustainable happiness is possible through focusing on positive emotions and happiness, being motivated and committed and focusing on increasing the number of positive experiences and increasing the social support we have. So, first of all we have to be honest about assessing how happy we are, and how happy we think that we could be. Lyubomirsky (2008) says that it is essential that we practice being grateful and positive and taking care of our bodies and souls through meditation, acting happy, exercising and giving ourselves the opportunity to be spiritual, as well as managing our stress and focusing on our coping strategies. We need to forgive ourselves as well as others, and that can be very difficult to do, because self-compassion is difficult, and we often have higher expectations of ourselves than we do of others. Seldon (2015) says that:

> the happier we become, the more energy we have, the more committed we feel and the more we engage with others. The less happy we are, the more energy is sucked out of us. Life becomes heavy and dull and even simple tasks become an effort.
>
> (Seldon, 2015, p71)

We need to try to move beyond happiness to joy by accepting ourselves and others and having a sense of belonging. This also involves having character virtues that help us to live fulfilling lives, strengthening our resilience, empathising and the ability to show compassion, focusing on our goals, giving to others which energises us, and being healthy in mind, body and emotions and maximising opportunities for happiness.

So, we need to think about what constitutes feelings of happiness and sadness, though this might seem obvious. Feelings of sadness and happiness are all on a continuum (Sand 2017). When we are sad we can be more tired than usual and lack energy but the furthest end of this continuum is deep lethargy and exhaustion, where we want the world to stop and not be here anymore or in the worse case actively wanting to die. We could feel a sense of foreboding, be tearful and wobbly and want to cry or even cry uncontrollably. Feelings of happiness can be on a continuum from light sensations, bubbles in our stomach, feeling enthusiastic, inner joy and warmth and even wanting to embrace someone or kiss or dance.

I have designed the assessment tool below (Questionnaire 5.3) to help you to assess feelings of sadness and happiness and how often they occur. Feelings of happiness could be as simple as:

- Getting a new edition of a magazine you enjoy.
- Someone saying something nice to you.
- Having something nice to eat.
- Time with friends and family.
- Someone recognising something that you have done, or a skill you might have.
- Having a long bath.
- Accomplishing something that you find difficult or completing a task that needs to be done.
- Eating something nice is very transitory, but eating that food with friends makes memories and is much longer lasting.

Once you have assessed how much happiness you have in your life, and what makes you happy, and to what extent, you can work on increasing how often these happen. So, for each part of the day think about whether anything has happened which makes you feel content or happy, and give it a score out of 10 for its impact on your happiness levels Then you can focus as much as possible on increasing these activities in your life (Sand, 2017).

QUESTIONNAIRE 5.3 Happiness and sadness assessment

Assess your sadness and happiness in relation to the highest score at each point on every day that you want to assess. Then plot your scores onto the assessment grids for the week. Try to think about what you did to dispel feelings of sadness and encourage feelings of happiness. Then assess your whole week in relation to your feelings of happiness and sadness and try to analyse your overall assessment of how the week has been for you.

Feelings of sadness	Score	Feelings of happiness	Score
More tired than usual	1	Feeling positive	1
Feeling of foreboding	2	Feeling that something good might happen	2
Lack of energy	3	Feeling bubbly	3
Feeling tearful	4	Feeling invigorated	4
Feeling wobbly and anxious	5	Feeling energised	5

Wanting to cry	6	Wanting to smile	6
Feeling distressed	7	Feeling passionate about something	7
Crying uncontrollably	8	Wanting to laugh	8
Deep unhappiness	9	Laughing	9
Exhaustion and wanting to sleep all the time	10	Having fun with others	10
Wanting to sleep forever and never wake up	11	Wanting to make others happy	11
Wanting to stop the world and leave your troubles behind	12	Feeling as if you could do anything	12
Feeling suicidal	13	Feeling joyful	13
Having suicidal plans	14	Wanting to dance and sing	14

Sadness assessment grid

	Mon	Tues	Weds	Thurs	Fri	Sat	Sun
Sadness highest score	3		6		7		
Positive actions	Mon – woke up tired and went to work and felt better Weds – feeling tired and miserable in the evening, had an early night Fri – argument with friend, felt better when we discussed how we felt						

Happiness assessment grid

	Mon	Tues	Weds	Thurs	Fri	Sat	Sun
Happiness highest score		7	5		10	13	
Positive actions	Tues – got involved with a new project Weds – did a work task well Fri – went out with friends, and despite the argument had a great night Sat – had a great first date						

Overall assessment for the week

Day	Comments
Mon	Felt tired when I woke up and did not want to get out of bed. Once I was at work I felt more positive.
Tues	Got involved with a new project and felt positive as a result.
Weds	Did a work task well and felt like I had accomplished something to a high standard. Felt tired and miserable in the evening though, so I had a bath and an early night and felt fine in the morning. Today had its highs and lows but overall it was not a bad day
Thurs	Usual day at work and a quiet evening in and I did not feel particularly positive or negative

Fri	Went out for a night out. I had an argument with a friend which really upset us both. However, we talked it through and we enjoyed ourselves afterwards and I had a great night overall
Sat	Had a great first date with someone who I had been interested in for a while. We arranged to see each other again which made me happy
Sun	Quiet day in doing chores and preparing for another week. Did not feel particularly positive or negative
Week assessment	Managed to achieve things at work, had a good night out with friends and started a new relationship. Overall assessment: a good week
What I have learnt and what I want to take forward	Work makes me happier than I realised and achieving things does make me feel better about myself. At times I do not feel that happy but it could be a good day overall. When I have arguments it is important to sort them out and then we can still both have a good evening.

Sadness assessment grid

	Mon	Tues	Weds	Thurs	Fri	Sat	Sun
Sadness highest score							
Positive actions							

Happiness assessment grid

	Mon	Tues	Weds	Thurs	Fri	Sat	Sun
Happiness highest score							
Positive actions							

Overall assessment for the week

Day	Comments
Mon	
Tues	
Weds	
Thurs	
Fri	
Sat	
Sun	
Week assessment	Overall assessment:
What I have learnt and what I want to take forward	

Having focused on our feelings of happiness it might be helpful to see how much balance we have in our lives in terms of physical, emotional, social and intellectual health, because we do not always think about what generates happiness in relation to all these areas. We can neglect one area, by focusing too much on another. So, if we work hard but are not intellectually stimulated, or focus on our physical health to the detriment of our social and emotional health we will not be happy. We need balance in all areas of our life.

We also need to have the impetus to take control over life's issues by having a strong self-concept, and Rungapadiachy (2008) sees this as being hierarchical in nature, with physical, social, emotional and intellectual self-concepts being part of this hierarchy. We need to have a strong **physical self-concept** in relation to our physical appearance, our body image and our physical strengths and weaknesses. Many people do not have this and feel disadvantaged by how they think people view them physically and therefore they lack confidence in how confident they feel in other areas of their self-concept. They become under confident in their **social self-concept**, and in their relationships with others which impacts on their interactions, roles, status, sense of autonomy, loneliness, dependence and interdependence with others. That in turn can impact on **emotional self-concept** and on feelings, such as anger, anxiety, fear, shame and joy, and on moods, such as feeling depressed or elated. Finally, our sense of **intellectual self-concept** can be impaired, and our ability to be receptive to new learning and thoughts, and to express ourselves in language that others can identify with can also be impaired. We need our thinking to be clear, rather than confused, and to solve any problems that arise in our lives. Therefore, it is imperative that we have a positive self-concept in relation to how we look, how we interact with others, how we are emotionally and how we think and learn. If we are not capable of having a positive self-concept this will minimise our ability to take control of our lives, and make the changes that we need to, in order to make a positive contribution to society and to making our lives as positive as possible. If we can see that any of these areas of self concept are weak in ourselves it is important to identify potential ways to strengthen these so that we can maximise our self-efficacy and the extent to which we can make change happen in our lives and our work environments.

I would suggest that you do the questionnaire below (Questionnaire 5.4) to see how balanced you in terms of your total health.

QUESTIONNAIRE 5.4 Assessment of total health questionnaire

Activity	Do already	Do more
Physical health		
• Plan regular exercise during your week		
• Take the opportunity to increase your exercise during the day when possible, for example walking upstairs rather than taking the lift.		
• Walk briskly for a short burst of time		
• Take a walk before bedtime		
• Go for a swim		
• Take part in fun activities – dance, swim, walk, sing, play sports		

- Eat regularly
- Eat healthily
- Sit down and enjoy a really good breakfast
- Take time to relax after a busy morning and enjoy your lunch
- Plan to take time to really enjoy your supper
- Eat calmly and in a relaxed way
- Seek medical help when you are ill
- Take time off sick when you are unwell
- Take all your annual leave entitlement
- Go away on holiday
- Take mini vacations and day trips
- Spend time away from phones, computers, social media
- Wear clothes that you like
- Get enough sleep
- Any suggestions....

Activity   *Do already*   *Do more*

Emotional health

- Look for things to make you laugh out loud
- Allow yourself to cry
- Spend time really enjoying music
- Watch a film or television for pure enjoyment
- Think about ways to decrease your stress levels
- Read for pleasure – short stories, magazines, books, poetry
- Take time to express your caring and affection for friends or family
- Take time to be sexual
- Tell yourself how well you have done when something was not easy
- Think about what situations, places, activities, things and people you find comforting and then actively think of ways to experience these more
- Practice saying no sometimes and think about what situations you need to do this more
- Practice receiving back from others – time, praise, gifts etc
- Listen to your thoughts and notice your beliefs, attitudes, values and thoughts
- Do something where you are not the expert or in charge
- Make quiet times in your life
- Take a break during the day
- Any other suggestions....

Activity	Do already	Do more
Social Health		

- Spend time with people whose company you enjoy
- Stay in contact with important people in your life, however far away they live
- Think about being in contact with *all* of your family (if appropriate)
- Entertain people at your home
- Spend time with children or animals
- Spend time outside and enjoy the feel of being outside
- Think about what is meaningful to you and find ways to explore these activities more
- Contribute time or money to causes you believe in
- Find a spiritual or community connection
- Take time to chat with work colleagues
- Give and receive support from others
- Any other suggestions…

Activity	Do already	Do more
Intellectual health		

- Feel genuinely stimulated intellectually by your job
- Enjoy a good discussion with friends
- Become involved with interests outside your job
- Reread favourite books, watch again programmes and films that you enjoy
- Be curious about things
- Develop a new hobby
- Write in a journal or a diary
- Focus on times when you feel positive and happy, and spend time doing these things more
- Any other suggestions….

Having balance in our lives is important for our wellbeing as is knowing what makes us happy. The Oxford Happiness Guide (Hills and Argyle, 2002) highlights the importance of a sense of wellbeing, self-esteem, a sense of purpose, social interest and humour. These all help our level of happiness. In terms of what we do we need to have a certain level of person activity fit (Lyubomirsky 2007). We all have things in our jobs and in our lives that we feel forced to do, and others that we feel guilty if we don't do them. If we don't put the bins out on a Sunday night we will miss the weekly rubbish collection which will cause all sorts of practical problems, as well as making us feel guilty. There could be monthly reports or statistical analysis of what we do at work which is mandatory. This is a JFDI or a Just Fliipping (or whatever seems most appropriate in the situation) Do It. We all have these parts of our jobs, and we might procrastinate, but they haunt us until they are done. Other things we feel guilty about, and we feel guilty until we phone that friend who is having a hard time, for example. More positive motivators are the activities that we enjoy, or those that are in line with our core values. In addition, some things come naturally to us, and we enjoy and value these activities. If we stop feeling guilty and do the JFDI activities that we need to, and we also have many activities in our lives that we actively enjoy and value, then we will be happier.

However, we also need to focus on exactly how we will make changes in our lives. Oettingen (2014) advocates the WOOP approach. We need to plan for realistic setbacks and how we intend to overcome them:

- Wish – what do we want to happen
- Outcome – visualise a positive result
- Obstacle – what challenges could arise
- Plan – to overcome the challenges

If we want to be more healthy (W) we might want to go running after work(O) however we realise we might be tired and hungry (O) so we need to plan to put our running shoes by the door and have a high protein snack on the way home from work (P). This is just a simple example, but this approach helps our positive intentions to become a reality in our busy lives.

It is crucially important that we focus on being positive, having a balance in our lives and being aware of the negative messages we give ourselves and what makes us happy and sad. Being positive prolongs our lives by 7–10 years (Fredrikson et al, 2008) because it promotes our mental and physical health.

Seligman (2006) says that pessimism is self-fulfilling, and when things turn out badly it becomes a catastrophe in our mind and makes us less likely to succeed in the future. Seligman says that the 3Ps of pessimism are **personalisation** when you believe the worst of yourself and take things personally, **permanence** where you believe the worst will be true forever, and **pervasiveness** where one thing going wrong impacts on every other aspect of your life. Seligman (2011) says that wellbeing is associated with positive emotions, engagement, interest, meaning and purpose. This involves having self-esteem, optimism, resilience, vitality, self-determination and positive relationships.

The brain is like Velcro for negative experiences and they stay with us and are difficult to detach ourselves from, whereas positive experiences ate like Teflon and slide away and do not stay with us as long. https://headstrongmindset.com/velcro-teflon-theory/.

In a previous article I have focused on the importance of being positive (Chambers, 2017) and the need to develop our own strategies for staying positive and realistically optimistic. We all need to work out what will work for us personally in terms of being positive and not listening to the negative voice inside our heads.

Fox (2012) says that pessimists become fixated on things going wrong, rather than optimists who look for signs of things going well. So, optimists see problems as challenges to overcome, whereas pessimists perceive problems as insurmountable and not within their capacity to control or overcome.

We need to focus on being the best version of ourselves as much as we possibly can. Achor (2011b) says that we need to avoid the "error of the average" where we only aspire to be at "normal" levels for everything. At some things we will excel. We need to focus on possibilities and opportunities to make this happen. Achor (2013) says that we need to imagine being successful and then build goals to get there and give ourselves positive messages rather than negative ones. If we only do what everyone else is doing, we will only achieve the same types of things. We need to create new strategies and ways of doing things. For example Freddie Mercury and Queen challenged existing ways that popular music had been happening. Queen's Bohemian Rhapsody was much longer than music tracks had been and included an operatic style section. If they had just accepted the norms of the time then we would not have been able to experience tracks like this.

Pamela Wible (2012) the primary care physician in Oregon, whose approach was discussed in Chapter 2) created an innovative family care facility. She is an excellent exemplar of making change happen in her community and her work environment, and she was able to see herself as an effective agent of change, and create the change that she wanted to see, in health care in her community. She clearly had a hardy personality, because despite how stressed and depressed she felt in her previous role as a doctor, she was able to take responsibility for creating the change she wanted to see in her life and in health care. She was therefore able to create a health care service which patients wanted. She was committed to solving the problems that she saw in the current service provision and had a strong sense of self-efficacy and an internal locus of control and created a change which led to a coherent service which made sense to her.

Pamela Wible (2012) experienced positive emotions, engagement and positive relationships, and accomplished a great deal with true meaning in relation to the health care services she developed. Her wellbeing and positivity shine through her book which details her experiences in setting up her ideal clinic. It is clear that her clinic would be a very positive place to work. So how can work environments become positive places to work, and foster a sense of wellbeing amongst those who work there, and why is it so important that employers create a positive work environment which does this?

Pamela Wible (2012) clearly moved away from feeling depressed and unable to derive any pleasure from her previous role as a doctor, to increasing her connection with others and creating a more person-centred health resource. She used her personal resources and her abilities as a physician to function at a high level, and therefore increased her feelings of happiness and satisfaction. She increased her wellbeing in terms of connecting with others, carrying on learning, being curious and active and giving something to her local community that they valued. Heidegger (1966) referred to the concept of gegnet in relation to wellbeing, which is a combination of dwelling and mobility. In other words, the ability to feel at home with ourselves combined with the ability to move forwards in our thinking. Wible (2012) must have felt a sense of confidence in her own ability to develop a service that met the needs of patients, as well as feeling the sense of drive to move forward and provide that very innovative "ideal" clinic environment.

Fredrikson (2009) says that positivity includes joy, gratitude, serenity, interest, hope, pride, amusement, inspiration, awe and love. She also says that we need a ratio of 3:1 positive to negative thoughts to be able to be sensitive and give to others. Then we can reach a tipping point (Gladwell, 2000) where we can make things shift towards the more positive. We need to actively focus on being positive and increasing our positive thoughts to make this happen.

Seppala (2016) says that in order to be happy we need to:

- Stop chasing the future and live in and enjoy the moment.
- Step out of overdrive, manage our stress and tap into our natural resilience.
- Manage our energy by creating times of calm.
- Get more done by doing more of nothing and be mindful and revisit the pleasure of having fun and being idle.
- Be good to ourselves and enjoy a successful relationship with ourselves by being less self-critical, focusing on our strengths and self-compassion.
- Show kindness and compassion to others and ourselves.

There are strong overlaps between positivity and happiness as can be seen in the table below (Table 5.4).

Table 5.4 Aspects of positivity and happiness

Positivity	Happiness	References
Choose to be positive Focus on positivity breeding positivity – virtuous circles Snack on joy and create and savour moments of joy Focus on realistic rather than over optimism Be assertive and be an advocate for others Recognise issues and deal with them Be better at decision making, clearer thinking and peripheral vision Counter negative messages to ourselves Avoid catastrophising and polarised views Create balance in our lives – physical, emotional, social and intellectual Be emotionally intelligent and emotionally agile and learn new skills Be grateful Aspire to be the best version of ourselves and avoid the "error of the average" Be kind and practice random acts of kindness Be open minded, engaged and curious Forgive others	Focus on happiness and what causes this in our lives Be hopeful, optimistic and future minded. Have positive values, positive emotions Being happy in the moment and creating happiness opportunities Have a sense of accomplishment Be a courageous leader. Use your strengths. Create a tipping point for change Being happy increases our resilience and problem solving. Persevering when there are challenges Be playful and have a sense of humour. Enjoy beauty, excellence and have a sense of spirituality Manage our energy and enjoy moments of calm. Have a strong self-concept and positive identity and social competence Essential for happiness Exercise self-control and be a loyal team player and connect with others Be passionate and enthusiastic Be honest, generous, genuine and kind. Be humble and modest. Open your heart Be curious and interested in the world and enjoy learning. Crucial to life satisfaction Be non-judgemental and merciful	Teater and Ludgate (2014), Fredrickson, (2009), Watson et al (1988), Hills and Aryle (2002), Lyubomirsky (2007) Sima (2022), Sand (2017), Style (2011) David (2018) David (2018), Seligman (2006b), Fox (2012), Gladwell (2000) Fox (2012), Style (2011) Fredrikson (1998), Fredrikson et al (2008) Isen (2000), Fredrikson and Branigan (2005) Garamoni et al (1992) Griffiths and Robinson (2009), Baylis (2009) Seligman (2011) Achor, 2011b) Ballatt and Campling (2011) Style (2011) Griffiths and Robinson (2009) Seligman (2011) Seligman (2003, 2006, 2011)

Summing up the connections between positivity and happiness there is a ripple effect of gratitude, happiness and positivity and this spreads to others and they are likely to be happier too. So random acts of kindness can be beneficial to ourselves and others.

If we are optimists, we are more likely to be healthy, less stressed, bounce back faster, have more persistence and spread joy. We can also make others' lives better. This is a quote from a patient about a student of mine, Jo, and a colleague:

> I never thought heartbreak could be mended in the Acute Assessment Unit – without surgery. These two ladies fixed my heart with laughter, joy and happiness. Although I don't want to come back here for treatment, they have made my stay memorable, which means that I might come back for check-ups.

Eleanor Roosevelt said "happiness is not a goal, it's a by-product". If we chase happiness, it is illusive, we need to live lives of purpose and meaning. We don't have to find happiness; it will find us. She goes on to say that:

> paradoxically, the one sure way not to be happy is deliberately to map out a way of life in which one would please oneself completely and exclusively... For what keeps our interest in life and makes us look forward to tomorrow is giving pleasure to other people.
>
> https://www.goodreads.com/quotes/1413647-
> happiness-is-not-a-goal-it-is-a-by-product-paradoxically

So, optimism and happiness are co-dependent and mutually reinforcing. They also have a real effect on our wellbeing.

The key difference between those who have a sense of wellbeing, and those who do not, is the ability to cope with life's problems and challenges, and to be happy and satisfied with life

We chose to work in health care because we wanted to care and if we are unable to do this our stress increases and this contributes to burn out and exhaustion. If we are not able to act compassionately our health and wellbeing deteriorates due to ethical distress (Mendes 2017) because our values are being compromised. So effectively our relationships with patients and clients are "sustaining, not draining". (Youngson 2012 p80).

Webb (2012) differentiates between people who are drains and those who are radiators. Drains are negative, apathetic and drain the enthusiasm out of us whereas radiators exude warmth, vitality and energy. Csikszentimihalyi (2002) says that flow is key to this because flow is the ability to be totally involved in the positive aspects of experiences. Some people have "autotelic personalities" and can create this positivity even in the most challenging of circumstances. They create opportunities out of challenges and create their own enjoyment. Rubin (2016) says that we need to create habits in our lives which are just instinctive, and we just do them regardless. She discusses the importance of meeting our own expectations, and not just trying to meet the expectations of others, so what do we want to achieve in life and how are we going to go about making these things happen? Rubin (2009) also says that we have to make an active choice to be happy boosting our energy, focusing on our relationships, aiming high, pursuing a passion and acting happy. In order to do this, we need to connect with others, be active, take notice and be curious, keep learning and give or do something nice for others. This increases our connections with others and links our happiness to that of the wider community (New Economics Foundation 2008). This has been used in some community and mental health settings but it has not been adopted in hospital settings to any great extent.

I have encapsulated the different components of wellbeing in the last book in Figure 5.1 (Chambers and Ryder, 2019, p 132).

In order to practice wellbeing we need to focus on our positivity and happiness in a meaningful manner and I have put together the following table (Table 5.5) to draw on themes, emotions and actions. You might want to think about these characteristics and how you can increase these in your personal and professional lives.

Having focused on positivity, optimism and happiness and how these are crucial for our wellbeing, the importance of taking a mindful approach will be discussed, and how to create opportunities to do this.

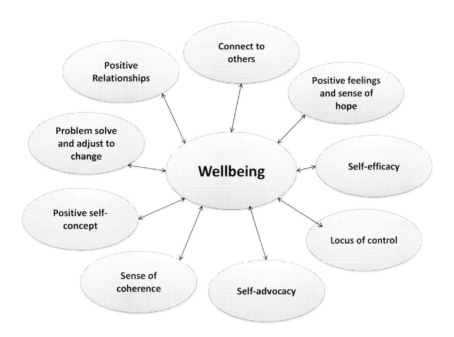

Figure 5.1 Characteristics of wellbeing (Chambers and Ryder, 2019, p132)

Table 5.5 Aspects of positivity, happiness and wellbeing

Themes	*Emotions and actions*
Positive emotions	Honesty, kindness, genuineness, generosity, savouring goodness, modesty, humility, finding positive meaning
Engagement	Playfulness, sense of humour, passionate and following passions, enthusiastic, be a radiator not a drain
Interest	Curiosity, loving learning, open minded, opening our hearts and minds, creativity
Meaning	Fairness, equity, common sense, dreaming about the future, spirituality
Purpose	Sense of purpose, perseverance, being a leader, being courageous
Self-esteem	Be good to ourselves, stop being so self-critical, increase our self-compassion, focus on our strengths, have a positive self-concept – physically, socially, emotionally and intellectually
Optimism	Be aware of beauty and excellence, be grateful and hopeful, be optimistic, be future minded and connect with the future
Resilience	Practice self-control and focus on self-awareness, stress management, focus on our natural resilience
Vitality	Manage our energy and motivation, create moments of calm and do nothing, practice mindfulness
Self-determination	Focus on our strengths and what we want to achieve, be a problem solver and a change agent, have a locus of control and a sense of self-efficacy and be a self-advocate, have a sense of coherence
Positive relationships	Non-judgemental, open minded, keep a sense of perspective, be a team player, be loving and allow others to love, be loyal, use our emotional intelligence, be cautious and discrete, forgive others and connect with others

Mindfulness and the window of tolerance

Mindfulness is present moment awareness when we pay attention to our thoughts, emotions and feelings as they are happening, and we can then adopt an attitude of curiosity and compassion. This can help us to deal with difficult emotions, fluctuations in our mood and physical pain. Then we do not react and get stuck on autopilot and our normal responses to emotional triggers. Mindfulness teaches us to:

- Be more present and engaged in everyday life, rather than being lost in thoughts about the past or worries about the future.
- Step out of autopilot so we can be more purposeful in our day-to-day choices.
- Notice our direct experiences (body sensations, emotions, thoughts) whether they be pleasant, unpleasant or neutral.
- Regulate emotions and ride the waves of intensity.
- Learn to respond rather than react to or avoid difficulties.
- Relate to ourselves and others with kindness, warmth and compassion (htpps://www.stmichaelshospital.com.pdf/programs/mast/mast-session1.pdf).

Mindfulness is perceived as a process of interrupting the cycle of pain, stress, reaction and suffering by focusing on acceptance, kindness and choice. When we experience primary suffering, this can lead to increased resistance which can lead to secondary suffering and increased mental and physical symptoms. We can put too much emphasis on constantly rethinking situations and catastrophising, and this increases our anxiety and fear. Mindfulness can reduce this secondary suffering and we need to focus more on self-soothing and calming and building resilience and making genuine choices. As Monson says "we can't direct the wind, but we can adjust the sails" https://www.goodreads.com/quotes/499597-we-can-t-direct-the-wind-but-we-can-adjust-the-sails. So we cannot change the stressors that life brings but we can alter our responses to these stressors.

As nurses we need to multitask all the time so that we can keep shifting our priorities as situations change. A study by Anthony et al (2010) found that intensive care nurses are interrupted between 2 and 23 times an hour, and this leads to negative outcomes and errors. However, this ability to flit from one priority to another and have butterfly or grasshopper thinking can mean that we never slow down and concentrate on the here and now. Sheridan (2016) says that if we calm down and concentrate for longer we pay more attention, increase our memory skills, boost productivity and reduce our stress levels. So, we all need to learn to be more mindful, and this involves being more present in the here and now. To practise mindfulness we need to focus on the moment in an intentional way, being present in the moment, and not being judgmental about where these feelings take us. Sometimes this involves a couple of minutes in the middle of very stressful situations, and sometimes this involves a longer pre-planned time. Focusing on mindful breathing can be helpful and Sheridan (2016) refers to the 3Ps whenever we approach a patient. We can **P**ause, take a breath and let go of being in "doing" mode. We can then be **P**resent by noticing our own body sensations, thoughts and emotions, accepting them for what they are. Finally, we can **P**roceed to doing what needs to be done and go back to "being" mode.

Chaskalson (2011) discusses the importance of mindfulness in reducing psychological distress, negative thoughts and defensive or aggressive responses. This can have an impact on addictive behaviour and can reduce blood pressure and hospital admissions for cardiac, cancer related and infectious diseases. Mindfulness is also associated with increasing attention span, and we can feel more in control, increase our emotional intelligence and have more satisfying relationships and better communication strategies. Gilbert and Choden (2013) highlight one of the challenges of mindfulness is that our minds so easily get pulled away from the present moment, by anticipating "what if" situations in relation to what could happen in the future, or what could have happened in relation to events that have happened in the past. Mindfulness can help us to witness from a distance the constant chatter and drama that goes on in our minds and analyse this less emotionally.

Siegel (2015) says that **hyperarousal** is the body and mind's response to perceived threat and our survival mechanisms kick in where we think it is better to be safe than sorry. When we cannot fight or flight we tend to freeze and shutdown. This leads to being overactive with unclear thoughts and being emotionally distressed. **Hypoarousal** creates tiredness through inactivity, and we become depressed, lethargic, numb and unmotivated. The optimum comfort zone where we are able to self soothe is our **window of tolerance** (Siegel, 2015). This is where we feel safe and supported and this further increases our window of tolerance. Our emotional resilience capabilities are increased, and this can widen our window of tolerance and prevent dysregulation. So, we need to balance our **drive systems** where we pursue and strive for achievement and our **threat systems** where we feel angry, anxious and are prone to self-criticism. We do this by using our **soothing systems** where we feel calm, safe, cared for and nurtured (Gilbert, 2010). We can deactivate our fight and flight responses and activate our soothing systems with a focus on our breathing which can stimulate or calm us in rapid and powerful ways.

Gilbert (2010) discusses emotional regulation systems where we switch between three systems to manage our emotions. These systems are firstly the **Drive** system which relates to what drives us and relates to our feelings of want, achievement and progress. Secondly, the **Threat** system which helps us detect threats and protects us. Feelings associated with this are anxiety, anger and disgust. Lastly, the **Soothing** system which helps us to manage our distress and promotes bonding, and that is related to feelings of contentment, safety, protection, trust and feeling cared for. Distress happens when there is imbalance between the systems. This is often associated with under development of our soothing system.

External threats are in our environments where deadlines and physical dangers can threaten us. However, there are also internal threats like threatening appraisals we make about ourselves, or any psychological events or emotions which can trigger physical symptoms. Compassion focused therapy has been developed to help with mental health issues which are maintained by feelings of shame or self-criticism. Feeling shame and self-criticism are very destructive emotions and the most powerful antidotes to these feelings are empathy and compassion. We need to be helped to normalise our experiences to reduce feelings of shame. This allows us to feel healthy pride, self-compassion and self-acceptance. In order to prevent the damaging effects of shame we need to build our own resilience so that we generally feel safe and in control and accept the things that we do not have the power to change. When mistakes happen we need to see them as teaching and learning events. (Cole, 2020). Corrigan et al 2011) state that focusing on the window of tolerance with people who have had severe traumatic events such as childhood abuse can increase emotional self-regulation and maximise the effects of pharmacological treatments.

Chen et al (2021) in their literature review of mindfulness interventions in relation to nursing students found that mindfulness significantly reduced symptoms of depression, anxiety and stress and enhanced students' positive benefits from mindfulness strategies. Lomas et al (2018) also carried out research with health care professionals and came to the same conclusions about the efficacy of mindfulness. Whitton et al (2019) found similar benefits with patients with mental health issues in a day hospital in Scotland where there was an eight-week intervention focusing on mindfulness enhanced wellbeing. Therefore, their results would indicate the importance of nursing educators adopting mindfulness interventions within nursing curricula. Focusing on self-compassion can help those of us who have experienced trauma, and are not sufficiently compassionate towards ourselves and are self-critical. Mindfulness is associated with higher levels of compassion satisfaction, quality of life and lower levels of burnout and secondary traumatic stress which are major components of compassion fatigue. Learning how to observe, describe and act with awareness and without self-judgement can reduce our negative responses and increase our social competence and general wellbeing (Magmanlac et al (2019).

However, it is important to acknowledge that intolerable work pressures and workloads, low morale, bullying and poor management cannot be rectified by stress management, resilience or mindfulness strategies and interventions. This merely shifts the blame on to individuals and means that organisations do not take responsibility for their poor work environment. Westphal et al (2015) state that work related interpersonal conflict in the emergency department led to higher levels of burnout, and they found that mindfulness reduced depression, anxiety and burnout, and taking other measures to reduce conflict at work was more helpful. The causes of the stressors are then reduced, reducing stress on the individuals involved, taking away the need for mindfulness interventions.

Mindfulness exercises can be challenging but if we focus on taking control back and increasing self-awareness, memory and concentration then we can become more engaged with life and can change how we think. We need to move away from constantly doing to being more in a "being mode" where we are consciously aware and living in the moment. This can reduce anxiety, stress, depression and sleep problems.

The mental health continuum recognises that we are all on a continuum in relation to our mental health with five zones of mental health. At the less positive end of the continuum we are in **crisis mode** when we have acute physical or psychological symptoms, or a lesser form of this can indicate that we are in **struggling mode** when we feel down or anxious and have poor concentration. Or we could be in **unsettled mode** where we are easily distracted, feeling out of sorts and not wanting to do our usual activities. We need to move on to being more in **thriving mode** where we feel positive and calm and then we can start to be in **excelling mode** and be joyful, energetic and focus on solutions. https://delphis.org.uk/mental-health/continuum-mental-health/.

So how do we focus on mindfulness. Firstly, we need to increase our awareness of what is happening at the moment and our breathing. We can then accept what is difficult in our lives and not judge ourselves for finding this difficult, so we show compassion towards ourselves. We can then notice the beauty around us, recognise the need to take a break before it is absolutely necessary, and focus on performing random acts of kindness and meditating on a daily basis. We need to make sure that we have created time and space and are comfortable prior to any mindfulness, relaxation or breathing exercises.

Various mindfulness exercises can be helpful:

- Focus on one constant stimulus for 10mins (a sound, your breathing, the edge of the desk, a candle flame).
- Our mind tends to be anywhere than in the present, and this is our mind functioning on autopilot.
- Whenever your attention wanders bring your focus back.
- What did you notice?
- Were you able to catch your autopilot?
- Where did your mind wander to?
- How long did you manage to stay with the stimulus alone (average 3–4 seconds only)?

- Can you try to work on increasing the time you continue to stay focused?
- We need to connect to our senses and concentrate on what we can see, hear and feel.
- Then we focus on our breathing and taking mindful breaths.
- Be aware of our bodies and the movements we are making.
- Be aware of our emotions and what we are feeling without judging ourselves for those feelings.
- Notice our thoughts, are they about current, past issues to the future and are they associated with worries or future plans. (Snyder 2014 p251)

We can then cut this down to a couple of minutes that we can incorporate into our usual working day. Or we could use this as a pre sleep meditation when we go to sleep at night.

Mindful seeing:

- Sit by a window and look out.
- Notice what you see and do not label things as a tree or a road but notice the textures and colours.
- Notice the movement of the grass or trees and the shapes things make.
- If you become distracted bring your mind back and think about the textures and colours.
- **Focus on your 5 senses**:
  - Notice 5 things you can see
  - 4 things you can feel
  - 3 things you can hear
  - 2 things you can smell
  - 1 thing you can taste

Alternatively, we can do a body scan and think about different areas of the body one by one from our toes upwards. This can be another way to practice mindfulness.

Practising mindfulness and not letting our negative thoughts take over can be essential in helping us to stay as positive as possible. However, increasing our emotional intelligence, and other intelligences, as well as our empathy can also have an impact on our positivity. Staying engaged and enthusiastic at work and in our personal lives can also be signs of our positivity, and this leads to even more positive thinking.

RECOMMENDATIONS FOR LEADERSHIP AS INDIVIDUAL PRACTITIONERS, LEADERS AND ORGANISATIONS

As has been discussed, positivity, happiness and wellbeing are all mutually reinforcing for ourselves, and we can be a catalyst for positive thinking in others. So, how can we take a lead on positivity as individuals and leaders and how can organisations foster this approach too?

Focusing on positivity and compassionate care as individual practitioners and leaders

As individuals we need to think exactly how we can increase our ability to be compassionate towards ourselves. There are various unhelpful ways in which we make things difficult for ourselves, and strategies which we could use to lower our anxiety (Table 5.6).

If we are as compassionate as possible towards ourselves, then patients in our care, their loved ones and our colleagues will benefit from this and we can be a more

Table 5.6 Strategies to help us to be positive and compassionate towards ourselves

Unhelpful thinking:	*Helpful strategies to reduce worry:*
• Black and white thinking and thinking of polarised options where only two possibilities are true. All or nothing thinking and wanting perfection • Disqualifying the positive • Emotional reasoning – making assumptions based on our feelings about what might be true and assuming we know how others are thinking and feeling • Personalising and taking things personally – blaming ourselves when there were other factors at play or blaming others when we were at fault • Over generalising based on single events • Maximising or minimising the importance of an action or a person's views • Jumping to conclusions – imagining that we know how others are feeling or trying to predict the future • Thinking that we "must" "ought" or "should" do things increases our feelings of guilt • Mental filtering – only taking notice of some types of evidence • Catastrophising, blowing things out of proportion or minimising the importance of things so they feel less important • Labelling ourselves or others in a negative way. • Making predictions that all will turn out in the worst possible way and we will not be able to cope.	• Talk it out • Write it out • Shrug it off – relaxation exercises • Breathe it away – breathing exercises • Sort it out – practical possible actions • Delay it – put it aside for a worry session at a later time • Work it off – physical exercise • Reverse it – think about taking the opposite approach and explore alternatives • Laugh it off • Distance it – how will this feel in a few years • Balance it – think about the good consequences and imagine those instead • Cancel it – think positively and do not let your negative thoughts drag you down • Exaggerate it – what is the worst that could happen • Win through it – imagine yourself being successful and feel good about it • Hold it – pause, think and take a fresh look • Escape it – notice something enjoyable around you, think yourself into the present. Expect to feel sad at times • Keep active, keep dancing and keep moving • Spend our money on experiences that will make us happy, rather than accumulating more things • Carry on learning • Have a strong sense of meaning and purpose which emphasises our values and character strengths and helps our wellbeing. That could mean having a job that does all those things. • Maybe get a pet • Enjoy nature • Eat healthily and think about our alcohol consumption • Remain spiritual and sexual and embrace our emotions • Look after ourselves and don't be a martyr but do things for others • Sleep as well as you can and have a morning routine that sets us up for the day

positive influence in our work environment. However, we also need to take a lead in ensuring that others do the same.

Goleman (2023a) says that if we hone our emotional intelligence skills, which are skills that can be learnt, this will advantage us in our personal and professional roles. When something triggers us we need to pause before reacting so that we can maximise our self-management and relationship management. We are more likely to be successful at work, and be a much more positive leader, if we have high emotional intelligence. If we are self-aware then we are more likely to possess many of the other emotional intelligence talents such as conflict management and empathy, and we are more likely to retain staff in our teams. There appears to have been a decline in how people manage their own behaviour in the last three years, however empathy levels do not appear to have declined in the same period of time. If patients, families and colleagues, as well as our organisational managers, are failing to control their own behaviour this puts a great deal of stress on us. However, if we also behave in a negative manner this will further exacerbate the situation. So self and relationship management is paramount in order to keep our teams in a state of high-level functioning, and for us to maintain our resilience.

Reis da Silva (2022) highlights the importance of "soft" skills which are the non-technical skills or personality traits which we use in our practice. These can be more difficult to define and measure than the "hard" skills such as venepuncture. However, as Reis da Silva says they:

> are the skills which are measured by every patient and relative. These include communication, compassion and patience, flexibility, adaptability, emotional stability, honesty, team-playing, work-ethic, time management, situation awareness and leadership. In a nutshell, emotional intelligence.
>
> (Reis da Silva, 2022, p 573)

Emotionally intelligent leaders are self-aware and empathetic. They also have high levels of self-regulation, and are aware of their personal values and are able to maintain, compose and demonstrate accountability. Their social skills including conflict resolution and communication skills foster team loyalty, and their high levels of motivation encourage optimism and motivate others.

An essential part of emotional intelligence is using our empathy appropriately. Goleman (2023b) says that there are three types of empathy that a leader can demonstrate. *Cognitive empathy* involves reading how others think and seeing their perspective and helps you to communicate with them in ways that resonate with them. *Emotional empathy* involves sensing how they feel which allows you to adapt your emotional tone to adjust to how they are feeling. Both of these types of empathy also work in the leader's best interests too. So, you can get the communication right from the start which reduces conflict, builds better relationships and takes less time. The third sort of empathy is "*empathic concern*" and this involves understanding how others think and feel, but also involves caring about them. This level of concern is what employees value most and this allows them to relax more because they know that their manager has their back and this inspires greater loyalty and a much reduced employee turnover. This again involves the best use of resources because staff turnover is very costly in terms of time and it destabilises teams and can encourage others to consider leaving too.

The pandemic has undoubtedly put stress on those working in health care, and morale is at an all time low (Ford, 2023a). More than 40% of staff in a study in 2023 said that their mental health was bad or very bad and that it was significantly worse than it had been during peaks in the pandemic. Strategies like restorative supervision can be successful in different aspects of nursing and health visiting (Kearney, 2023) and if we do not take time to care for ourselves then we cannot help others (Ford, 2023b). Resilience based clinical supervision had been set up for a critical care outreach team in Northumbria before the pandemic and this continued through the pandemic. It was difficult to carry on these meetings due to social distancing and being able to be physically together, so these meetings continued virtually. This safe space to discuss their emotions and focus on self-care enabled staff to move on from feeling threatened and anxious, to focus more on compassion and mindful approaches and being aware in the moment. Attendees were appreciative of the restorative element of the supervision, despite being sceptical at first, and were really positive about the sessions. If this type of intervention was rolled out more extensively this could increase the level of compassion in the organisation as a whole (Markham et al 2022). In another initiative a nurse lifeline had been set up nationally on weekday evenings to support nurses who were struggling (Griffiths, 2023). Hoyle (2023) talks about people being burnt out and stresses the importance of us knowing our tipping point, and being aware that perfectionists are more at risk, and many nurses do take on too much and want to do everything to a high level. If we are not sleeping well and are using negative coping strategies such as eating, smoking, drinking alcohol more than we were before, it is important that we recognise this and take action.

As leaders we need to demonstrate ethical and inspirational leadership. Ethical in terms of being honest, equitable, impartial, respectful and competent (Gillon, 1994). Also, to make sure that we are values-based in what we do. This involves selflessness, integrity, accountability, objectivity, openness, honesty and leadership (Nolan 1995 cited in Palfrey et al, 2006). Also, we need to be inspirational and be able to motivate others towards change and encouraging best practice (Table 5.7)

Focusing on positivity and compassionate care as organisations

There are many strategies which we need to use within our teams and these need to be also promoted by our employers at an organisational level. Key approaches which might be helpful at organisational level are:

- Reflection, and restorative supervision which focuses on what has happened in practice and developing coping strategies (Wallbank, 2013).

Table 5.7 Characteristics of ethical and inspirational leadership (Chambers and Ryder, 2012, p70)

Northouse 2009	Gillon 1995, in Palfrey 2006	Nolan Committee 1995, in Palfrey 2006	Westwood 2010	Wedderburn Tate 1999
Character of the leader		Selflessness Integrity	Courage and confidence	Welcomes challenge Resilient Intuitive about when to trust people and information Does not always know that they are a leader
Actions of the leader			Communication and negotiation Coaching Creativity Cheer (or compliments)	Encourages work/life balance Concentrates on objectives Gives and receives compliments
Goals of the leader	High levels of competence	Leadership	Consistency Clarity Connection	Political astuteness
Honesty of the leader	Respect Honesty	Openness Honesty		Emotional stability, and IQ. IQ is not necessarily the most important attribute
Power of the leader				Accepts they cannot always win
Values of the leader	Equity Impartiality	Objectivity Accountability	Compassion	

- Compassionate resilience – responding positively to adversity through self-compassion in challenging situations.
- Values-based employment and recruitment (NHS Constitution 2015) based on the values of respect, dignity, everyone counts, compassion, quality and the 6Cs – care, compassion, competence, communication, courage, commitment (DH, 2012).
- Encouraging being flexible in empathetic responses so that empathy can be turned on and off as the need arises, rather than being anxious in empathetic responses where we can be left feeling unable to deal with the pain of someone else 's situation.
- Appreciative enquiry which focuses on what is going well rather than on what is going less well (Cooperrider and Srivastva, 1987).
- Setting a clear and compelling vision for expected knowledge, values and behaviours is a realistically optimistic and motivating organisational approach. Encouraging an optimistic culture where people acknowledge setbacks and see these as temporary means they often try even harder to overcome obstacles in the future.

I have summed up strategies for resilience-based approaches below (Figure 5.2).

Finally in this chapter I want to sum up my thoughts about different strategies to promote positivity in ourselves, but also as leaders within the team. As I say, leaders can be at any level within an organisation, and we need to take a lead in promoting positivity with our colleagues and in our teams. However, these strategies also need to be promoted at organisational level (see Table 5.8).

This chapter has focused on the importance of remaining positive and engaged at a personal and professional level, as individuals and as members of the teams we

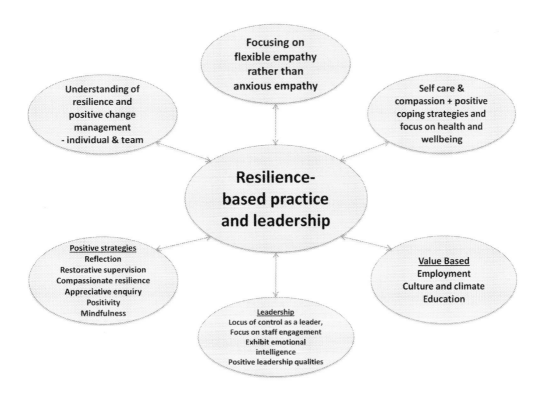

Figure 5.2 Resilience based practice and leadership (Chambers and Ryder, 2019 p104)

Table 5.8 Individual, team leader and organisational goals to promote positivity

Individual Goals	Team Leader Goals	Organisational Goals
Emotional intelligence/brilliance and empathy	Emotional intelligence/brilliance	Coach practice supervisors and assessors in promoting emotional intelligence
Positive self-concept and be proud of who you are	Show empathy about issues that colleagues face	Help students to cope with new environments
Positive and enriching relationships and communications with patients, loved ones and colleagues	Look for hidden messages	Help employees to reduce the impact of change
Practice self-compassion and feel at home with yourself and have a positive relationship with yourself	Focus on Team learning, shared goals and problem solving	Promote compassionate environments for patients and staff
Self-determination/efficacy and self-motivation, and internal locus of control with the right amount of arousal (within your window of tolerance)	Help employees to reduce the impact of change	Encourage compassionate teamworking and supportive environments with positive social climates and inspired colleagues
Choose to be realistic optimistic, hopeful, positive and happy and focus on sustainable happiness	Focus on teamworking and team communication and positive relationships	Value the art as well as the science of nursing and focus on qualitative aspects of care and not just quantitative targets
Be a radiator not a drain	Reduce the impact of changes on staff	Encourage team learning and problem solving
Be playful and maintain your sense of humour and snack on joy	Be a resonant and relational leader	Promote cultural intelligence, and understanding cultural contexts encourage new solutions
Be the best version of yourself and avoid the error of the average	Be transformational and relationship focused as a leader and encourage engagement	Encourage culturally competent compassion – awareness, knowledge, competence, sensitivity, values and principles
Be engaged and motivated and persevere	Be someone that your colleagues can trust	Avoid taking victim blaming approaches
Practice mindfulness and be serene and reflect on situations	Focus on role modelling positive values	Reduce regulation and over monitoring and encourage employees to take a lead on quality assurance
Stress tolerance and resilience and treat adversity as a challenge to overcome	Role model compassion to patients and colleagues	Discourage colleagues just feeling driven to work and encourage work engagement
Anger and conflict management and predict and de-escalate conflict	Respect and encourage diversity	Encourage harmonising passion where employees want to do a good job and enjoy their work and lives
Change management and flexibility and plan for change (WOOP wish, outcome, obstacle, plan)	Be charismatic and energised	Reduce job demands and increasing resourcing wherever possible to reduce work overload
Be grateful, humble and kind	Predict and de-escalate conflict	Focus on values-based recruitment and appraisals based on values – fairness, equity, openness and a sense of community
Reduce negative messages to yourself, catastrophising, and having polarised views	Inspire and encourage motivation	Encourage job engagement, job crafting
Focus on increasing what makes you happy and have a balance in your life (physical, emotional, social and intellectual)	Spot disengagement and try to develop strategies with your colleagues to mitigate this	Investigate reasons for high staff turnover, sickness, low motivation and motivation in a positive and not blaming way
Get JFDIs (just flipping do it) done quickly	Ensure that norms of reciprocity stay intact and that the psychological contact between employees, managers/ and organisations remain positive	Encourage a high person/job fit at recruitment
	Help employees to reduce the impact of change	Give constructive and positive feedback at appraisals
	Encourage Schwartz rounds and debriefing after traumatic situations	Carry out engagement training and engagement surveys.
	Carry out exit interviews to learn about why colleagues want to leave and their suggestions for improving the team environment.	Promote individual and group restorative supervision, and not just clinical supervision
	Focus on values-based recruitment and appraisals based on values – fairness, equity, openness and a sense of community	Encourage Schwartz rounds and debriefing after traumatic situations
	Give constructive and positive feedback at appraisals	

work in. In order for this to happen we need to be self-aware and empathetic towards our colleagues. We need to focus on enhancing our emotional intelligence and emotional brilliance, and our other intelligences, including cultural competence. We also need to focus on being compassionate towards ourselves and being mindful in our thinking, and practice mindfulness in whatever way works for us. We need to understand the links between being positive and being engaged and enthusiastic, and focus on being realistically optimistic, positive and happy in order to enhance our own wellbeing. Then we can take a lead in encouraging others to do the same and in promoting similar approaches with colleagues, in our teams and in our organisations.

The final chapter will draw together conclusions about stress management, resilience and positivity in relation to remaining compassionate in the challenging and stressful work environments where we all work.

REFERENCES

Achor S. (May 2011a). *The Happy Secret to Better Work*. www.ted.com/talks/shawn_achor_the_happy_secret_to_better_work.

Achor S. (2011b) *The Happiness Advantage*. London: Virgin Books.

Achor S. (2013) *Before Happiness*. London: Virgin Books

Anthony K, Wiencek C, Bauer C, Daly B, Anthony M. (2010) No Interruptions Please: Impact of a No Interruption Zone on Medication Safety in Intensive Care Units. *Critical Care Nurse*, 30(3): 21–29.

Avolio B, Bass B, Jung D. (1999) Re-Examining the Components of Transformational and Transactional Leadership Using the Multifactor Leadership Questionnaire. *Journal of Occupational and Organizational Psychology*, 72: 441–62.

Bakker A, Demorouti E. (2008) Towards a Model of Work Engagement. *Career Development International*, 13(3): 209–23.

Bakker, A. (2009). Building Engagement in the Workplace. In R. Burke, C. Cooper (eds.). *The Peak Performing Organization*. Oxon, UK: Routledge.

Bakker A, Albrecht S, Leiter M. (2011) Work Engagement: Further Reflections on the State of Play. *European Journal of Work and Organizational Psychology*, 20(1) 74–88.

Ballatt J and Campling P. (2011) *Intelligent Kindness: Reforming the Culture of Health care*, London: The Royal College of Psychiatrists.

Bar-On R, Parker J.(eds.) (2000) *The Handbook of Emotional Intelligence: The Theory and Practice of Development, Evaluation, Education and Application – at Home, School and the Workplace*. San Francisco, CA: Jossey-Bass.

Baylis N. (2009) *The Rough Guide to Happiness*. London: Rough Guides Ltd.

Blanch J, Ochoa P, Caballero M. (2018) *Over Engagement, Protective or risk Factor of Burnout?* DOI:10.5772/intechopen.81746.

Bradberry T. (2016) *11 Signs That You Lack Emotional Intelligence*. https://www.linkedin.com/pulse/telltale-signs-you-lack-emotional-intelligence-dr-travis-bradberry (Accessed 13/9/23).

Bradberry T.(2017) *Why You Need More Emotional Intelligence*. huffpost.com. https://www.huffpost.com/entry/why-you-need-more-emotional-intelligence_b_5952a975e4b0326c0a8d0bd2 (Accessed 26/1/23).

Brand T. (2007) *An Exploration of the Relationship Between Burnout, Occupational Stress and Emotional Intelligence in the Nursing Industry (Thesis)*. The University of Stellenbosch. https://scholar.sun.ac.za/server/api/core/bitstreams/7f316faa-364b-4bd3-aa23-06af93b17b01/content (Accessed 13/9/23).

Brown Brené. *Empathy vs sympathy*. https://www.youtube.com/watch?v=1Evwgu369Jw (Accessed 13/4/23).

Brummelhuis L, ter Hoeven C, Bakker A, Peper B. (2011) Breaking through the Loss Circle of Burnout: The Role of Motivation. *Journal of Occupational and Organizational Psychology*, 84(2): 268–87.

Campling P. (2013/14) Intelligent Kindness: Reforming the Culture of Health care in the Wake of the Francis Report. *Journal of Holistic Health care*, 10(3): 5–9.

Cankir B, Arikan S. (2019) Examining Work Engagement and Job Satisfaction Variables in their Relations with Job Performance and Intention to Quit. *Journal of Business Research – TURK*, 11(2): 1133–50.

Chambers C. (2017) Accentuate the Positive. *Community Practitioner*, 90(9): 48–49.

Chambers C, Ryder E. (2012) *Excellence in Compassionate Nursing Care – Leading the Change.* London: Radcliffe Publishing.

Chambers C, Ryder E. (2019) *Supporting Compassionate Health care Practice.* Abingdon: Routledge.

Chapman M. (2001) *Emotional Intelligence Pocketbook.* Alresford: Management Pocketbooks.

Chaskalson M. (2011) *The Mindful Workplace: Developing Resilient Individuals and Resonant Organizations with MBSR.* Chichester: John Wiley and Sons Ltd.

Chen X, Zhang B, Jin S, Quan Y, Zhang X, CUI X. (2021) The Effects of Mindfulness-based Interventions on Nursing Students: A Meta-analysis. *Nurse Education Today*: 98:104718 doi: 10.1016/j.nedt.2020.104718.

Chirkowska-Smolak T. (2012) Does work engagement burn out? The Person-job Fit and Levels of Burnout and Engagement in Work. *Polish Psychological Bulletin*, 43(2): 76–85.

Clancy C. (2014) The Importance of Emotional Intelligence. *Nursing Management*, 21(8): 15.

Cole E. (2020) *Expanding the "Window of Tolerance": Supporting Children's Ability to Cope With Anxiety.* https://www.psychologytoday.com/gb/blog/lifespan-psychology/202004/expanding-the-window-tolerance (Accessed: 13/9/23).

Cooperrider D, Srivastva S. (1987) *Appreciative Inquiry in Organizational Life.* In: Pasmore W, Woodman R. (eds.) (1987) *Research in Organizational Change and Development.* 1:129–69, Greenwich: JAI Press.

Corrigan F, Fisher J, Nutt D. (2011) Autonomic Dysregulation and the Window of Tolerance Model of the Effects of Complex Emotional Trauma. *Journal of Psychopharmacology*, 25(1): 17–25.

Csikszentmihalyi M. (2002). *Flow: The Classic Work on How to Achieve Happiness.* London: Rider.

David S. (2018) The Tyranny of Positivity: A Harvard Psychologist Details our Unhealthy Obsession with Happiness *Big Think* + https://bigthink.com/plus/the-tyranny-of-positivity-a-harvard-psychologist-details-our-unhealthy-obsession-with-happiness/ (Accessed 2/3/2023).

Delphis (2020) *The Mental Health Continuum is a Better Model for Mental Health.* https://delphis.org.uk/mental-health/continuum-mental-health/ (Accessed 13.04.2023).

Denner L, Thompson L, Chambers B, Jackson D, Cooke H, Magill L, Bubb J, Miller J, Harries M, Atkins S. (2019) Observing Everyday Interactions to Uncover Compassion in Care. *Nursing Times*, 115(1): 54–57.

Department of Health (DH). (2012) *Compassion in Practice: Nursing, Midwifery and Care Staff: Our Vision and Strategy.* London: Department of Health.

Ford M. (2023a) Mental Health at Perilous Low, Warn Nursing Staff. *Nursing Times*, 119(2): 6–9.

Ford S. (2023b) If Nursing Staff are not Cared for, They Cannot Care for Others. *Nursing Times*, 119(2): 4.

Fox E. (2012) *Rainy Brain, Sunny Brain*. London: Arrow Books.

Fredrickson B. (1998) What Good Are Positive Emotions? *Review of General Psychology*, 2(3): 300–19.

Fredrickson B. (2009) *Positivity.* Oxford: Oneworld Publications.

Fredrickson B. (2013) *Love 2.0: Creating Happiness and Health in Moments of Connection.* USA: Hudson Street Press.

Fredrickson B. L., Branigan C. (2005). Positive Emotions Broaden the Scope of Attention and Thought-Action Repertoires. *Cognition and Emotion*, 19(3): 313–32.

Fredrickson B, Cohn M, Coffey K, Pek J, Finkel S. (2008) Open Hearts Build Lives: Positive Emotions, Induced Through Loving-kindness Meditation, Build Consequential Personal Resources. *Journal of Personality and Social Psychology*, 95(5): 1045–62.

Furnham A. (2008) *Management Intelligence: Sense and Nonsense for the Successful Manager.* Hampshire: Palgrave Macmillan.

Garamoni G, Reynolds C, Thase M, Frank E, Fasiczka A. (1992) Shifts in Affective Balance During Therapy of Major Depression. *Journal of Consulting and Clinical Psychology*, 60(2): 260–66.

Gilbert P. (2010) *The Compassionate Mind*. London: Constable and Robinson.

Gilbert P. and Choden (2013). *Mindful Compassion: Using the Power of Mindfulness and Compassion to Transform our Lives*. London: Constable and Robinson Ltd

Gillon R. (1994) *Philosophical Medical Ethics*. In: Palfrey C, Thomas P, Phillips C. Health Services Management: What are the Ethical Dimensions? *International Journal of Public Sector Management*, 19(1): 57–66.

Gladwell M. (2000) *The Tipping Point*. London: Little Brown Book Group.

Goleman D. (1996) *Emotional Intelligence: Why It Can Matter More Than IQ*. London: Bloomsbury.

Goleman D. (2022) *2022: The Year for More Emotional Intelligence*. https://www.linkedin.com/pulse/2022-year-more-emotional-intelligence-daniel-goleman/?trk=eml-email_series_follow_newsletter_01-hero-1-title_link&midToken=AQEtkru62bnmlw&fromEmail=fromEmail&ut=0nBD_TUEYzNq41 (Accessed 02.03.2023).

Goleman D. (2023a) *Is Emotional Intelligence on the Decline?* https://www.linkedin.com/pulse/emotional-intelligence-decline-daniel-goleman/?midToken=AQEtkru62bnmlw&midSig=31qaFMJz6zmqE1&trk=eml-email_series_follow_newsletter_01-newsletter_content_preview-0-readmore_button_&trkEmail=eml-email_series_follow_newsletter_01-newsletter_content_preview-0-readmore_button_-null-3nu5a0~le5v4243~ag-null-null&eid=3nu5a0-le5v4243-ag (Accessed: 17/02/23).

Goleman D. (2023b) *Connecting Emotional Intelligence and Mindfulness*. www.linkedin.com/pulse/connecting-emotional-intelligence-mindfulness-daniel-goleman/ Accessed 14/07/2023.

Goleman D, Boyatzis R, McKee A. (2002) *The New Leaders: Transforming the Art of Leadership into the Science of Results*. London: Sphere.

Goleman D, Boyatzis R. *Emotional and Social Intelligence Leadership Competency Model*. https://www.keystepmedia.com/emotional-social-intelligence-leadership-competencies/ (Accessed 04/03/2022).

Gordon R. (1952) *Doctor in the House*. London: Michael Joseph.

Griffiths P, Robinson M. (2009) *The 8 Secrets of Happiness*. Oxford: Lion Hudson plc.

Griffiths T. (2023) We Understand What You are Going Through and We are Here to Listen. *Nursing Times*, 119(2): 15.

Gudykunst W, Hammer M. (1983) *Basic Training Design: Approaches to Intercultural Training. Vol 1*. New York: Pergamon. Cited in Berry J, Poortinga Y, Breugelmans S, Chasiotis A, Sam D. (2011) *Cross-Cultural Psychology: Research and Applications*. Cambridge: Cambridge University Press.

Gutermann D, Lehmann-Willenbrock N, Boer D, Born M, Voelpel S. (2017) How Leaders Affect Followers' Work Engagement and Performance: Integrating Leader-Member Exchange and Crossover Theory. *British Journal of Management*, 28(2): 299–314.

Hamidizadeh A, Hasan K, Fatemeh H. (2014) Is Workaholism Antecedent of Burn out? *European Journal of Academic Essays*, 1(8): 1–9.

Headstrong Mindset LLC (2020) *Velcro and Teflon Theory*. https://headstrongmindset.com/velcro-teflon-theory/ (Accessed 13/4/2023).

Heffernan M, Quinn Griffin M, McNulty R, Fitzpatrick J. (2010) Self-compassion and Emotional Intelligence in Nurses. *International Journal of Nursing Practice*, 16(4): 366–73.

Heidegger, M. (1966) *Conversation on a Country Path About Thinking*. In: Anderson J, Freund E. (trans) *Discourse on Thinking*. New York, NY: Harper and Row.

Hein S. (1996) *EQ for Everybody: A Practical Guide to Emotional Intelligence*. Clearwater, FL: Aristotle Press.

Hills P, Argyle M. (2002) The Oxford Happiness Questionnaire. A compact scale for the Measurement of Psychological Well-being. *Personality and Individual Differences*, 33(7): 1071–88.

Hoyle A. (2023) Feeling Burntout? Here's How to Come Back From the Edge. *The Times. Body and Soul*. 28 Jan. 2023 p243.

Hurley J, Linsley P. (2012) *Emotional Intelligence in Health and Social Care: A Guide for Improving Human Relationships.* London: Radcliffe Publishing Ltd

Isen A. M. (2000) *Positive Affect and Decision Making.* In: Lewis M, de Haviland-Jones J (eds). (2000) *Handbook of Emotions, 2nd edn.* New York: Guildford Press.

Kearney R. (2023) Supporting Staff Wellbeing with a Focus on Health Visitors. *Nursing Times,* 119(2): 22–26.

Koppula R. (2008) Examining the Relationship Between Transformational Leadership and Engagement. Master's Thesis. 3482. San Jose State University. https://scholarworks.sjsu.edu/etd_theses/3482 (Accessed 13/9/23).

Leiter M, Price S, Laschinger H. (2010) Generational Differences in Distress, Attitudes and Incivility Among Nurses. *Journal of Nursing Management,* 18(8): 970–80.

Leiter M, Laschinger H, Day A, Gilin-Oore D. (2011) The Impact of Civility Interventions on Employee Social Behavior, Distress, and Attitudes. *Journal of Applied Psychology,* 96(6): 1258–74.

Lomas T, Medina J, Ivtzan I, Rupprecht S, Eiroa-Orosa F. (2018) A Systematic Review of the Impact of Mindfulness on the Well-being of Health care Professionals. *Journal of Clinical Psychology,* 74(3): 319–55.

Lyubomirsky S. (2007) *The How of Happiness.* London: Piatkus.

Lyubomirsky S. (2008) *The How of Happiness*: *A Scientific Approach to Getting the Life You Want.* New York: The Penguin Press.

Magmanlac J, Ocampo N, Manibo J. (2019) The Quality of Life and Mindfulness Among Helping Professionals *Asia Pacific Journal of Education, Arts and Sciences,* 6(4): 13–26.

Mangi R, Amanat A, Jalbani A. (2013) Occupational Psychology in Higher Educational Institutions: A Study in Pakistan. *European Scientific Journal,* 9(32). https://www.researchgate.net/publication/330349701_OCCUPATIONAL_PSYCHOLOGY_IN_HIGHER_EDUCATIONAL_INSTITUTIONS_A_STUDY_IN_PAKISTAN (Accessed 13/9/23).

Markham S, Jennings T, Brunsden S. (2022) Building *Resilience* and *Compassion* during COVID-19 *BACP Workplace.* https://www.fons.org/resources/documents/RBCS/Building-resilience-and-compassion-during-COVID-19.pdf (Accessed 13.04.2023).

Marques J. (2007) Leadership: Emotional Intelligence, Passion and …What Else? *Journal of Management Development,* 26(7): 644–51.

Maslach C, Schaufeli W, Leiter M. (2001) Job Burnout. *Annual Review of Psychology,* 52: 397–422.

Mendes A. (2017) How to Address Compassion Fatigue in the Community Nurse. *British Journal of Community Nursing,* 22(9): 458–59.

Minor L. (2018) *When Health Professionals Have Empathy, Patients aren't the Only Ones Who Benefit.* https://scopeblog.stanford.edu/2018/10/08/when-health-professionals-have-empathy-patients-arent-the-only-ones-who-benefit/ (Accessed 13/9/23).

Monson T, Quote. https://www.goodreads.com/quotes/499597-we-cant-direct-the-wind-but-we-can-adjust-the-sails (Accessed 13.09.23).

Morse J, Bottorff J, Anderson G, O'Brien B, Solberg S. (1992) Beyond Empathy: Expanding Expressions of Caring. *Journal of Advanced Nursing,* 17(7): 809–21.

New Economics Foundation (2008) *Five Ways to Wellbeing: Communicating the Evidence.* https://neweconomics.org/2008/10/five-ways-to-wellbeing.

NHS Leadership Academy (2014) 'Health care Leadership Model: The Nine Dimensions of Leadership Behaviour'. https://www.leadershipacademy.nhs.uk/wp-content/uploads/2014/10/NHSLeadership-LeadershipModel-colour.pdf (Accessed 30/11/22).

NHS (2015) *NHS Constitution for England.* www.gov.uk/government/publications/the-nhs-constitution-for-england (Accessed 13/9/23).

Nolan Committee. *Standards in Public Life* (1995) In: Palfrey C, Thomas P, Phillips C. (2006) Health Services Management: What are the Ethical Dimensions? *International Journal of Public Sector Management,* 19(1): 57–66.

Northouse P. (2009) *Leadership: Theory and Practice.* London: Sage Publications.

Nursing & Midwifery Council (2018) *The Code.* London: NMC.

Nyatanga B. (2019) When Words Make a Difference in Palliative Care. *British Journal of Community Nursing,* 24(7): 347.

Oettingen G. (2014) *Rethinking Positive Thinking: Inside the New Science of Motivation.* London: Current.

Papadopoulos I. (2018) *Culturally Competent Compassion: A Guide for Health care Students and Practitioners.* Abingdon, Oxon: Routledge.

Priyadarshi P, Raina R. (2014) The Mediating Effects of Work Engagement: Testing Causality Between Personal Resource, Job Resource and Work-related Outcomes. *International Journal of Indian Culture and Business Management,* 9(4) 487–509.

Quinn S. (2020) Compassion, the Life Blood of the NHS. *Oxford Brookes Poetry Centre.* https://weeklypoems.brookes.ac.uk/2020/03/.

Rayton B, Yalabik Z. (2014) Work Engagement, Psychological Contract Breach and Job Satisfaction. *The International Journal of Human Resources,* 25(17): 2382–400.

Reis da Silva, H. (2022) Emotional Awareness and Emotional Intelligence. *British Journal of Community Nursing,* 27(12): 573–74.

Roosevelt E, Happiness quote https://www.goodreads.com/quotes/1413647-happiness-is-not-a-goal-it-is-a-by-product-paradoxically (Accessed 6/4/23).

Royal College of Physicians (2017) '*National Early Warning Score*'. https://www.rcplondon.ac.uk/projects/outputs/national-early-warning-score-news-2 (Accessed 30/11/22).

Rozanski A, Bavishi C, Kubzansky L, Cohen R. (2019) Association of Optimism With Cardiovascular Events and All-Cause Mortality. A Systematic Review and Meta-analysis. *JAMA Network Open,* 2(9): e1912200. https://jamanetwork.com/journals/jamanetworkopen/fullarticle/2752100.

Rubin G. (2009) *The Happiness Project.* London: Harper Collins Publishers.

Rubin G. (2016) *Better Than Before: Mastering the Habits of Our Everyday Lives.* USA: Crown Publishers.

Rungapadiachy D. (2008) *Self-awareness in Health Care.* Basingstoke: Palgrave Macmillan.

Salovey P, Mayer J. (1990) Emotional Intelligence. *Imagination, Cognition and Personality,* 9(3): 185–211.

Sand I. (2017) *The Emotional Compass: How to Think Better about Your Feelings.* London: Jessica Kingsley Publishers.

Seldon A. (2015) *Beyond Happiness.* London: Hodder & Stoughton

Seligman M. (2003) *Authentic Happiness.* London: Nicholas Brealey Publishing.

Seligman M. (2006) *Learned Optimism: How to Change Your Mind and Your Life.* USA: Vintage Books.

Seligman M. (2011) *Flourish.* London: Nicholas Brealey Publishing.

Seppala E. (2016) *The Happiness Track: How to Apply the Science of Happiness to Accelerate Your Success.* London: Harperone.

Sheridan C. (2016) *The Mindful Nurse: Using the Power of Mindfulness and Compassion to Help You Thrive in Your Work.* Galway, Ireland: Rivertime Press.

Siegel D. (2015) *The Developing Mind (2nd Edition). How Relationships and the Brain Interact to Shape Who We Are.* New York: Guildford Press.

Sima R (2022) Want to Feel Happier? Try Snacking on Joy. *The Washington Post* https://www.washingtonpost.com/wellness/2022/11/17/feel-happier-joy-flourishing/ (Accessed 2/3/23).

Snir R, Harpaz I. (2004) Attitudinal and Demographic Antecedents of Workaholism. *Journal of Organizational Change Management,* 17(5): 520–36.

Snowden A, Stenhouse R. (2016) *Emotional Intelligence May Not Make You a Better Nurse Says Report.* The Conversation. https://theconversation.com/emotional-intelligence-may-not-make-you-a-better-nurse-says-report-59713 (Accessed 13/9/23).

Snyder M. (2014*) Positive Health: Flourishing Lives, Well-Being in Doctors.* Bloomington, IN: Balboa Press.

Sparrow T, Knight S. (2006) *Applied EI: The Importance of Attitudes in Developing Emotional Intelligence.* Chichester: John Wiley and Sons Ltd.

Spence J, Robbins A. (1992) Workaholism: Definition, Measurement, and Preliminary Results. *Journal of Personality Assessment,* 58: 160–178.

Style C. (2011) *Brilliant Positive Psychology.* Harlow: Pearson Education Limited

Teater M, Ludgate J. (2014) *Overcoming Compassion Fatigue: A Practical Resilience* Workbook. USA: PESI Publishing & Media.

The Boston EI questionnaire. https//geminicapital.ie/wp-content/uploads/2021/12/The-Boston-EI-Questionnaire.pdf (Accessed 13/04/23).

Trepanier S, Fernet C, Austin S. (2013) Workplace Bullying and Psychological Health at Work: The Mediating Role of Satisfaction of Needs for Autonomy, Competence and Relatedness. *Work and Stress*, 27(2): 123–40.

Wallbank S. (2013) Recognising Stressors and Using Restorative Supervision to Support a Healthier Maternity Workforce: A Retrospective Cross-sectional, Questionnaire Survey. *Evidence-based Midwifery*, 11(1): 4–9.

Walsh M. (2019) *Embodiment – Moving Beyond Mindfulness.* Unicorn Slayer Press.

Watson D, Clark L, Carey G. (1988) Positive and Negative Affectivity and their Relation to Anxiety and Depressive Disorders. *Journal of Abnormal Psychology*, 97(3): 346–53.

Webb L. (2012) *How to be Happy: Simple Ways to Build Your Confidence and Resilience to Become a Happier, Healthier You.* Chichester, West Sussex: Capstone Publishing Ltd.

Wedderburn Tate C. (1999) *Leadership in Nursing.* London: Churchill Livingstone.

Westphal M, Bingisser M, Feng T, Wall M, Blakley E, Bingisser R, Kleim B. (2015) Protective Benefits of Mindfulness in Emergency Room Personnel. *Journal of Affective Disorders*, 175: 79–85.

Westwood C. (2010) *How to Succeed as a Nurse Leader.* https://www.nursingtimes.net/archive/how-to-suceed-as-a-nurse-leader-21-03-2010/ (Accessed 13/9/23).

Whitton T, Buchanon G, Smith S. (2019) How a Mindfulness Intervention Can Improve Patients' Mental Wellbeing. *Nursing Times*, 115(7): 48–51.

Wible P. (2012) *Pet Goats & Pap Smears.* Oregon: Pamela Wible Publishing.

Youngson R. (2012) *Time to Care.* New Zealand: Rebelheart Publishers.

Zaluski W. (2017) On Three Types of Empathy: The Perfect, the Truncated and the Contaminated. *Logos i Ethos*, 2(45): 1–16.

https://www.stmichaelshospital.com.pdf/programs/mast/mast-session1.pdf (Accessed 05.02.2021).

6

How can I take a lead on compassionate practice, stress management, resilience and positivity in my team?

- Introduction
- Discussion – main points and evidence with exercises, aide mémoires and questions

  - Leading with compassion
  - Individual leadership
  - Team leadership and compassionate leadership
  - Educational leadership
  - Organisational leadership
  - Using the RESPECT toolkit to take a lead.

- Recommendations for leadership as individual practitioners, leaders and organisations.

  - Focusing on leadership in compassionate care, stress management, resilience and positivity as individual practitioners and leaders.
  - Focusing on leadership in compassionate care, stress management, resilience and positivity as organisations.

INTRODUCTION

This chapter focuses on how we can make a difference in terms of taking a lead on compassionate care and what skills and attributes we need as a leader. We need to harness our natural wish to practice in a compassionate manner and focus on what led us to want to work in health care. We can then take a lead on using patient situations to teach others about best care and challenge others in a positive manner to deliver person centred compassionate care. We can then focus on ways to use our energy and motivation to reenergise our teams and inspire and motivate our colleagues and students. Then we can reach that "tipping point" (Gladwell, 2000) where situations, and care, can be moved forward in a positive way, despite the challenges of today's health care environment. In order to do this we need to have a positive team, educational and organisational culture. We will then draw all this together via the RESPECT toolkit (Chambers and Ryder, 2019) which can be used by individuals and teams to address issues within their working environment and how this can enhance compassionate health care practice.

The format will be:

- Case studies
- Discussions

DOI: 10.4324/9781315106861-6

- Pointers which encourage personal strategies
- Recommendations for leadership as individual practitioners, team leaders and organisations

DISCUSSION

Case Study 6.1

Kerry's focus on encouraging social interaction and change

I had arranged to accompany the lead community matron and she explained that she only had one visit to carry out but that it was likely to be time consuming because the patient does not like to be rushed and that she tries to give him plenty of time. The patient is male and aged 65 years and lives alone. He has COPD and should be on oxygen but due to the fact that he smokes and is a hoarder the environment is too challenging for oxygen to be stored in the home. She explained that he had been offered help with stopping smoking and he had also been offered help with clearing his home but he had declined both, and it is his choice to live in this way.

The environment was very challenging, and the Matron had difficulty manoeuvring herself and her equipment amongst the stored boxes and papers. A small clearance had been made to allow access to the man who seated himself directly at the end of the hallway facing the entrance, so he could see who was in his home. The door was unlocked when we arrived and this, together with the challenging environment, I found alarming. I struggled to get inside the space as the Matron was already there. She was only able to carry out a limited assessment due to the restricted space. I acknowledged the man from a distance, and he agreed to me being there. After 30 minutes of standing in a confined space the man agreed to me squeezing past him to a larger clearing with a chair next to him, and he agreed that I could sit there.

This changed the whole visit, and I was now able to engage with the man who I had never met before. I asked him general questions about himself and his family and friends. He said he was divorced and had two sons who he has not spoken to for a considerable amount of time. He did not know where they live, and he had no interest in resolving this situation. He had a passion for old cars and he had worked in a timber yard for 50 years. The house was his parents' and they were hoarders and he had moved in with them following his divorce. Since they had died, he had never got round to having the house cleared. He said that he does not like being told how to live. I replied that is his home, and if he is safe and comfortable then that is his choice. He smiled and said that he liked me.

I explained that the local council had a service called prescribe a friend, and that this is a free service and is made up of volunteers who are there to help people who are lonely. They will visit people for a cup of tea and a chat and they might well have shared interests, for example cars. The man really liked this idea and immediately agreed to the matron referring him to this service. The matron then broached the subject of having more space created, and although he appeared reluctant at the start he then agreed after understanding that the referral to the befriending service might be rejected due to the limited space and his hoarding.

On return to the office the matron was very happy with the outcome of the visit and was able to contact the local council about having space made in his home. This had been offered many times before but had always been declined.

The man had now agreed that they could assist him and the referral was then made for prescribe a friend.

I finished the day feeling very positive about having made a difference to this man, if only for today, because he could change his mind again by the time the matron went back. I used my social skills to assess the situation myself, rather than just listening to others' opinions. Sometimes we all have different connections with people and I could tell that the silence in the home while the matron was completing her paperwork was making the man uncomfortable. When I spoke to him, and we spoke about his interests and I asked if there was anything we could do to help him, he seemed to perk up. I do not think that he had felt friendliness for a long time and he was isolated and lonely.

Since our visit the matron has told me that the man is still enthusiastic and his home has been cleared of a huge amount of clutter and they have seen a slight improvement in his COPD, possibly by more air circulating and windows being able to be opened. Sometimes a social situation being improved can have a huge impact on a person's wellbeing, and viewing someone holistically can be the most important part of nursing.

Kerry makes some excellent points here. She developed her own relationship with this patient, and her different strategies made headway in a way that had not been possible in the past. She was non-judgemental, empathetic and built a trusting relationship and used her active listening and questioning skills to build on his interests and motivations. Instinctively she used a motivational interviewing RULE approach (Miller and Rollnick, 2002 and 2012) and **resisted trying to make everything right**, **understood** his perspective, **listened** and **empowered** him to take control in the ways that he found acceptable. This approach was discussed in Chapter 2 but it is interesting to see this strategy in action. What is really impressive is that although Kerry is a qualified nurse now, at the point that she wrote this she was only in the first year of her nursing programme. She had not heard about motivational interviewing as a strategy but her high skill set gleaned from years as a health care assistant enabled her to use her extensive communication skills. She thought creatively, and this enabled the man she was visiting to make crucial changes in his life.

Case Study 6.2

Jen's focus on end-of-life care when the patient was alone at home

One night I joined the night nursing team in my local district nursing service. It was a really beneficial shift and it really made me think about what had happened. The main patient that will remain with me was a gentleman who was dying. He lived in a very grand block of flats but we had received a call at around 10:30 pm from the worried warden stating that Mr X was known to be in the palliative stage of his illness and his family had disconnected from him and did not wish to support him through his end-of-life period. The warden had just been in to check on him and was concerned as he was muddled, agitated and seemed to be in pain. We said that we would go and assess him and we reprioritised our already busy schedule.

When we arrived, the warden met us at the front gates and seemed quite distressed herself. After reassuring her we were taken to Mr X. When we arrived, he was distressed. He appeared to be hallucinating and was reaching out for objects that were not there. The room smelt of urine and, on inspection, his pad was full. The qualified nurse and I provided personal care and then re-assessed him. Although he was marginally less agitated, he now seemed to be grimacing more and showing signs of discomfort. The nurse asked my opinion of how I felt he was and what treatment I felt he should have. We discussed this, and both concluded that he needed some Midazolam for the restlessness and some Morphine for the pain. This was administered to him once all checks were made. We also checked he had enough stock of medications and checked his end-of-life plans to ensure that we were complying with his wishes. These were all luckily clearly laid out on the bedside cabinet.

After ensuring he was settled, we left the room. The discussion then led to when we should next visit. The warden, who had found him in distress, stated that she could return in 2 hours, but that should an emergency happen she may not be able to do this. We gave her our telephone number and she said that if she could not return that she would let us know and we would visit or find another person to visit. The warden called again to say he was in distress again at around 2am and so we visited again to assess and administer another subcutaneous dose of each drug. The warden stated that she would now sit with him for a while and would ring us if she was further concerned. No more calls were received during our shift and so we handed the up-to-date information to the day staff for them to assess and see if he needed further treatment. They were going out to assess him on their first visits.

I personally feel that, in this situation, the dilemma was that the patient was dying alone. He had no family that wanted to be present during this episode of need. The warden was restricted with time for him, as she had other patients to see. And we ourselves had a very busy schedule but were available should another emergency arise. The dilemma here was how we were going to know if he was in pain and how this was going to be ascertained. By working with the warden and her priorities, we devised a satisfactory plan. For me though, I struggled knowing that he was dying alone. I did not know the reasoning behind the family not being present, but it made me feel sad for the patient. We did, however, have other patients to see and they also needed our help. And so the dilemma was not about what care we should give, but how often that may be required and how we were going to accommodate that. Fortunately, we did not receive any other emergency call-outs and so were able to return to him on the second call out. This made it easier to assess him as we had already met him previously and had a base line of his health status. The NMC Code (2018) talks about the importance of being compassionate to others during this stage of someone's life, being their advocate and responding to their needs. I feel that we did everything possible to ensure that he did not die in pain, and we ensured that he had follow up care to continue that process. He died the following day. Due to the lack of family support, I feel that we adapted to the situation and provided him the best care that we could at this time.

I feel that our interactions with the warden and Mr X were appropriate and met his needs, both from a physical and an emotional perspective. He had made his wishes clear and I feel that we assessed all of his needs and responded accordingly.

I will continue to uphold this practice and remember to look at the situation individually and not generically. Yes, in an ideal world, we would all have family surrounding us. But there are, and will be many more, that do not have this ideal and so our care plans need to adapt to that individual and make it the best possible situation for them in that circumstance.

Jen again is now a qualified nurse but was only in year 1 of her nursing programme when she wrote this. Both Kerry and Jen were experienced health care assistants in district nursing teams so had a great many transferable skills when visiting patients in their homes. Jen was empathetic about her patient's end-of-life needs and the fact that his family did not want to be there to support him. The district nursing team supported him as much as they could within their busy caseload, and were compassionate and supportive to the patient, but the warden of the flats where he was living was also very supportive.

Both scenarios demonstrate a highly compassionate holistic approach to patient needs as first year students. However, as qualified nurses now both Kerry and Jen need to take a lead on compassionate care. How can we be not just excellent practitioners, but leaders in excellent and compassionate care?

Leading with compassion

Being compassionate to patients is infinitely easier if we work in a compassionate team and a caring organisational culture. West and Chowla (2017) say that compassionate leadership for compassionate health care services involves:

- Attending – paying attention to staff and "listening with fascination".
- Understanding – shared understanding of what they are facing.
- Empathising – understanding the needs of others.
- Helping – taking intelligent action to serve or help.

In order for staff to thrive they need to have:

- A sense of belonging in an inclusive and compassionate organisational culture.
- Competence which allows for growth, skill development and career progression.
- Autonomy and control with fair and employee centred practices (West et al, 2015).

This involves feeling part of a team where there is a recognition of individual people's value, effective induction, ongoing social interaction and supervisory support. This also requires a positive culture and leadership which focuses on making people feel valued and where there is positivity, mutual respect and staff engagement. There needs to be equality, diversity and inclusion in a positive workplace which supports wellbeing and is inclusive of everyone. In order for a high-quality care culture there needs to be:

- An inspirational vision of high-quality care.
- Clearly aligned goals at every level with helpful feedback.
- Good people management and employee engagement.
- Continuous learning and quality improvement.
- Enthusiastic team working, cooperation and integration (West et al, 2018).

Leadership needs to be authentic, open and honest, humble and curious, optimistic, appreciative and compassionate (West et al, 2015). Leaders need to create positive emotion and a positive culture and be optimistic, have a sense of humour, be compassionate and care for staff. For example, this could be through providing Schwartz round opportunities (Schwartz, 2012). Managers and leaders also need to deal with aggression and poor performance in employees.

Radcliffe (2020) describes a time when he accompanied a friend to have a scan. His friend was anxious because of past experiences when he had a scan which was uncomfortable and painful because of the necessary movement and positioning issues. When he expressed this to the clinician they did not minimise or ignore his concerns, but asked what had helped in the past, and asked what they could do to help. They then carefully listened to his responses and said that they would explain this to their team. Other team members then came in and asked more questions, rather than perceiving him as being difficult. This thoughtfulness probably saved time because he was not distressed in the scan which would have caused delay, and it enabled the clinicians to be more in control of their day, as well as having a powerful impact on all those concerned.

De Zulueta (2013) says that even ten years ago there is a tension between efficiency and patient-centred care where economics and resource constraints meant that health care professionals felt alienated and struggled to perform healing roles so patients felt abandoned and anxious. Nyatanga (2013) calls for a whole systems approach for compassion saying that compassion breeds compassion, but the opposite is also true. He says that:

> a compassionate government is needed, along with compassionate schools, hospitals, hospices, universities, cities, media and communities. It is only when evidence of compassion is viewed in this wider lens that people – nurses included- will start to live, breathe, eat and drink compassion; and this no doubt will be transmitted into caring for all patients.
>
> (Nyatanga, 2013, p 299)

It is important also that communities take a lead in supporting people on a population wide basis. Abel and Clarke (2020) use the example of Frome in Somerset which has taken a lead on compassionate approaches as a community to help address individual issues and loneliness amongst those who live there (Case Study. 6.3). They advise a call to action for all people, or a manifesto for compassionate communities. This involves:

- As individuals – everyone having a caring responsibility for those around them and celebrating diversity and rejecting repression.
- Education – based on emotional literacy, dealing with difficult emotions, creatively using imagination and sharing information.
- Business and media – environmental care, rejecting corruption and support of those who are leading challenging lives.
- Religion – spiritual expression, celebrating multi faith approaches, and not coercing others to acquiesce to our own beliefs.
- Politics – rejecting oppression and violence and promoting cultural diversity.
- Health and welfare – this does not rely only on the statutory health and social care services. We all have a responsibility here.
- Environment – avoiding environmental damage and concern for animals and the planet.

Case Study 6.3

Frome Compassion Project

In Frome they have reduced hospital admissions by 30% for people with three or more long term conditions and this is a genuine £2 million cost saving for the NHS as well as most importantly creating a really positive caring and compassionate community (Health Connections Mendip https://healthconnectionsmendip.org/our-model/videos/). Funding was agreed as an innovation project but this brought financial benefits to the NHS. For every £1 spent on the scheme, where costs are rising elsewhere, there has been a £6 saving for the NHS.

Firstly, they started by mapping the local resources which already existed and then analysed where the real and perceived gaps in provision were. They then developed a directory of resources and put this information on a health connections website which was developed. Health connectors are paid members of staff, and they are social prescribers which is a vital part of their role. Medical advice and guidance is given as necessary and health care assistants are involved with one to one discussions and group facilitation. The SBAR approach is used to assess needs looking at **Situation, Background, Assessment and Recommendations** (Institute for Health care Improvement).

Health connectors train volunteers who are called social connectors and there are 500 so far and this is increasing. They cascade messages down and this creates a ripple effect through one to one and group discussions.

There are complex care and MDT meetings on Mondays and Fridays which are held every week. They involve social services, district nurses, mental health practitioners and GPs, and individuals with the greatest needs are targeted. There is a social worker on site one day each week. There are also frequent discussions with the discharge liaison nurses at the hospital focusing on those with complex discharge planning issues. There is a strong relationship across the interface of primary and secondary care.

Exercise groups, social get togethers, befriending services, talking cafes, where people can meet up and make friends and meet social connectors, are all part of the newly devolved scheme. Advice and support is available, from grass cutting services and blue badge support helpers, and families are contacted to ask for their help with internet shopping, home deliveries and much more.

There are also On Track groups to help people to focus on what is important for them, and to help them set goals and keep on track with these and self-manage their health conditions. This is through a focus on weight management, eating advice, exercise, pacing themselves, sleep, smoking cessation etc.

Younger people's experiences are also heard, and creative approaches are used to enhance peer support. Groups such as carer support, macular degeneration, stroke and other long term conditions groups. dementia, healthy walks and leg ulcer groups have also been created.

The scheme focuses on having one foot in primary care and one foot in the community. These creative and innovative approaches have rejuvenated practice. Furthermore, the project has helped develop healthier and happier individuals and a compassionate community which cares for individuals who are most vulnerable and isolated. Individuals feel part of the community and get their lives back and this reduces loneliness. This also helps keep people out of hospital. It is driven by the community and what individuals feel is most important to them.

So, we need to make community connections and create environments where people can share experiences through talking cafes, men and women sheds, wellbeing forums and happiness labs. Gardening groups, choirs and local existing groups are all central to this. Wellbeing forums can include people in professional roles in health and social care like care navigators, social prescribers, health care practitioners, patient participation group committees, Age Concern/UK, Citizen's Advice, town employees, church members, school leaders, Home-Start and Crosslink. Approaches to encouraging wellbeing in schools and communities from the cradle to the grave need innovative and joined up thinking.

It is essential for us to understand the importance of compassion in the care environment and how much people remember when they have felt cared for. Not feeling rushed, a calm tone of voice, eye contact, empathy, being present with the patient are all crucial tools in our compassion toolbox. Kate Granger was a champion of the importance of this and introduced the "Hello, my name is…" approach which has been widely adopted. She was a doctor who was diagnosed with a terminal illness, and she was shocked to be on the receiving end of dehumanising care and she made it her mission to try to bring about change (Picard, 2016).

We need to encourage others as well as ourselves to look for similarities between ourselves and patients in our care and listen without judgement to deepen our compassion. We also need to search within ourselves for areas in our lives where we lack compassion, trust, forgiveness and acceptance, and explore the reasons for this and work on our feelings. Finally, we need to carry out random acts of kindness (Weaver, 2016). This focus on compassion has a positive impact on us physiologically by lowering our blood pressure, increasing our immune responses and creating greater calmness and this impacts on us psychologically. It also creates a ripple effect of compassion and kindness. We need to work on eliminating variations in care and use leadership to promote a culture where compassion is central. By working in partnership with patients and loved ones, as well as others in our team, to respond to what really matters to patients and colleagues we can ensure that the right education and CPD is in place, and challenge inconsistencies and unacceptable practice. We need to celebrate excellent care, and not just notice poor care. This is often not measured or valued but it is essential to those in our care (Radcliffe, 2014). Showing compassion saves time because we really listen to our patients, and this improves outcomes and helps people to become more resilient. This in turn reduces future financial investments and costs. We need to start with caring for ourselves, so we can care for others, and show care for our colleagues and our managers who might not have any positive messages given to them on an ongoing basis.

Sometimes it is a matter of working out the different ways that we need to develop and learn in order to take a better control over our lives. Leffert et al 1998, cited in Petersen and Seligman, 2004) identify different internal development assets which link to character strengths. These are:

- a strong commitment to learning through achievement, engagement in school or study or reading for pleasure. This links to character strengths such as a love of learning, persistence, curiosity and citizenship.
- Positive values – caring, equality and social justice, integrity and responsibility. These link to character strengths of kindness, fairness, integrity and self-regulation.
- Social competencies – interpersonal and cultural competence, peaceful conflict resolution and planning and decision making. These link to character strengths, of hope, and open-mindedness, love and social intelligence, self-regulation and leadership.
- Positive identity – personal power, self-esteem, sense of purpose and a positive view of personal future. These link to character strengths of creativity, spirituality and hope.

So, it is important that we continue to develop ourselves through our commitment to learning, our personal values, social competencies and positive identity in order to maximise our character strengths of kindness, fairness, hope, creativity and wanting to carry on learning about life. These all link to positivity which will be discussed in greater detail in the next chapter. However, all these attributes contribute to our wellbeing and our ability to care for others.

The New Economics Foundation (Aked et al, 2008 and Michaelson et al, 2012) says that "wellbeing can be understood as how people **feel** and how they **function**, both on a personal and a social level, and how they **evaluate** their lives as a whole" (p6). They make the point that people might **feel** happy or anxious in terms of their emotions but these are often transient emotions which might not reflect their overall wellbeing, how their function in life or how they would evaluate their lives as a whole. How they **function** might be more about how connected they feel to others, or how competent they feel in life in general. Whereas they might **evaluate** their life in relation to the best possible life they could imagine. If someone is flourishing we would see them as having a high level of wellbeing and being able to function well and having positive feelings. Someone who was struggling in terms of wellbeing would have negative feelings and not function well in their lives. This could be connected to whether they have a sense of autonomy and control over life, as well as having a sense of purpose in life. Positive feelings can also help people to respond more positively to life's challenges and build on their personal resources and capabilities. So, happiness can increase people's capacity for doing well in life. The New Economics Foundation model for wellbeing (Michaelson, 2012) identify **external conditions**, such as income, employment status and social networks as acting together with **personal resources** such as heath, resilience, optimism and self-esteem. These both help a person to have **good functioning and satisfaction of needs**, so that they are more likely to be autonomous, safe and secure and connected to others and **experience good feelings** on a day-to-day basis such as happiness, joy, contentment and satisfaction. It is important to appreciate that we need to make a choice to be happy, but this needs to become a habit, not just an occasional experience. Happiness like optimism is a magnet for others and attracts others to feel the same.

The New Economics Foundation (2008) go on to suggest five ways to improve our wellbeing, which also increases our ability to be resilient:

- Connect with others – at home, at work, in our local communities etc because this enriches our lives on a daily basis.
- Be active – whatever physical exercise suits your mobility and fitness.
- Take notice and be curious – try to notice the beauty in our lives and savour the moments we enjoy, because this helps us to appreciate what matters most to us.
- Keep learning – learning new things can make us more confident and can be fun.
- Give – do something nice for someone, smile, give some time to others, this increases our connections with others and helps link our happiness to that of the wider community.

Martin Seligman (2011) in *Flourish*, his book on wellbeing and happiness, takes a positive psychology approach and says that wellbeing has five elements. These are **positive emotion**, **engagement**, **meaning**, **positive relationships** and **accomplishment**, which he explains under the mnemonic PERMA:

- Positive emotion – happiness and life satisfaction are key components of enjoying a pleasant life.
- Engagement – so how involved do we feel in what we are doing. If we are really engaged in something we might not even realise that we are enjoying what we are doing. This could be because being that engaged means that thoughts and feelings are often absent at the time of the activity.

- Meaning – there needs to be something that makes an experience have a coherence for us that outlives the time of the event itself. In addition, this needs to have some meaning and coherence for others too, which is measured independently of positive emotion, engagement, accomplishments and relationships.
- Accomplishment – the need to gain something is important here, but it might not be for the purpose of success in its own right, it might be because of the enjoyment of taking part. For example, some bridge players only feel that they have accomplished something important if they have won, whereas others might feel that they have accomplished something if they have learnt something which will help them to improve in the future. Feeling positive about the experience will therefore vary from one person to another in terms of what they feel that there was to accomplish, and whether they managed to do this.
- Positive relationships – Seligman (2011) makes the point that very little that is positive is solitary and that loneliness is a disabling condition and that we live longer if we have people to share our problems and experiences with. Our relationships with others tend to be what makes an experience more enjoyable.

All these elements of wellbeing are important from a leadership perspective and showing gratitude, being engaged in what we do and maintaining relationships all promote wellbeing. We need to try to find meaning in what we do and, if it is helpful, make lists of what we have achieved and what we feel most proud of. These can all form part of the culture of a work environment which promotes wellbeing amongst those who work there. It is easy to take for granted the small things in life which are just "ordinary" and these things can be less noticeable.

Having thought about the importance of leading with compassion we can go on to think about our own role in taking a lead.

Individual leadership

Case Study 6.4

Andrew's focus on promoting dignity

Whilst on my placement I was carrying out regular hourly observations. As part of the physical observations, it was necessary to monitor a patient's respiration rate for one minute. Whilst monitoring Jane's (pseudonym) respiration rate I noticed that her respiratory rate was increasing. After the minute was completed, I asked her if she was ok and she told me she felt uncomfortable as she felt I was staring at her chest. She stated she knew I was only looking at her chest for monitoring purposes but it still made her uncomfortable because of my gender. I reported this back to my mentor who then spoke to the patient who again stated that she knew it was for the purpose of monitoring and had no concerns about me.

I can understand how Jane felt and I am glad she did not perceive what I was doing as inappropriate. After this event I sat with my mentor and we discussed ways that we could resolve this concern and ways to address it in the future. Taking physical observations is a vital aspect of nursing as it allows us to calculate an early warning score which gives a good indication of how a patient's organs and systems are working. This allows for timely intervention if necessary and allows us to monitor recovery. It is important to monitor a patient's respiration rate for a full minute as during that time it can increase or decrease and give a different score which would prompt us to investigate further. It is also important to treat our patients with decency and respect. This allows them to feel safe and trust staff carrying out their care.

After speaking with my mentor, we tried a strategy which allowed me to still monitor Jane's respiration rate but did not cause her the discomfort she was feeling before. The new idea was to take the patients wrist as if we were checking her heart rate but instead, I would count her respiration rate. This indirect way of viewing her chest still provided a good visual picture. This worked very well and when I checked with Jane, she found this much more comfortable.

Since this situation arose, I have implemented this when taking observations with female patients as I believe it improves the care I provide for them. It was invaluable having my mentor there to support me and Jane, and to help me improve my standard of care and this shows that feedback from both our perspectives can result in a more positive outcome.

Andrew has demonstrated great self-awareness when he could have felt vulnerable and criticised. He has taken the patient's feedback very positively and escalated that to his mentor and together they experimented with a new approach to reducing Jane's anxiety. This demonstrates great maturity and professionalism, and has allowed him to move on and carry out care in a different way with patients who might not have felt as able to be as assertive. This would be a real teaching moment for Andrew in his coaching role, both with male and female health care practitioners. We can get so blunted by everyday practice that we fail to see that staring at someone's chest is just not normal in everyday life. It is also possible not to think as clearly about how we can maximise people's dignity, we just carry on doing what we usually do. It is crucial that we try to focus on making positive changes whenever we can and respond with a "**yes, we can do this**" rather than find reasons why we cannot adapt and change. It would have been so easy for Andrew to just respond with giving a rationale for **why** he needed to assess Jane's respiratory rate, rather than to think of the **how** it could be carried out in a less embarrassing manner.

If we are resilient and can bounce back after stressful events then our teams are more likely to be resilient too. Having a positive outlook is important because this empowers us to meet challenges effectively. It is possible to develop resilience and positivity, and it is important that we do so. An example is an American hockey team who had excellent results throughout the season but when they were eliminated in the first round of the national playoffs the team could not cope with the pressure and collapsed under it. Their team coach said that individual resilience was the biggest indicator of team resilience, and this was particularly true in the core leadership part of the team. It is important to develop optimism as an individual, and CBT and NLP (neurolinguistic programming) are particularly helpful in this by disrupting negative thoughts and reframing these from different perspectives. We can then think of alternative strategies and learn from situations. We can learn how to be optimists.by learning new cognitive skills and embracing a more dynamic approach to life and seeing the potential benefits of any given situation. Optimists tend to expect positive outcomes and therefore believe that they will succeed and have higher coping abilities. By helping individuals to develop optimism organisations can create and sustain highly resilient teams through hope and self-talk. Resilient teams are not demoralised by adverse situations and accept them as happening and do not focus on the past and what has been lost; they focus on the positives for the future. Resilience and optimism should exist together because they feed on, and reinforce, each other. So, optimism leads to resilience and resilience leads to further optimism.

Boynton (2022) talks about the importance of soft skills like emotional intelligence, communication and person-centred and relationship skills. These include trust, self-awareness self-control, assertiveness and respect. Team skills like collaboration and teamwork and the ability to lead and follow, being adaptable and being able to switch between leading and following are also important. Creighton and Smart (2022) say that an effective leader accepts their leadership role, calls for help appropriately and constantly monitors situations, makes decisions, inspires the team and resolves conflicts. We can be very damning of soft skills and see them as being just touchy-feely things that we do when we have time to be warm and fuzzy. However, using these skills oils the wheels, and helps relationships to thrive and for everyone to feel more positive, so they are even more crucial in today's stressful environment.

Schein and Schein (2018) discuss humble leadership which values all members of the team as individuals and creates trusting and open relationships with each member of the team. Humble leadership is the opposite of heroic leadership which focuses on the team being dependent on one individual leader. The emphasis of humble leadership is on building trusting and open relationships in the team and using experiential learning to develop strong team dynamics.

Higgins and McBennett (2007) discuss the "petals of recovery" which promote resilience. These petals can overlap but they involve:

- Positive self-image and identity
- Spiritual connection
- Relationships
- Trust in self
- Self determination
- Meaning
- Voice
- Confidence and control
- Personal resourcefulness
- Hope.

For these to exist we also need to be:

- Compassionate
- Resilient
- Able to manage ourselves
- Positive
- Ready to take a lead on compassion
- Emotionally intelligent and self-aware
- Mindful
- Problem solving.

Emotionally intelligent (EI) leaders are able to understand themselves and manage their emotions and their relationships and have emotional capabilities. We can expand our emotional intelligence in a way that we cannot do with our intellectual intelligence. We can use different competencies and leadership styles depending on the circumstances. There are ways we can enhance our emotional intelligence by using different leadership styles (See Table 6.1):

Table 6.1 Leadership styles and emotional intelligence

Leadership styles	Approach	EI competencies	Positives	Negatives
Visionary / Authoritative	Motivation and commitment to common goals "This is what I see, I want you to see it too and I need your help to get there"	Self-confidence empathy transparency, catalysing change	In almost every team especially when things are difficult. Probably the most effective style and has a positive cultural influence	In a team with more experience this does not work so well
Coaching	Focus on self-development and genuine interest, long term goals, new ways of working, communication and flexibility	Empathy, developing others, self-awareness	When people are aware of strengths and weaknesses and want to be coached	When people are resistant to change and learning or there is an ineffective coach
Affiliative	Emotional bonds and harmony, communication, flexibility to create new ways forward "Let's work together on this"	Empathy, conflict management, collaboration, relationship building	Good all-round approach, harmony, morale and communication and can heal breakdowns in trust	Can fail to give clear direction. Best used with another style due to emphasis on praise rather than on poor performance
Democratic	Consensus through collaboration. Encourages ideas and a say in decisions	Team leading, collaboration, influence, conflict management, communication	Trust, commitment, flexibility, high morale. Uses the experiences and views of all	Inappropriate in crises or when team members lack experience, knowledge or competence
Pace setting/ Coercive	Expects excellence and self-direction. "Don't ask questions, just do it" and "keep up"	Drive to achieve, initiative self-control and conscientiousness	If people are self-motivated, skilled and need minimal direction. Can work with other styles.	Less emphasis on empathy & self-awareness, anxiety, endless demands and a lack of clear direction
Commanding	Demands immediate compliance and can resort to threats	Influence, achievement, initiative	Useful in a real emergency but should be used with great care and used alongside empathy and self-control	Inflexible, seeks tight control, rarely issues praise & frequent criticism, pride, morale and satisfaction

Different combinations of these leadership styles are needed in different circumstances and a pick and mix approach is helpful. The coercive pace setting style tends to have a negative impact with leaders being discouraging and demotivating and this alienates their team members and does not help them to improve. Authoritative leaders tend to have a vision for their service and communicate this to others, but the trick is to take others with them and this is not always the case. In order to work towards better care and patient experience all members of the team need to be engaged in how best to enhance care. (https://app.goodpractice.net/#/open-university/s/zn0qxby2qc). The organisations which are most successful at leadership focus on emotional intelligence competencies, so we all need to focus on ways to lead with emotional intelligence.

Youngson https://www.youtube.com/watch?v=jU_hCYXOFrI focuses on the 12 practices for compassionate connection with patients. These are:

- Take care of your attitude through positive body language and speech.
- Make a human connection and maybe ask them what they would be doing today if they were not there and invite them to share their concerns and fears.
- Take care with introductions explaining who you are and what your role is.
- Express your intention to care and that you are there to help them.
- Meet patients at their level and be at the same level as them so that they are not intimidated, and they can express their concerns.
- Ask the patient how they are feeling so that they feel heard.
- Make past traumatic events explainable so that they feel that they will be avoided this time.
- Lead the patient one step at a time in manageable chunks.
- Put the patient in charge and ask their permission to do things.
- Acknowledge the patient is an expert in themselves and ask what has been helpful in the past, and what they found difficult.
- Be a healing presence and use your tone of voice and non-verbal communication in a therapeutic way so that they feel that they have been cared for with compassion.
- However, in order to be able to do this we need to focus on our personal and professional lifestyle and then we can focus on our team being a positive place to work. So, some questions to ask yourself are:

Personal lifestyle:

- Are you getting sufficient sleep and is this good quality sleep?
- Are you able to eat healthily most of the time?
- Can you do the exercise and physical activity which you think is important for you?
- Can you work out what your main priorities are, and can you achieve these?
- Are you taking enough annual leave, and can you take time away from your normal worries and work when you want to?
- Do you have any interests and hobbies, and can you make time for those?
- Do you reflect on your personal and work scenarios, and maybe practice yoga or meditation, and attend to your spiritual needs?
- Do you have a network of friends, and do you give and seek support from family and friends as necessary?

Professional lifestyle:

- Do you set realistic goals, vary your work routine when possible and take short breaks as possible?
- Have you thought about your communication skills recently, and how you can be a stronger advocate for those in your care, as well as your colleagues?
- Do you support others in your team and help you and them not to focus too much on negative experiences, grieve appropriately when you lose a patient, and support each other?

Organisational issues:

- Do you do your best to encourage a positive culture in your team, and encourage good, healthy and supportive interpersonal relationships?
- Do you ask others about how they feel about the organisational culture where you work?
- Could you focus more on participatory decision making in relation to patient care?
- Do you access and encourage others to take up psychological wellbeing training as available?
- Are you a strong leader and do you encourage this in others?

To be a great leader we have to want to make a difference and want people in our team to take a lead too. We need to influence and not want to exert power and control and have a passion for what we do. We need to be trusted and earn the respect of our team. We also need to focus on compassionate leadership, demonstrating compassion for our patients and our colleagues. As Alverez says "the point is not to pay back kindness but to pass it on" (https://quotefancy.com/quote/1555192/Julia-Alvarez-The-point-is-not-to-pay-back-kindness-but-to-pass-it-on).

Clouston (2015) refers to the importance of knowing what is urgent, and what is important. We often get distracted by what is urgent which takes our attention away from what is important. The nonurgent and non-important tasks we need to avoid, delegate, say no to, or cancel from our to do list. The urgent but not important things can be interruptions that prevent you from achieving your goals, so try to say no or delegate these. The urgent but not important tasks are important goals that can become urgent if not dealt with. So, when you can, these need to be scheduled in make sure these happen. The urgent and important tasks are critical activities, some of which can be planned for, and others cannot. We need to plan for those we can and leave time for those we cannot plan.

I try to take this approach myself and organise as far ahead as I can to allow myself time to cope with last minute urgent demands on my time. I plan student meetings into my diary a few weeks in advance, which makes it easier for students and their practice assessors to meet the requirements of the programme in relation to meetings with me. Of course, these sometimes need to change, but I try to allow flexibility in my diary to accommodate these last-minute changes due to sickness, low staffing on the day etc. As I am in control over my diary I often have more planned than others would ever plan for me, and that can lead to not having time to do the admin tasks that I need to complete in relation to each student straight afterwards, so I end up with a list of tasks to do at the end of the day. This is not ideal, but it is part of working with students and mentors who have busy working lives and not enough staff. What I struggle most with is procrastination of important work, through focusing on the small but less urgent work. This is so common, and I know that we all struggle with this. Because we are busy doing really valuable tasks, and are not sitting reading a magazine, we can justify not getting round to writing assignments, or for me writing this book. That then increases our stress because big tasks hang over us and cause us more stress. We feel so much better when we have made headway on a big task. We all want to achieve that wonderful sense of accomplishment without having focused on the nitty gritty of actually doing it.

So, we need to appreciate that we are doing very well to cope with busy and stressful events in our lives and be compassionate to ourselves when our lives are less organised than we might have hoped for. We need to focus on self-care when we can by:

- Taking time for relaxation and having opportunities to indulge our sense of humour.
- Dealing with emotions in a healthy manner.
- Responding to the emotions of patients, colleagues and others in our lives.
- Staying true to own feelings where possible.
- Using problem solving and seeking social support when necessary.
- Distancing work from home when focusing on our home lives, and this can be harder for those who work from home, as many are continuing to do since the pandemic.
- Accessing more mental health support for depression, anxiety etc when necessary, and encouraging others to do the same.
- Utilising strategies for insomnia, stress management, building higher self-esteem, and the appropriate use of humour.
- Accessing specialist support if suffering from long COVID, or at times of acute or ongoing physical or emotional symptoms.

I have summed up compassionate leadership from an individual perspective with possible SMART goals below (Table 6.2). Try to develop your own.

Table 6.2 Promoting individual compassionate leadership in ourselves and others

What to achieve (Specific)	Why this is important (Relevant)	How will this be achieved (Attainable)	How will you know that you have achieved this (Measurable and Timely)
To maximise my resilience	In order to bounce back when possible	Reflect on situations that have increased my stress	Discover learning for future situations. Reflect on the way home and make a time within the next week to implement change
Increase my EI and self-awareness	Essential for responding to feedback	360 degree feedback from others	Positive feedback from nursing and MDT colleagues and students
Focus on communication and relational skills	Essential for patient contact and teamworking	360 degree feedback from others	Positive feedback from nursing and MDT colleagues and students
Become adept at flexible leading and following	Encouraging leadership in others	Ability to switch between leading and following	Encourage others to lead and delegate to you at times and supervise this at others. Have an ongoing timetable to encourage leadership opportunities
Focus on conflict management awareness	Conflict can be prevalent in work settings	Help others to spot conflict building up	Good conflict prediction and de-escalation. Discuss scenarios in team huddles
Be a humble leader	Heroic leadership is no longer appropriate	Help others and value what they do	Positive feedback strategies in place. Reflect on leadership opportunities regularly.

(Continued)

270

Table 6.2 (Continued) Promoting individual compassionate leadership in ourselves and others

What to achieve (Specific)	Why this is important (Relevant)	How will this be achieved (Attainable)	How will you know that you have achieved this (Measurable and Timely)
Show compassion to yourself	In order to be compassionate to others you need to be compassionate to yourself	Give positive feedback to yourself as you would to others and plan self-care activities	Think about holistic lifestyle activities and record reflection on what has gone well. Carry out self-care activities every week and reflect at the end of each day on what has gone well
Coach others	In order to help others to develop professionally	Analyse different coaching strategies and ask students about how they learn best	Positive feedback from students and new members of the team
Organisational influence as appropriate	To enhance the workplace culture	Ask team members for what they find positive and challenging about working in the team	Escalate concerns in response to individual and team feedback. Regular discussions to assess how team members feel about the working environment.
Focus on kindness	Showing kindness encourages others to be kind.	Pass kindness on and encourage others to do the same	Positive relationships in workplace
Focus on what is important	It is easy to focus on the urgent rather than important	Be clear about the important goals that you have and block out time for these	Keeping track of on term goals and timetable these into your life.
Deal with own issues as they arise	Ensure that your own health issues are managed	Assess your levels of stress, anxiety and low mood	Ensure that you carry out activities that improve your health. Ongoing timetabling of health enhancing activities.
Radiate positivity	Positivity radiates positivity	Do not be a drain and deplete others' energies, focus on positivity	Feedback from others

These are all strategies that are much easier said than done, but all we can do is try to focus on our individual leadership and support of others, and compassion for ourselves. We need to be role models for others in how we deal with our stress, and that is an important part of leadership. However, we also need to take a part in team leadership and the focus will be on this now.

Team leadership and compassionate leadership

A team leader does not need to be in a management role, and more junior members of the team can be leaders too. We need to be engaging transformational leaders (Alban-Metcalfe and Alimo-Metcalfe, 2018) and the authors cite the transformational leadership model (Alban- Metcalfe and Alimo-Metcalfe, 2006) which focus on:

- Servant leadership – supporting others and encouraging them to be leaders in meeting the needs of patients in their care.
- Working in partnership to focus on reducing barriers to communication and sharing of ideas.

- Respecting others' views, concerns and experiences.
- A culture that encourages all to challenge the status quo and think of new ideas.
- A culture that supports individual personal development and learning from mistakes and using these as learning opportunities.

There are many differences between top-down managers and leaders:

- Top-down managers take credit rather than giving it.
- Tell people what to do rather than taking a collaborative approach in getting work accomplished.
- Generate fear rather than inspiring others and creating enthusiasm.
- Drain people rather than growing them.
- Keep hold of power and control and know how to accomplish things but do not show others how to do the same.
- Uses "I" rather than "we".

Whereas team leaders:

- Are courageous and make difficult decisions when necessary and challenge others.
- Are effective communicators.
- Are generous and praise others.
- They thank others.
- Are humble and will help others and do not always know best.
- Are self-aware and know their strengths but also their developmental areas.
- Treat others as they would want to be treated.
- Are passionate and enthusiastic.
- Are positive.
- Are authentic and honest.
- Are approachable.
- Are accountable and do not blame others.
- Have a sense of purpose.
- Show some vulnerability.
- Are genuinely pleased to see others develop, have good eye contact and communication skills and remember small details about others and form connections
- Look for areas of agreement not areas of conflict.
- They put people before processes.

West and Markiewicz (2016) say that the key elements for effective teamworking are:

- A clear agreed vision with challenging objectives
- Role clarity
- Positivity, optimism, cohesion and compassion
- Effective communication and constructive debate
- Enthusiastic and supportive within the team and across teams and MDTs.

We need to be confident leaders, so that others can believe in us and sometimes this involves a certain swan like approach where we are paddling like mad out of sight but appearing confident and serene. We can be really concerned about a patient in our care who is deteriorating fast, and in an unanticipated way, but if we seem worried and panicked this worries the patient and adds to their stress. I remember as a first-year student nurse I was in charge on my first set of nights on a surgical ward and a post operative patient with a very large abdominal wound coughed and said, "Oh look what I have just done". I looked under the covers and his whole wound was wide open. I somehow remembered something in my introductory block about keeping exposed bowel damp and asked for wet dressings and asked for the doctor to be contacted and I stood with him holding his wound together and reassuring him that all was under control. I was actually terrified, but sometimes being confident is about being brave, and you cannot be brave unless you are scared. The 6Cs (Department of Health, 2012) rightly have courage as one of the core values of compassionate practice and I was definitely using a lot of courage on that night. The patient went back to theatre as an emergency, made a good recovery and went home. Years later though when I was a staff nurse that same patient approached me in a corridor and thanked me for what I did on that night. He said that he was so frightened but as I had seemed so calm he believed that he would be fine. He had no idea how worried I was, but he remembered me because of how calm I had been when he was having a crisis. An important message is that patients remember us for what we do, and how we behave, and how we make them feel, and we need to be remembered in relation to positive experiences.

The 6Cs form the Compassion in Practice strategy and they focus on the values for compassionate practice. These values of care, compassion, courage, communication, commitment and competence should be exemplified throughout health and social care environments. So, they should form part of recruitment, appraisals and training for all those working within those care environments, not just nursing staff (Department of Health, 2012)

Hougaard et al (2020) says that compassion on its own is not sufficient and that compassion needs to be combined with wisdom. There are two axes ranging from indifference to compassion and from ignorance to wisdom:

- Ineffective indifference (ignorant and indifferent) – lacking interest and concern for others.
- Uncaring execution (wise but indifferent) – putting results before people's wellbeing.
- Caring avoidance (ignorant but compassionate) letting empathy be a barrier to compassion by not doing the tough parts of leadership like giving hard feedback.
- Wise compassion (wise and compassionate) – getting tough things done in a human way by balancing concern for others with needing to meet tough objectives. This involves taking tough action when needed but with genuine caring for people's feelings and wellbeing.

In order to be wise and compassionate we need to have genuine self-compassion and adopt daily compassion practices because compassion is a trainable skill. We also need to check our intentions and put ourselves in others' shoes and then have assertive, candid and transparent discussions with others, and recognise that being clear is also about being kind because concealing tough criticism is not kind, it is misleading. I use this all the time with my students, and I believe that students should be the best practitioners that they can be, and that their patients need and deserve this. It is not enough to be just good enough, they need to be exemplary. In order to do this, I always use Daloz's (1986) model of mentoring relationships where high support is combined with high challenge. So, I tell them all the time how inspiring and excellent they are, but I also encourage them to challenge their own thinking about how they practice. One student who I had been trying to encourage to do just that sent me an email saying, "I am grateful that you pushed me to complete everything to the standard you knew I was capable of achieving". That clearly demonstrated how her self-awareness and self-belief had increased through the year and her clear insight was impressive.

I like this quote: "leaders are developers, team builders, imaginers, culture caretakers, roadblock removers and inspirers. Their success depends on enabling the success of others" (Leadership First www.leadershipfirst.net). This is the very essence of compassionate leadership. Goleman (2022) says:

> For most positions, especially leadership, the relevant cognitive or technical skill set is a threshold ability – one you need to get and keep the position. But what makes someone a standout in that position is due in large part to emotional intelligence. A growing body of research now strongly supports the benefits for any organisation of having emotionally intelligent leaders and employees.
>
> (Goleman, 2022 https://www.linkedin.com/
> pulse/2022-year-more-emotional-intelligence-daniel-goleman/?
> trk=eml-email_series_follow_newsletter_01-hero-1-title_
> link&midToken=AQEtkru62bnmlw&fromEmail=
> fromEmail&ut=0nBD_TUEYzNq41)

Bauer-Wu and Fontaine (2015) in their compassionate care initiative, focus on the wellbeing of clinicians and they highlight the importance of having compassionate care role models and catalysts. They also state the importance of being the best version of ourselves which involves resilience, mindfulness, interprofessional collaboration and a healthy work environment where people are engaged and there is a focus on creating a compassionate place to work. Waddington (2016) in her study of university culture highlights the importance of kindness, kinship and compassionate relationships to combat the toxic workplaces that often exist in higher education, and sometimes in health care environments I would suggest.

Atkins and Parker (2012) say that compassionate leadership involves four behaviours:

- Attending – This means being present with and focusing on others – "listening with fascination". Kline (2002) says that most of us think that we are good listeners, but many of us are not, and that we all need to focus on listening to a deeper level. West et al (2015) says that "listening is probably the most important leadership skill, and compassionate leaders take time to listen to the challenges, obstacles, frustrations and harms colleagues experience as well as listening to accounts of their successes and joys".
- Understanding – This involves taking time to properly explore and understand the situations people are struggling with. This involves valuing and exploring conflicting perspectives rather than leaders simply imposing their own understanding.
- Empathising – This involves mirroring and feeling colleagues' distress, frustration, joy, etc, without being overwhelmed by the emotion and becoming unable to help (West and Chowla, 2017).
- Helping – This involves taking thoughtful and intelligent action to support individuals and teams. Removing obstacles that get in the way of people doing their work (e.g. chronic excessive workloads, conflicts between departments) and providing the resources people and services need (e.g. staff, equipment, training) are the most important tasks for leaders (McCauley and Fick-Cooper, 2020).

So why is compassionate leadership so important? Research shows that compassionate leadership has wide-ranging benefits for both staff and organisations:

- If we work in supportive teams with clear goals and good team leadership, we have dramatically lower levels of stress (West et al, 2015). Compassionate leadership increases staff engagement and satisfaction, resulting in better outcomes for all organisations, including improved financial performance, or in the case of health care a better use of resources (West, 2021, West and Dawson, 2022).
- In NHS trusts where staff report the absence of such leadership, staff also report higher levels of work overload and less influence over decision making (West et al, 2020) and poorer outcomes for patients (West and Dawson, 2022, West et al, 2011).
- Staff who are treated with compassion are better able to direct their support and care giving to others (Goetz et al, 2010). This results in higher quality care and higher levels of patient satisfaction (West and Dawson, 2022, West et al, 2011). Where staff generally report the absence of compassionate leadership there are lower levels of patient satisfaction (West et al, 2020) and there is poorer quality of care (in the acute sector) and higher patient mortality (West and Dawson, 2022, West et al 2011).
- Trzeciak and Mazzarelli (2019) make a compelling case for 'compassionomics', the knowledge and scientific study of the effects of compassionate health care. Their research reviews hundreds of published studies which show that compassion is the most powerful intervention in health care. Compassionate health care is beneficial for patients through improving clinical outcomes; for health care systems by supporting financial sustainability; and for health care professionals, through lowering burnout and promoting resilience and wellbeing.

West et al (2015) highlight the importance of collective leadership, which involves all members of the organisation taking responsibility for the success of the organisation as a whole. This involves a focus on continual learning and improvement of patient care, rather than on focusing on the development of individual leadership capability. There needs to be high level dialogue and analysis to develop shared understanding about quality concerns and strategies to address these. Everyone needs to be a leader and take collective responsibility in developing safe, effective, high quality and compassionate care (West et al 2020, West et al 2021). This involves planning, commitment and tenacity and ensuring that there is an ongoing focus on nurturing leadership and the culture of the organisation.

The Kings Fund (2011) highlight the importance of not having "hero" type leaders who everyone turns to for decisions. Some of these charismatic type leaders are negative examples who have carried out barbaric acts, for example Hitler. We might not like to think that they are charismatic, which we see as a positive trait, but without their charisma they would never have managed to persuade others to conform to their personal agenda. Other people are positive role models and make excellent decisions, but there is a leadership vacuum when they are not on shift or busy elsewhere. No one person can always be right, and within health care now there is a move away from individual decision making to MDT decision making and protocols. For example, in an arrest everyone involved is asked if they agree with stopping resuscitation, and in long term decision making the MDT is crucial in making decisions. This is an approach which came about as a result of changes in the airline industry following a plane crash in 1977 where it was found later that the First Officer had challenged the decision of the captain of the plane, but he was not listened to and a terrible crash involving two 747 planes resulted and 583 people were killed. Health care leadership has been transformed as a result and collective leadership means that all members of the team should feel like they have a leadership role, and the best leaders foster this culture.

A few points about compassionate leadership:

- Compassion can be defined as "a sensitivity to suffering in self and others with a commitment to try to alleviate and prevent it" (Gilbert and Choden 2013). We can experience compassion in different ways: we can feel compassion for other people; we can experience compassion from others; and there is also the compassion we can direct towards ourselves.

- Compassionate leadership involves a focus on relationships through careful listening, understanding, empathising and supporting others This enables those we lead to feel valued, respected and cared for so they can reach their potential and do their best. There is clear evidence that compassionate leadership results in more engaged and motivated staff with high levels of wellbeing, which in turn results in high quality care (West et al, 2020).

- How do compassionate leaders behave? They empathise with their colleagues and seek to understand the challenges they face; they are committed to supporting others to cope with, and respond successfully to, work challenges; and they are focused on enabling those they lead to be effective and thrive in their work. Compassionate leaders do not have all the answers and don't simply tell people what to do. Instead, they engage with the people they work with to find shared solutions to problems.

- For leadership to be compassionate it must also be inclusive. Compassion blurs the boundaries between us and others, promoting belonging, trust, understanding, mutual support and, by definition, inclusion (West et al, 2020). This creates an inclusive, psychologically safe environment in which diversity in all forms is valued and team members can contribute creatively and enthusiastically to team performance.

- It is evident that the NHS has struggled over many years to sustain inclusive, people-centred cultures. Ross et al (2020 in their research found that it is local action in teams, departments and organisations (big and small), where the work to create these types of cultures is most effective, because that is where the people are. Developing compassionate leadership approaches helps leaders hold crucial conversations about inclusion, ensuring they hear and reflect deeply on what staff are telling them and then take necessary action to help address inequalities and discrimination in the workplace.

- Compassionate leaders also acknowledge the humanity of all those they work with and acknowledge the stress that they, and others, are experiencing. Wheeler (2023) gives an example of a pilot of a plane she was travelling in when an engine exploded. The pilot had to carry out an emergency landing and he came through to the main cabin afterwards and said that he had been scared, and he was sure they were too. He explained what had happened and congratulated the passengers on staying calm and following instructions. As a result, the passengers all started to relax, because he had acknowledged all the feelings that they were all experiencing, allowing them to deal with these emotions, and he congratulated them for their response to the frightening situation. So, preparing for the emotional reactions to stress and change and acknowledging these, and focusing on these at times can be part of compassionate leadership.

The importance of creating caring cultures is discussed by the Foundation of Nursing Studies (2015) (https://www.youtube.com/watch?v=cZyN_UZvYnQ&feature=youtube). Competence and caring work together, and are not mutually exclusive, and they are both needed to create and maintain a compassionate culture. Staff need to be asked what it feels like to work where they do because they feel heard and listened to, and as a result patient care is enhanced. Values and beliefs form the basis of attitudes and behaviours, and we learn from what happens in practice. If we take responsibility for improving practice, this enhancement continues. Effective leadership involves listening, being enthusiastic and working within teams to enhance care. Change takes time and we need to celebrate small changes and wins (Shuttleworth, 2015). For safe and effective care staff need to feel valued and engaged and work within a caring culture.

Maben et al (2012) discuss how due to limited resources, poor leadership and an uncaring culture health care practitioners can focus more on the "poppets" who they have more empathy for and were easier to like. This was to the detriment of those who were harder to like and were perceived as demanding and difficult. This second group felt that they were likely to be moved around as "parcels". Therefore, patients went out of their way to be seen as easy to care for. This needs to be challenged by more senior members of the team, as well as every member of the team. There needs to be high support/high challenge conversations (Daloz, 1986) and transformational leadership in order for high quality care to thrive and this can transform the care environment (Murray et al, 2012).

Meeting people's core needs at work is important in supporting their wellbeing and motivation. Compassionate leaders constantly strive to understand and meet the core needs of the people they work with (West et al, 2015).The Health and Care Select Committee recently conducted an inquiry on workforce burnout and resilience in the NHS and social care (House of Commons Health and Social Care Committee 2021 https://houseofcommons.shorthandstories.com/health-and-care-staff-burnout/index.html). It concluded that burnout is a widespread reality in today's NHS and has negative consequences for the mental health of individual staff, which has an impact on their colleagues and the patients and service users they care for.

Recent studies in relation to doctors, nurses and midwives including those in training, have shown that wellbeing, flourishing and work engagement of health and care staff is affected by eight key factors which can be organised into three core needs (see below). Meeting the core needs of health and care staff can help transform their work lives and in turn, the safety and quality of the care that they deliver (West and Coia, 2019).

West et al in The Kings Fund report "The Courage of Compassion" (2020) discuss the stresses of the COVID-19 pandemic on nurses and midwives. They say that nurses and midwives have three core needs to ensure wellbeing and motivation and minimise workplace stress. These are:

- Autonomy – having control over their work lives and be able to act consistently within their core values.
- Belonging – to feel connected, valued, respected, supported and cared for by colleagues.
- Contribution – to be effective at work and deliver outcomes.

In order for this to be the case they made eight recommendations focusing on:

- authority, empowerment and influence – influencing cultures, processes and decisions.

- justice and fairness – psychologically safe cultures with proactive and positive approaches to diversity, inclusion and equity.
- work conditions and work schedules -minimum standards for working conditions.
- teamworking – effective MDT teamworking for all.
- culture and leadership – compassionate leadership and nurturing cultures to ensure high quality and continually improving compassionate care.
- workload – tackling chronic excessive work demands that exceed capacity, compromises safety, high quality care and staff health and wellbeing.
- management and supervision – effective support, reflection, mentorship and supervising to ensure that all can thrive.
- learning, education and development – ensuring that processes are in place to ensure that there is learning and development throughout careers which promotes equitable outcomes throughout (West et al, 2020).

West and Bailey (2019) say that the five myths about compassionate leadership are that if you are compassionate:

- There will be a loss of commitment to purpose and high quality performance.
- Tough performance management and conversations will not happen and might be labelled as bullying.
- That we will always take the easy and consensus way forward rather than putting patients and communities first.
- The status quo will not be challenged and radical changes that are needed by patients and communities will not take place.
- Teamwork and system working will be controlled by whoever has the power and is most ruthless.
- Compassionate leadership is about focusing on the collective good, rather than on individual agendas. Therefore, inappropriate power and control over resources which are inconsistent with the values of our health services are not challenged.

Creighton and Smart (2022) say that teamworking issues are linked to nursing care and omissions and this can lead to mistakes and to poor care. The SBAR (Situation, Background, Assessment, Recommendation) method is commonly used to communicate in a structured way particularly when a patient is deteriorating. It is important to recognise that any tool is not perfect, and only as good as the practitioner using it, and we need to use our own clinical expertise to do a reality check. However, having clear communication strategies means that the escalation of concerns happens in a timely way. Communication is the most important aspect of teamworking, and self-awareness is key to communication and we need to have a team culture that reinforces self-awareness. Creighton and Smart (2022) say that successful teams have had the correct training, have a common goal, use communication methods and have designated roles that all team members understand. Training, reflection and simulation or role modelling are key, as are knowing and working within our limitations, being self-aware and promoting mutual respect and support pf colleagues and patients.

Clinical supervision can be detrimental if it is abusive with derogatory attitudes which demean, humiliate and threaten the individual, or where the views of the other person are ignored. Restorative supervision increases resilience in relation to the negative impacts of work, and reduces burnout and enhances physical and mental health, empathy and compassion and increases the quality of patient care. Group clinical supervision can increase resilience through increasing confidence, regulating emotions, enhancing coping strategies, managing expectations and developing self-awareness, as individuals and as a team.

Restorative supervision is a kind of clinical supervision that supports reflective practice which can help build our resilience by focusing on our experience, sustaining our wellbeing and motivation at work. This model has shown to reduce stress and burnout and increase compassion satisfaction (Griffiths, 2022) Restorative supervision is based on the principles of the Solihull approach (Solihull, 2015) as well as motivational interviewing and leadership theories. This involves psychological support, listening, supporting, challenging thereby increasing coping strategies, especially in stressful circumstances. It helps individuals to think and understand at a deeper level and this helps their decision making. Restorative supervision increases how valued we feel and how we function, and our work satisfaction and more effective work life balance helps reduce stress and burnout. Benefits for the organisation include better service outcomes, retention of staff, patient and practitioner satisfaction and better team dynamics. A London trust invested time and resources so that restorative supervision supervisors were trained based on the Wallbank model (Wallbank, 2016) and supervision was then offered to nurses, midwives and allied health professionals. For this to take place there needed to be organisational commitment and motivation which supported the trust's wellbeing agenda.

Organisational commitment is also necessary to implement any sort of supervision, whether one to one, group based or virtually through Teams etc. In 2020 Health Education England https://london.hee.nhs.uk/reflective-writing-role-reflection-developing-resilience (cited in Agnew, 2022) commissioned a programme of virtual resilience based clinical supervision for mental health and learning disability nursing. This was perceived as being important for all nurses transitioning to newly qualified roles, but this has never really been adopted widely. Schwartz rounds are a form of group reflection and are carried out in a multiprofessional environment involving clinical and non-clinical staff. Group clinical supervision focuses on our emotional responses to work situations. Elements of mindfulness and reflective discussion, underpinned by the principles of compassion focused therapy, (Gilbert, 2010) are integral to this process.

Schwartz rounds (https://www.theschwartzcenter.com) are a forum for clinicians to reflect on what they did in a specific situation, and how they felt about what took place, what the patient and their loved ones might have thought, their professional competence and what could have improved. This is a supportive MDT environment where emotions can be expressed and strategies revisited, particularly in relation to the emotional and social aspects of care. We need to remain uncertain in relation to how we feel about our actions and explore our uncertainties in a confidential forum where these can be discussed in a supportive way. It is however really important to encourage team debriefing after particularly distressing situations.

George (2017a) says that nonclinical managers are more likely to have a more controlling leadership or management style which is at odds with supporting caring professionals. Compassionate and collegiate style leadership is needed to enhance staff wellbeing, and this would move away from seeing staff stress and individual mental health issues as being a personal deficit. This thinking should form part of the training of senior NHS managers. In another article (George, 2017b) says that managers need help with dealing with their own emotions and the emotions of others and in demonstrating compassionate leadership; the Schwartz rounds (https://www.theschwartzcenter.com) can help staff in the caring professions to cope with the emotional aspects of their roles.

Practice Action Learning Sets are encouraged within some settings, such as care for people with dementia. Russell et al (2022) refer to Driscoll et al's (2019) principles of clinical supervision and highlight important aspects of learning sets:

- A safe space for self-care and promoting resilience
- Peer support and being part of a team learning culture

- Shared perspectives and reflections from a range of care settings
- Structured facilitation so that all members contribute
- Developing knowledge and skills and therefore practice
- Using reflection to unpick complex care situations
- Role modelling for newer members of the team.

Compassionate teams do not happen by accident and exist within the wider context of the organisation. Our actions and behaviours are shaped by our experiences and values, and often by those of our colleagues too. The organisational health care system context is also crucial in terms of the practices, opportunities and limitations which reinforce or challenge our actions and behaviours.

Egan (2019), a New Zealand doctor, says that the reality of emergency care can feel very stressful for health care personnel, and they often do not feel like a place of healing. She advocates an appreciative inquiry approach where positive parts of emergency care are focused on for all staff to encourage a thriving, rather than a surviving approach which leads to greater excellence. The dimensions of this approach are:

- Appreciation and gratitude
- Self-care
- Having fun
- Knowledge and wisdom
- Shared achievement
- Shared humanity, kindness and compassion
- Human connection
- Making a difference.

https://acem.org.au/getmedia/70a19d7e-e5e6-4c10-8fff-b8987969d983/1120-Johanne-Egan.

Maben and Bridges (2020) discuss the stress that health care practitioners have been under throughout the COVID-19 pandemic and the importance of team support, of employees feeling valued, and of a focus on wellbeing and resilience. Practitioners who are struggling can feel that they are "not resilient enough" and can feel judged when this is not fair or acceptable. They say:

> let this be an opportunity to fully recognise the inherent stresses and emotional strain that nurses bear on behalf of society and ensure support, not only through the crisis but after it is all over. When health care is back to "normal", ongoing support for nurses' wellbeing will remain critically important. While COVID-19 places particularly high stress on nursing, there is very little in the guidance presented here that was not relevant to staff wellbeing " pre-COVID" and when the pandemic is over, we look forward to the guidelines being used to establish better support for nurses and nursing in the future.
>
> (Maben and Bridges 2020, p2748).

This of course has not happened and nurses and care staff have been expected to just carry on despite a huge backlog of care needs and health care staff strikes against a backdrop of depleted, demoralised and damaged staff.

Helping colleagues to understand potential triggers that can result from past events and can cause emotional stress is important. End-of-life situations have a great capacity to do this and there need to be opportunities for increased support, supervision and debriefing. When a new person joins the team, they are not used to the traumatic situations that other team members have strategies to cope with. It is important that we help colleagues to self-care and understand how past events could affect their emotions now, that we cannot be perfect, and none of us feel happy all the time. We need to be able to deal with unhelpful thought patterns, where we criticise ourselves, thinking that we are a failure and encourage taking time out for relaxing and quietening down, learning to self soothe. Maybe through yoga, breathing exercises, meditation and mindful approaches we can regulate our emotions and talk to ourselves kindly. We do not want to anaesthetise ourselves through using alcohol or medications, we need to focus on self-care instead.

Warr and Nielsen in Diener et al (2018) say that people with increased wellbeing tend to perform better at work, and that teams which are positive and happy tend to also perform better.

Miles (2023) discusses the importance of professional nurse advocates (PNAs) in district nursing teams to reduce burn out and improve patient care. This could be through facilitating restorative supervision sessions which allow staff to step back and consider the challenges of practice and possible strategies to move forward. The focus is on the A-EQUIP approach (NHS, 2017). This involves the following functions:

- Formative – focusing on training on and development.
- Normative – focusing on quality assurance and supporting staff to be confident and competent and consider near misses and errors and ways forward in terms of accountability and effectiveness.
- Restorative – focusing on emotional support, listening resilience, wellbeing and restorative supervision.
- Personal action – focusing on everyone seeing their role in quality improvement and assurance.

With this approach learning and development needs can be identified which enhance patient care, as well as reducing staff stress and enhancing wellbeing. As they say this "improves attendance, retention, innovation and quality of patient care" (Miles, 2023, p 136)

Having focused on team leadership it is also important to also discuss the important of educational leadership in order to sustain our ongoing learning and development.

Educational leadership

Case Study 6.5

Coaching and support related to a cardiac arrest

A long-term patient on the intensive care unit who was in his forties suffered a cardiac arrest which necessitated prolonged resuscitation and this was unfortunately not successful. The senior registrar who was in charge of the arrest predicted that the small ICU staff available would understandably find this physically exhausting as the resuscitation needed to carry on for so long. He also knew that they would be finding this emotionally very hard too because the staff knew him so well. So, he put out a call for available staff from nearby wards to come to help. One of my students responded to the call. The registrar asked if she had witnessed an arrest before, and if she had carried out resuscitation. She said no to both, and she was visibly very worried by the whole process. The registrar then coached her about what was needed, and how to carry out cardiac compressions. She felt very supported and left the arrest feeling much more confident. It is essential that teaching takes place in a calm supportive environment, especially when stress levels are high and confidence is low. The student was very grateful for the support she received.

The registrar was calm throughout the arrest and looked for times when members of staff were physically tired or distressed and calmly managed the whole situation. When the time came to stop resuscitation, he checked for agreement from all staff present and enabled the patient's end of life to be managed with dignity and care. He then arranged a debriefing session for those present to discuss their feelings and their sense of shock and distress. This was a highly sensitively managed situation, and I heard about this from two students. Firstly, the student who came to help, and secondly from an ITU based student who was very upset by this patient's death. However, she felt that she had been given the opportunity to accept the situation and move on before going home to an empty house at the end of her shift.

It is essential that teaching and coaching is carried out in a sensitive way, taking into account the knowledge base and skills of the person who is being taught. This situation was highly emotive and it would have been so easy for this arrest to have left members of staff feeling deskilled, underconfident and distressed after this unsuccessful resuscitation. The registrar treated this arrest as a teachable scenario for some, and supported members of the ITU in managing their feelings afterwards. Both students used this scenario as reflective opportunities, one in relation to coaching, and the other from a leadership role modelling perspective. Teachable scenarios are very effective ways to teach, at the time and in reflective discussions afterwards. I use this scenario in discussions with other students and both students will remember the day for the rest of their professional careers. So, this is a very powerful way to demonstrate educational leadership and coach others.

Outreach teams can be very supportive of students who need more knowledge base concerning medicines and assessment. Students feel underconfident when going with the outreach team to assess the needs of patients who have deteriorated rapidly. More confident specialist nurses who are skilled at educational support stress the student's positives and reassure them so that they feel able to develop this knowledge. Therefore, outreach team experience can be a very positive learning environment for students who are finding structured assessment challenging.

I find that students who are a long way out of their comfort zone in placements can feel really underconfident. The more advanced in their studies they are the more difficult this can be. There are expectations that third year students should have a certain level of expertise, but this is not the case when this is their first placement in an acute or community trust. Documentation is different and students from the community are used to case management but not bay management, and vice versa. Students whose home base is Theatres, Recovery, Outpatients, Endoscopy often also have the same transition shock, even if they have worked in the same hospital for some years. Students from acute care settings can also feel the same crisis of confidence if their placement is in the community where the care io more isolated. Sometimes these students can be criticised and judged, and this makes them feel even less competent and competent. Practice assessors need to start by discussing where their strengths and skills lie and then ask them what they see as their learning needs. Then they need to assess their skills in line with their new speciality and build their confidence and focus on their learning. In a busy practice setting this does not always happen and students are left to run a bay of acutely unwell patients. Patients are then vulnerable as is the student and other members of the team too. It is easy for us all to underestimate the knowledge and skills that we use every day in an area that is familiar to us, but experienced practitioners who are new to this environment do not necessarily have these skills. Students, and other new members of the team can then have a real crisis of confidence when they could quickly develop if they are supported and treated with kindness.

Boo (2022) says that kindness enhances learning and better educational outcomes. The brain is a social organ and learning is optimised when it takes place in a supportive environment. In addition, if learners feel stressed their distress can prevent learning taking place. Therefore, kindness is necessary for learning to take place. Resilience is boosted and we are less susceptible to anxiety which limits our thinking, and how we act and behave. Boo (2022) highlights research from 50 universities worldwide where kindness has been incorporated into the curriculum and grades and student wellbeing has been enhanced. Students being more kind to their peers and encouraging less confident students has increased intellectual insights and cooperation in group work. "Furthermore, when previously there was a considerable academic attainment gap between black and ethnic minority students compared to white students, following the introduction of kindness into the curriculum, this gap ceases to exist." (Boo, 2022, p 56)

Kindness has been perceived as being irrelevant in some roles, but treating patients with kindness enhances clinical outcomes and reduces errors, and colleagues interacting kindly enhances wellbeing (Youngson, 2012). Kindness has also been viewed negatively in leadership and management because there has been some misunderstanding of the nature of kindness. Kindness does not mean being submissive and fawning, but requires self-assurance and strength of character; it involves genuine concern about the wellbeing of staff, but does not hide poor performance and challenges this. Boo (2022) says that "if someone is attempting to hide poor performance by being nice, that is not kindness. Genuine kindness requires honesty, transparency and willingness to do what is possible to reduce suffering and promote wellbeing for everyone" (p75). Therefore, kindness can be hard and distressing and can take courage, which might explain why it is not as prevalent as it might be. So Boo (2022) identifies the need for "intelligent, courageous and fierce kindness." (p92). We all need to promote this individually, and in our team and educational leadership, so that we can treat patients, colleagues, peers, students and employees with kindness.

Teaching practitioners to take the initiative and be creative and courageous and find solutions is important. For example, helping a post operative patient to shower for the first time can involve the health care practitioner being in the wet room, and potentially getting wet, in order to help a patient wash. Treating this situation with innovation and humour, perhaps involving plastic bags over shoes, is excellent practice and other colleagues can benefit from this role modelling.

Xanthopoulou et al (2012) say that even staff who enjoy their work can have times when they feel less enthusiastic and fulfilled. Psychological strategies which develop our wellbeing include how we perceive events, maintaining a sense of humour and hope and balancing our skills with the challenges life and work bring. However, leadership training that helps cultivate our strengths can boost individual wellbeing which can make a big difference to us on an individual level and be of benefit to the organisations we work for.

Stainer et al (2022) highlight the problems raised by practice supervisors and practice assessors due to the COVID-19 pandemic. The pandemic caused huge additional pressures for all staff, and this impacted on the learning environment and how students were assessed and supported. There were restricted learning opportunities in many practice environments making assessment more difficult. There were also stressful new procedures, the use of PPE and challenging risk assessments to cope with. Clinical environments suffered excessive pressures and were extremely busy, and potentially unsafe. In addition, there was staff sickness and shortages increasing pressure on teams and making supernumerary status for students impossible. However, there were also some very positive aspects in relation to student learning, with greater learning opportunities and innovative practice, and the increased workload meant that learning was increased. Some assessors and supervisors found teaching and supporting students at this time enjoyable and students gained a great deal from their experiences. Some important messages come from this. Stainer et al (2022) highlight the importance of dedicated time for supervisor and assessor training and opportunities for protected time to share their experiences. They also highlight the importance of signposting wellbeing resources and considering student stress in relation to their wellbeing and focusing on new ways of working between practice and educational services. They also suggest more streamlined practice assessment processes where possible.

From the educational perspective in supporting students both as a module tutor as an academic assessor and practice tutor with students in multiple trusts through the pandemic, I would agree with all these points. Students have taken part, and taken a lead, in practice situations that have been highly traumatic and would never have happened in non-pandemic times. They have facilitated patients having to say goodbye to loved ones over the phone and using tablets to make these happen. They have also had to break bad news to loved ones at home who were unable to visit their dying relatives, friends and partners. They have found new ways of adapting their practice and enhancing their communication skills due to using PPE and have supported experienced colleagues who were devastated by experiences in practice. I have been amazed and inspired by students' experiences and they have felt that they have learnt a great deal. Debriefing and others' focusing on their wellbeing has not always happened, but often it has, with a team approach being taken to support all involved. Assessment in practice has taken place virtually through online meetings and these have generally worked very well, despite the challenges of very sporadic internet access at times. Relationships with students have been good with new strategies developed to support them, and quality assurance strategies have not been compromised. Supporting students and helping them to develop their thinking, practice and leadership through reflection on practice scenarios has enabled them to see how exemplary their practice has been. They have used their experiences in practice assessment interviews which has enabled them to gain well deserved marks for their excellent practice. Some of their scenarios have been deeply traumatic to hear and read, and it has enabled some very thought-provoking discussions. and increased supportive conversations, to take place. Students have been so very impressive in their person-centred and compassionate practice and discussions with their practice assessors have been supportive. I have always thanked practice assessors and supervisors for their support of students and helped students to understand how excellent their practice has been.

Smith et al (2016) discuss the model for compassionate care in practice which came from the work in the Leadership in Compassionate Care Programme at Edinburgh's Napier University. The model focuses on caring conversations, flexible person-centred risk taking, seeking and responding to feedback, knowing yourself and others, valuing others and being transparent and creating spaces that help people to discuss and constructively challenge care. The article highlights the importance of:

- Developing strategies in questioning care practices that are not compassionate.
- Undertaking regular and focused reflective activities for students to explore their drivers, values and perspectives of compassionate care.

- Actively integrating theory with practice so that in the practice and university setting students can consistently develop their compassionate caring.
- Facilitating an understanding of emotional intelligence which helps to increase self-compassion and resilience.

The Work, Relax and Play (WRAP) programme focuses on optimum wellbeing and was designed by two paramedic lecturers to address complex issues related to wellbeing in health care students (Geis, 2022). A positive social environment was created where exercise and relaxation were encouraged alongside information about healthy eating, and this was found to helpful in helping students to manage workload stress.

Newly qualified nurses need additional support through preceptorship programmes and support strategies and Gibbons and Newberry (2023) found that online coaching and wellbeing support helped newly qualified nurses to focus on practicing self-compassion and encouraged them to ask for help and speak out about their concerns. They could then perceive their feelings of vulnerability as demonstrating courage, and that self-compassion would be helpful to them, and their feeling and experiences could then be validated. Sharing and listening to the experiences and feelings of others helped them to put their experiences in context and helped them to reframe their thinking and develop strategies for the future. Greenwood (2022) talks about how we can all feel elements of imposter syndrome and feel that we are unworthy of our status or success. Newly qualified nurses can feel this and we can feel this as we move into different roles. We can be full of self-doubt and inadequacy, and have feelings of impending failure because we do not feel that we have the skills and ability to carry out our new role. Shifting the focus away from ourselves and what others might be thinking, and increasing our feelings of owning and embracing our new role can help with feelings of inadequacy. Again, reflecting with others, clinical supervision and peer support can be helpful.

It might be useful to encourage discussion on burnout and resilience so that all members of the team have a higher level of awareness about these crucial areas of wellbeing. Questions to ask ourselves in relation to burnout (B) and resilience (R) could be:

- Am I still interested in aspects of my work and do I feel challenged by my work in a positive way? B
- Do I still enjoy my work and my role and do I feel engaged with what I do at work? B
- Do I feel energised and passionate about my work and do I feel this is the only sort of work I would be happy doing? B
- Can I generally cope with my workload and work pressures? B
- Do I talk about work in a positive way? B
- Can I relax after work as easily as I could in the past and do I have enough energy for my leisure and social interests? B
- Am I exhausted by my work and do I feel worn out, emotionally drained and tired even when I arrive for work? B
- Do I do my work mechanically and do I feel disconnected or sickened by anything at work? B
- Do I find it difficult to cope with stressful events and do I bounce back as quickly as I have in the past after difficult situations? R
- Is it hard for me to recover from situations, or do I cope with them as well as possible, and get over setbacks as well as in the past? R
- Can I cope with what comes my way and can I adapt to changes in my life? R

- Can I see the funny side of things? R
- Does stress make me stronger and do I see myself as a strong person who can cope with challenges and difficulties?
- Can I stay focused and positive when under pressure? R
- Can I achieve my goals, and not be phased by minor setbacks, and develop strategies to overcome difficulties?

These are based on aspects of the Oldenburg Burnout Inventory which assesses burnout, (Demerouti 2008) and the Brief Resilience Scale which is a self-reported and self-perceived tool assesses an individual's ability to bounce back (Smith et al, 2008). The Connor Davidson Resilience Scale again measures the ability to bounce back, but over the preceding month (Davidson, 2018).

It is essential to link our compassion with emotional intelligence and fostering resilience and effective coping strategies. Ballatt and Campling (2011) say that kindness is most effective when coupled with intelligence, hence their focus on intelligent kindness. A team approach needs to promote virtuous circles rather than vicious ones (Campling 2013/2014 and this should be facilitated as organisations and in the support of students. Competencies and proficiencies focus on skills to achieve such as medicines management knowledge and other practical skills. Practice assessment documents focus on these plus reflections on practice. However, students also need to be encouraged to focus on their self-awareness and emotional intelligence and how they give and receive feedback. When they are nearing the end of the course they also need to focus on their leadership, how they challenge poor practice, and take a lead on excellent and compassionate practice, and encourage resilience, positivity and wellbeing.

So, can we teach compassion? I think that is essential that we teach and role model compassion. Shaw (2022) promotes the Clinical Learning Environment Relationship Model (CLERM) which is based on the CLES (Clinical Learning Environment and Supervision Scale) (Saarikoski et al 2008 and Saarikowski and Strandell-Laine (2018) where the importance of a positive culture in the practice environment is highlighted with a sense of team spirit and constructive cooperation and positive leadership within the team. Shaw's CLERM model (2022) focuses on the **student** and their needs and experiences seen through the **lens** of compassion, emotional intelligence, promotion of resilience and intelligent kindness. The support for the student comes from the **learning environment** and the support from the practice assessor, the whole team, the practice tutor and learning environment team. The ward manager needs to be promoting a culture of education within the team. However, the **organisation** needs to be supportive in terms of sufficient resourcing too.

Psychological wellbeing includes positive feelings, self-value, self-confidence, goals of life, engagement, and a sense of belonging (Su et al, 2014) which enables the student to thrive and grow rather than survive in their placements. The supervisory relationship has a profound effect on the student in terms of the quality of the learning environment. This is about the quality of feedback and the supervisory relationship which includes interaction, mutual respect and a positive attitude as well as a focus on promoting learning and reducing the theory practice gap. In order to do this the learning and teaching styles of the learner and the coach need to match. A student needs to be asked how they learn best, for example are they visual learners or do they learn by doing. The VARK model (Fleming, 2006) focuses on Visual, Auditory, Reading/Writing and Kinaesthetic learning so do we learn by seeing, hearing, reading or writing or through doing? Or using another model Honey and Mumford (1986) focus on whether we are activists, reflectors, theorists or pragmatists. In other words, do we learn by doing, watching and thinking, understanding the theoretical perspective or

Table 6.3 Promoting team compassionate leadership

What to achieve (Specific)	Why this is important (Relevant)	How will this be achieved (Attainable)	How will you know that you have achieved this (Measurable and Timely)
Culture where everyone leads	Everyone should feel able to lead the team	Do not encourage over reliance on heroic leadership	All members of the team feel able to make suggestions which are then acted on
Encourage servant leadership	Care of patients needs to be central	All members of the team should be working for excellent care	Positive feedback from patients and loved ones and easy feedback mechanisms
Focus on excellent communication	This makes for a positive environment	Use scenarios to help team members to discuss communication	Positive feedback from patients and all members of the team concerning communication
Positive attitude	Focus on positive and appreciative communication	Focus on feedback that is constructive and helpful	Ask patients and team members what it feels like in the care environment. Then act on the feedback.
Combine compassion with wisdom	Both are essential for high quality care	Wise compassion combines tough objectives with concern for others	Team members are able to focus on quality of care and outcomes. Act on quality indicators and the feelings of team members and patients
Support and challenge	Both are required for excellent care	High support combined with high challenge	Ongoing feedback mechanisms. All team members respond positively to feedback
Encourage engagement	All team members need to feel engaged	Empathy and valuing others key to culture	Ongoing low staff turnover and high morale reported
Best use of resources	Resources are key to high care	Compassionomics is the best use of resources	Compassionate managers, happier staff and happy patients with better outcomes. Ongoing discussion about best use of resources and care with compassion
Collective leadership	Humble leaders encourage others to be leaders too	Do not focus on heroic senior level leadership but on everyone taking a lead.	All staff make suggestions. Suggestions are acted on and team members feel valued
Caring culture	Essential for excellent care	Need to focus on creating and sustaining caring cultures	Ongoing evaluation on what constitutes a caring culture for patients and staff.

(Continued)

Table 6.3 (Continued) Promoting team compassionate leadership

What to achieve (Specific)	Why this is important (Relevant)	How will this be achieved (Attainable)	How will you know that you have achieved this (Measurable and Timely)
Cultural competence	Inclusive environment essential for good care	Encourage team to understand diversity and cultural competence	All team members and patients feel included and valued and cultural needs met on an ongoing basis.
ABC approach	Key to compassionate leadership	Focus on autonomy, belonging and contribution	All team members feel able to act and that their contributions are valued. Autonomous staff who feel valued on an ongoing basis.
Supervision	Key to safe and excellent practice	Restorative supervision as well as clinical supervision	Individual and team approaches as appropriate. Ongoing reflective practice encouraged
Schwartz round approach	Help staff to process their emotions	Encourage staff to focus on how they feel after events	Management see the value of Schwartz rounds and these are held regularly
Encourage debriefs	Helps staff to cope with traumatic events	Hold debriefs after every significant and distressing incident	Perceived as essential after traumatic events. These take place after every particularly distressing event.
Avoid victim blaming	Important that individuals do not feel blamed	Staff are not blamed for not being "resilient enough"	Strategies are put in place to resolve organisational issues. Staff feel listened to when feeling under stress on ongoing basis

by putting learning into practice. If we take a theorist approach, when they are practical learners, or learn best by seeing what is happening, this will make their learning much more difficult. So, understanding learners' learning needs is crucial.

The wider spheres of influence, responsibility and indeed accountability are essential in enabling this positive learning environment. We need to ensure that whilst recognising the importance of individual professional accountability we do not reinforce the victim blaming approach which abdicates responsibility and accountability at team and organisational level. Baines (2023) reports on a survey of nurses where 60% of respondents said that the NHS had forgotten some or all the lessons learnt from the Mid Staffordshire and Francis enquiry (Francis, 2013). Respondents in the survey said that they were ignored or subjected to bullying and harassment from senior managers if they tried to raise concerns about inadequate resourcing. Baines (2023) says "one respondent identified their hospital culture as one of "toxic resilience", where there was an acceptance of chaos and short staffing, and where those who challenged this were labelled as "unable to cope"" (Baines, 2023,p 9).

Table 6.4 Promoting educational compassionate leadership

What to achieve (Specific)	Why this is important (Relevant)	How will this be achieved (Attainable)	How will you know that you have achieved this (Measurable and Timely)
Understanding student needs and learning styles	Reduces student and new team member feeling under confident and feeling set up to fail	Focus on student learning styles. skills, experiences and strengths as well as their expectations and what they need to achieve	Students report that their learning needs and styles have been understood at the start and ongoing through their placements
Encouraging compassionate care and compassion approaches to colleagues	Compassionate care and compassionate relationships and teams is crucial to patient and staff wellbeing	Teach compassionate care and cultural competence. Also, appropriate use of humour with patients and colleagues	All staff feel cared for and valued and positive feedback on care from patients and their loved ones
Promote resilience	To counter burnout	Signpost wellbeing resources	All members of the team feel supported
Promote intelligent kindness	Combining wisdom with compassion encapsulates the science and art of nursing	Integrate theory with practice and encourage caring conversations	All team members understand the need to combine evidence-based practice with compassionate care
Foster a positive learning environment	Students and new team members learn best in a positive environment so that time is used to best effect	Prioritise training opportunities and not just mandatory training. High support but also high challenge	Students give positive feedback on the learning environment
Encourage virtuous circles	Avoid vicious circles which demotivate staff and encourage least good care	Challenge less compassionate care and escalate concerns appropriately	All staff confident to escalate concerns and positive change is encouraged
Encourage reflective practice	Reflection enables us to learn from experiences and transfer this learning into new situations	Regular discussions on perspectives on compassion and values and drivers	All staff focus on their reflection on action and encourage this in others
Focus on emotional intelligence	This enables us to reduce the chances of conflict and helps us to give and respond to feedback in a positive manner	Encourage self-awareness and self-management, relationship awareness and relationship management	All staff focus on self-awareness and self-management and relationship awareness and management in their interactions with patients and colleagues
Avoid toxic resilience	Victim blaming is unhelpful and this leads to higher sickness and staff turnover	Do not accept under resourcing and seeing others as "not coping"	A supportive, not a victim blaming approach is taken in relation to team members' stress levels
Encourage creativity in teaching and learning	Practice is complex and learning should be ongoing as new situations arise.	Use teachable moments and scenarios. Focus on new ways of working and developing best practice e.g. use of PPE. Encourage creativity, taking the initiative and finding solutions	Creative approaches are used to stimulate learning and positive feedback given in relation to these.

(Continued)

Table 6.4 (Continued) Promoting educational compassionate leadership

What to achieve (Specific)	Why this is important (Relevant)	How will this be achieved (Attainable)	How will you know that you have achieved this (Measurable and Timely)
Encourage staff to maximise learning opportunities	Individual learning is crucial in creating learning teams	Encourage preceptorship. Teach and coach when patients are critically unwell and in distressing situations. Encourage feedback from study days etc	Learning is maximised in all situations in practice, including when a patient deteriorates fast
Ensure that there are debriefing opportunities after distressing situations	Staff going home without debriefing increases stress and distress and sickness and turnover rates increase	Initiate Schwartz rounds when possible. Debrief at the end of shifts, at ward rounds and team huddles	Debriefing opportunities carried out when there have been traumatic and challenging situations and team members see these as helpful

So, having discussed the importance of taking a lead educationally, we need to develop our thinking further in relation to understanding the organisations where we work, and how we can actively influence our organisations when possible.

Organisational leadership

Case Study 6.6

Excellent care in Barchester Cherry Blossom Manor care home

Cherry Blossom Manor is a Barchester care home in Bramley, Hampshire. My mother is a resident there and the care is always excellent. It is a very visually attractive building which feels like home, and the outside area and grounds have beautiful flowers and themed decorations at key points in the year. There are different places to be, with a lively café area and a cinema/pub room. Innovative activities keep residents socially engaged, and the activity team and other members of staff facilitate these. However, what is particularly impressive is that everyone from the administration team, to the domestic, activity, catering and gardening teams are excellent with those who live there. Carers and members of the nursing team, day and night, are all person-centred, problem solving and caring. Everyone appears to like working there and there is a very low staff turnover rate. As I do not work there I do not know for sure but this appears to come from managers and senior nursing staff who are highly engaged with residents and staff. There appears to be a clear attitude of valuing residents as well as staff. The manager, deputy manager and head of care all know each resident, as does every member of staff. This does not happen by accident and the organisational culture is very positive and caring with high standards of care being seen as essential at all times.

Members of staff approach residents who have dementia and are having a bad day in a sensitive and caring way. For example, one resident who was clearly agitated was outside with two members of staff who were engaging with her and pointing out flowers and birds, and following her when she did not want to talk. A good sense of humour, used appropriately, can also help to build trusting relationships and seeing carers and nurses laughing with my mother is always good to see. One senior carer has developed a good relationship with my mother which can at times be cajoling in terms of encouraging her to take a shower or take her medications. My mother responds well to her approach and likes her and knows her name. The nurse who is often on at night when, despite best efforts, she can fall, has a different relationship with her. They laugh together when my mother has fallen and my mother refers to her as the friend who has come to help her back on her feet. Another senior nurse has a different approach again and is very compassionate, but they can all encourage my mother to do what is best at that time using their different communication skills. One other resident who has advanced dementia is visited daily by her husband. He said one afternoon that she had just had her breakfast and explained that, as she does not sleep well, they give her breakfast when she wakes up and they adapt the day to her waking periods. He also said that the night staff talk to her and engage her in activities when she is awake at night. This was very impressive to hear.

One day when we arrived one of the residents was sitting at the reception desk looking at a daily paper. She clearly felt as if she was in charge so I asked her a question and she said that she would ask her assistant. Her "assistant" was the receptionist who was working alongside her, and she builds good relationships with residents. I know at times my mother has gone to sit with her too.

The culture of the organisation, led by managers and senior staff, enables each member of staff to be creative in their approach. This makes for a happy environment for residents and staff.

A positive workplace culture creates a positive environment for service users, staff and those who come into contact with the service, for example loved ones, visiting professionals and lay people. However, many workplace cultures have a strong negative impact on the wellbeing of those who work there. Staff are overworked, there is no empathy, recognition, valuing, socialising or fun. There are a lot of unnecessary rules that make no sense to those who work there, people do not help each other, and there is no encouragement to succeed and managers do not listen (Bradberry, 2019 https://www.linkedin.com/pulse/how-cutthroat-work-cultures-suck-life-out-you-dr-travis-bradberry/). The NHS culture and leadership programme focuses on compassionate and collective leadership and advocates a 3-stage approach:

- Discover – identify the culture of the organisation
- Design – develop collective leadership strategies
- Implement – collective leadership strategies.

It is important to practice the art as well as the science of health care. Compassion is strongly linked to the practice of how we do what we do, and therefore the art of how we care for patients in our care. The emphasis can be on evidence-based practice, where clinical judgement making is the only thing that matters, and how this is carried out is perceived to be much less important. However, as I have said before people forget what we say and do, but not how we make them feel, and in many situations they will remember this for the rest of their lives and we only get one chance to make this right. Trzeciak and Mazzarelli (2019) say that compassionomics is the hypothesis that there is science in the art of medicine. Compassion for patients is highly therapeutic, and also highly cost effective. It radically enhances patients' lives and makes for more fulfilling careers for health care professionals. Trzeciak and Mazzarelli's (2019) highly insightful book on compassionomics makes a powerful argument for compassionate care having significant physiological and psychological health benefits, and compassionate approaches also motivate patients to self-care and become more engaged. In addition, compassion is vital for high quality care and prevents depersonalisation, which increases the chances of health care practitioners making mistakes. There are many examples given about how compassionate care is financially advantageous. Medical errors are costly financially, as well as physically and emotionally costly for those involved. Patients who are satisfied with their care because they feel cared for, are more likely to value their care and not make complaints which are time consuming and take time away from other care. Compassionate physicians also order less investigations and refer less, and patients are more likely to be concordant with their care and do better and heal faster. This has been discussed in greater detail in Chapter 1.

Radcliffe (2022a) says that the best nurses stay curious, listen and ask questions. They feel like they never know enough, and do not luxuriate in their expertise, or feel like they are experts. We are never experts in the lived experience of patients in our care and we should be learning from patients, students and colleagues throughout our nursing careers. We need to stay humble and carry on learning and acknowledge that although we are skilled in some aspects of care, we need to continuously learn. If we are real experts we know the limits of our expertise, and our knowledge and skills need to carry on developing and then our expertise will carry on growing.

Radcliffe (2022b) in another article discusses how nurses have been "forever altered" by their experiences through the COVID-19 pandemic. He says that nurses have been "parachuted into clinical areas with which they were unfamiliar, or being stretched way beyond safety, in terms of loss, despair, isolation, relentless pressure. (Radcliffe, 2022b, p17) Being "forever altered" is a long term and permanent response, and health care organisations that are predominantly interested in only outcomes, and not the wellbeing of their employees, are culpable in not supporting their staff and not focusing on trying to reverse long term effects of experiencing traumatic practice situations.

In patient-centred care environments (Shaller, 2007 cited in Goodrich and Cornwell, 2008):

- Senior managers feel directly responsible for patients and staff and their experiences.
- Senior managers make sure that they are actively informed about the quality of care that is on offer and visit wards and units and talk to staff and patients in lifts, corridors and clinics.
- Training on patient safety and quality improvement takes place and committee meetings focus on listening to and learning lessons from individual care reviews and what individuals and groups of patients say.
- Resource strategies are developed to improve communication and quality of care so that staff understand the strategic goals and their role in achieving them.
- Patients and families participate in hospital committees and decision making at all levels.
- Different ways of receiving feedback from the patients' perspectives are used – for example, mystery shoppers, patient surveys, open days, focus groups and phone surveys.
- There is a supportive work environment for staff and the physical care environment is as high quality as possible.
- Innovative use of innovative technology to provide information to patients and families.

Boo (2022) highlights stress at work and how this reduces productivity and creates physical and mental ill health. If a work environment is kind employees feel safe, and more likely to offer feedback, speak honestly and be creative. This in turn enables better problem solving and learning from mistakes, a safer environment, less likelihood of future problems and high levels of team performance and innovation and creative and collaborative problem-solving strategies and solutions,

Ball et al (2022) carried out a review of literature in relation to what keeps nurses in nursing and they identified several key nurse retention themes:

- Job satisfaction
- Work life balance
- Relationships and support
- Achieving care excellence
- Adequate staffing and resources
- Sense of control and being heard
- Opportunities to develop
- Pay and reward.

Ball et al (2022) also say that "more nurses could be retained by:

- Having compassionate and caring leaders.
- Fostering team cohesion to support nurses' well-being and professional development.
- Providing adequate staff and resources to allow nurses to deliver excellent care.
- Supporting nurses at different career stages and recognising the need to adapt what is on offer according to the workforce profile; for example, mentorship and education packages may be most effective for new starters, while flexible pension provision and job redesign could help retain the older workforce.
- Paying and rewarding staff fairly, which provides tangible signs of how they are valued.
- Investing in tailored education programmes and continuous development to enhance nurses' skills and career prospects.
- Reducing stress, burnout and job dissatisfaction, which are risk factors of nurse turnover.

(Ball et al, 2022, p 41)

Discussion has taken place about the increased workload which has resulted in high levels of stress brought about by nursing through the pandemic. Squires et al (2022) say that primary care staff are still experiencing high levels of stress due to staff illness and isolation against a background of unmet patient need and patients' fears and denials about COVID-19. This has had an impact on the mental health of many patients, as well as health care professionals. Late in 2022 there were still high numbers of acutely unwell people and others suffering from long COVID, and in 2023 there are still delays in accessing secondary care, alongside challenges in accessing primary care, staff strikes and staff being needed to administer the COVID-19 vaccination service. If staff are supported this empowers them and helps their coping strategies and resilience, but it also enables them to pass on this understanding to patients and their loved ones. Possible team organisational SMART goals focusing on compassionate leadership are below in Table 6.5. You could adapt these to use in your own practice area as appropriate.

Table 6.5 Promoting organisational compassionate leadership

What to achieve (Specific)	Why this is important (Relevant)	How will this be achieved (Attainable)	How will you know that you have achieved this (Measurable and Timely)
Leading by example and role modelling compassionate leadership	All staff need to understand compassionate leadership	A central focus at induction and this should be a central focus on mandatory training and unit-based discussions	All members of the team able to apply compassionate leadership to their practice
Adapt care where possible to encourage meeting patient needs	Care of patients needs to be central	All members of the team should be working for excellent care	Positive feedback from patients and loved ones and easy feedback mechanisms
Design and implement collective leadership strategies	This makes for a positive environment	Use scenarios to help team members to discuss leadership	Positive feedback from patients and all members of the team concerning leadership
Create a positive workplace culture for patients and staff	Focus on positive and appreciative communication	Focus on feedback that is constructive and helpful	Ask patients and team members what it feels like in the care environment. Then act on the feedback.
Combine clinical decision making and evidence-based practice with person-centred compassionate care	Both are essential for high quality care	This combines the art and science of nursing	Team members are able to focus on quality of care and outcomes. Act on quality indicators and the feelings of team members and patients
Be supportive of staff and encourage opportunities for debriefing	This enables staff to deal with the feelings brought about by challenging situations	Ensure that debriefing is normal practice after traumatic incidents	Staff report that they have had the opportunity to discuss their feelings after difficult events.
Encourage motivation to focus on self-care and focusing more on being engaged with care	All team members need to feel healthy and engaged	Self-care and engagement key to culture	Ongoing low staff sickness and turnover and high morale reported
Encourage staff to stay curious, humble and carry on learning	Ongoing learning crucial to practice	Encouraging a culture of ongoing learning and coaching	Appraisals indicate ongoing learning and students and new members of the team feel supported.
Create a focus on high level communication and all staff being involved in achieving strategic goals	High standards of verbal and written communication and goal setting essential for good care	Create opportunities for team discussions on communication and including these in goal setting	Team members are evaluated on their communication skills and all staff feel involved in strategic goal setting.
Involve patients and loved ones and actively seek feedback	Essential for excellent care	Need to focus on creating and sustaining caring cultures	Ongoing evaluation on what constitutes a caring culture for patients and staff.

(Continued)

Table 6.5 (Continued) Promoting organisational compassionate leadership

What to achieve (Specific)	Why this is important (Relevant)	How will this be achieved (Attainable)	How will you know that you have achieved this (Measurable and Timely)
Encourage ways to increase job satisfaction, work life balance, a sense of control and being heard.	High morale is essential for positive cultures and self-care is crucial for this	Encourage team to discuss ways that they maintain balance in their lives	All team members and patients able to help others to maintain a healthy balance in their lives.
Create a caring and compassionate culture where there is a focus on team cohesion and support	Key to compassionate leadership	Focus on compassion and team working in everyday work.	All team members feel able to act as a teamplayer and support others.

Using the RESPECT toolkit to take a lead

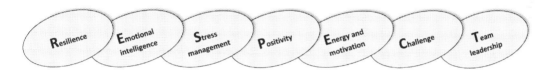

I developed the RESPECT model (Chambers and Ryder, 2019) to encapsulate the key areas of leadership that all the books on compassionate practice have led me to think about. (Chambers and Ryder, 2009, 2012 and 2019).

This stands for:

- Resilience – bending but not breaking
- Emotional intelligence – self and relationship awareness, self and relationship, management and empathy
- Stress management – awareness and strategies
- Positivity – optimistic attitudes to trigger positive emotions
- Energy and motivation – turning challenges into opportunities
- Challenge – being that "tipping point" to challenge the culture
- Team leadership – compassionate and challenging and being conflict aware.

According to Seligman (2002), the three pillars of study of positive psychology are positive emotions, positive traits (virtues, personal strengths and skills) and the positive institutions that facilitate the development of these emotions and traits. So, the thinking in this and the other books is based strongly on the principles of positive psychology.

Extensive discussion has taken place around the importance of all these important principles throughout this book:

- Resilience (Chapter 4)
- Emotional intelligence (Chapter 5)
- Stress management (Chapter 3)
- Positivity (Chapter 5)
- Energy and motivation (particularly in relation to engagement in Chapter 5)

- Challenge (in the recommendations for personal, team and organisational leadership in all chapters)
- Team leadership (see above in all chapters and conflict management in Chapter 4).

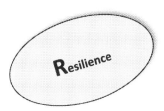

Being **resilient** personally, professionally, as teams and as organisations is key to managing the stressful issues we deal with in today's challenging environment. However, this does not mean taking a victim blaming approach where we lay all issues on the individual. This means that we stigmatise those who are finding the stress more difficult to navigate, and perceive them as people who are less able to cope. Often the solutions are at team and organisational level, and responsibility and accountability need to lie there.

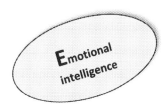

Emotional intelligence is key to us managing situations in a way that does not increase the stress on others, especially as their attitude and behaviour could be contributing greatly to our stress. As discussed already it is at times when we are feeling most judged and criticised that our emotional intelligence needs to be at emotional brilliance level. Taking an emotionally intelligent approach gives us the greatest chance of success in de-escalating conflict and giving constructive feedback in a way that is most likely to be acted on positively. We need to be self and relationship aware and manage ourselves and our relationships with empathy and understanding. We need to make positive connections with those at work and communicate at our highest level. Style (2011) says this involves:

- Recognition – giving positive feedback, thanks and celebrating success
- Friendship – supportive and close relationships at work
- Positive structures and support – from managers and colleagues
- Positive teamwork – team spirit
- Building trust – listening to others
- Generosity – time, praise, support (giving and receiving)
- Look at what works – rather than focusing always on what needs solving
- Understand the role of optimism and pessimism – optimists are good at problem solving but pessimists can be more realistic in challenging situations. We need both, but overall we need realistic optimists or optimistic realists.

If we think about our three longest social interactions in our work day, how in tune and connected did we feel with that person? If our connections are absent or compromised, we are unlikely to feel positive about our work. We need to look for ways to connect with others in our working day and take opportunities to re-engage in our normal work contacts. We also need to communicate as equals, using assertive rather than submissive or aggressive communication strategies (Fredricksen, 2009).

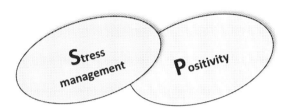

Stress management and **positivity** have been discussed in depth and we do need to be able to manage our stress in our home and work lives to enable us to remain as calm and focused as possible. However, this also involves a certain amount of positivity, hope and optimism.

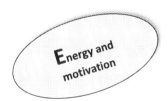

Energy and **motivation** are also key to developing strategies which pass this motivation on to others. The importance of virtuous rather than vicious circles has been discussed, and how feelings are highly contagious, and we can easily infect others with our negativity. However, we can also encourage others to be more positive too. Being energetic and motivated means that we are committed to being the best that we can possibly be. We need to actively look for ways to enhance the service we provide, and enjoy the challenge of doing this. For this to be the case we need to be motivated and really enjoy our role and feel that we are generally providing a good service. We can then use our energy to turn the constraints of our jobs into problem solving and opportunities to be more creative. This results in enjoying the challenges that our role brings, and being satisfied that we are making a difference. In that way we experience a sense of "flow" (Csikszentmihalyi, 2002) which is related to joy, creativity and total involvement in our work and life in general.

So, how can we reenergise our teams and help with their motivation? Eaton (2010) discusses how a personal commitment to change is related to a perceived high level of dissatisfaction with a low perceived personal risk and this gives the highest personal motivation to creating change. A moderate chance of success would be brought about by either a high level of dissatisfaction with a high personal risk, or a low level of dissatisfaction and a low personal risk. However, a high personal risk and a low level of dissatisfaction will rarely bring about someone wanting to initiate change. So as leaders we need to focus on areas where there is maximum dissatisfaction and reassure members of the team that making changes is not going to make them unpopular, or if this could be the case that they will have support.

Another important point is that we need to avoid creating resistance, which is a natural response to change (Youngson, 2016). The motivational interviewing approach is helpful here (Miller and Rollnick, 2002 and 2012). Listening, understanding and empowering are all essential and not giving solutions but trying to ask others for their ideas, so they do not just resist your ideas. Youngson (2016) discusses being an inner activist and focusing on compassion and a non-judgemental attitude, and increasing connections with others. This involves not focusing on persuasion and being the expert, but listening to the wisdom of others, and not focusing on problems but taking an appreciative inquiry approach where you look at what does work, and what actually matters to patients.

Deutser (2018) discusses purposeful as opposed to accidental culture and the fact that some organisations have a culture which does not drive forward innovation or enhanced performance. Therefore, this lack of purpose can result in gradual slippage in an accidental way. So, a culture needs to be positive and purposeful and then values can be sustained and developed through behaviour, processes and actions. It is important that we recognise the culture of our environment, and where that helps to enhance patient care, or where it accidently enables slippage and gradually eroding practices.

Positive psychology principles are again helpful here (Style, 2011), with the emphasis on focusing on the strengths of those who work there which encourages engagement. This also involves encouraging variety and newness which also encourages us to be engaged and energetic This involves having clear goals, job clarity and getting that essential "flow" which helps us to use our skills, and encourages team members to be autonomous (Style, 2011). Then, all team members can take more control over their role and working lives.

This positive psychology approach differentiates between the following sorts of lives (Seligman, 2016):

- A "pleasant life" where we think constructively about the past and are optimistic and hopeful about the future. This makes us happier in the present and creates positive emotions.
- A "good life" means that we are absorbed in activities and tasks which we find gratifying and this links to good character and lasting happiness.
- A "meaningful life" where we use our character strengths and virtues in the service of something larger than us. That could be in our work role, or in volunteering or caring in our home lives.

> An old Cherokee Indian told h.is grandson, "My boy, there is a battle between two wolves inside us all. One is Evil. It is anger, jealousy, greed, resentment, inferiority, lies and ego. The other is Good. It is joy, peace, love, hope, humility, kindness, empathy and truth". The boy thought about it, and asked "Grandfather, which wolf wins?". The old man quietly replied, "The one you feed".
>
> (Youngson, 2012, p 94)

So, we can either feed the wolf of ego or the wolf of compassion, either individually, within teams or across the organisation. Feeding the ego wolf can lead to a toxic workplace culture and this is very common. Not feeding the compassion wolf has a negative impact on individuals and organisational culture and values. Frost et al (2006) highlight three lenses of compassion. Firstly, compassion as interpersonal work, which recognises that noticing, feeling and responding to those who need compassion takes some time and effort. However, small actions can make big differences for all involved and this does not always feel like work. Secondly, compassion as narrative where understanding others' perspectives have an impact, and an example is given of how

Reuters supported loved ones of employees who died in the 9/11 atrocities. Thirdly, compassion as organising, which involves coordinating a compassionate response which can involve structural and organisational change, for example Reuters adapted their systems post 9/11 to ensure that they could track information focusing on the whereabouts and wellbeing of their employees. Lilius et al (2011) calls for formal roles to institutionalise compassion and formal programmes to maximise peer support and support strategies for people in need (http://www.academia.edu/26719043/compassion_revealed_what_we_know_about_compassion_at_work_and_where_we_need_to_know_more_?email_work_card==title).

So, to use another analogy, we need to be a radiator, not a drain (Webb, 2012). Drains, drain the energy of others, whereas radiators radiate energy. We can probably all recognise the drains in our lives, but we need to respond by carrying on radiating energy and positivity. We need to be the best versions of ourselves, being kind to ourselves and recognising our positive points. In order to do this, we need to understand our emotions, find the positives in situations, anticipate problems and enhance our coping strategies. We need to be able to diffuse stress and negative emotions, through our use of positivity and humour. This increases our ability to be altruistic when life is difficult for others.

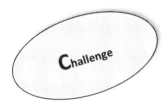

However, in terms of **challenge** we do need to be that tipping point. Gladwell (2000) states the law of the few, and says that it takes very few people to change the mindset of an organisation. Messages and emotions are like wildfire, and they spread quickly if they have a "stickiness factor" which makes them memorable. Gladwell (2000) says "that the world can seem like an immovable, implacable place. It is not. With the slightest push – in the right place – it can be tipped" (Gladwell, 2000, p259). We need to be instigators in a change of mindset and reach that tipping point. By doing this we can make the world a more compassionate place.

Edmund Burke said in the 18th Century that "all that is necessary for evil to prevail is for good men to do nothing" (www.brainyquote.com/quotes/edmund_burke_377528). So, we can either accept that substandard approaches are a necessity in our resource challenged environments, or we can take an active part in challenging these and take a lead in making our work environments as good as they can possibly be.

It could be argued that whilst the Mid Staffordshire inquiry into unacceptable levels of care (Francis 2013) highlighted where the problems actually lay, there would have been many concerned practitioners and staff who could have done more to escalate concerns. There are many reasons for this inaction in terrible situations like this, fear of reprisals and needing to keep on working, being unsure who to contact and how, or just simply not having the confidence and courage of our conviction. This is why the 6Cs (Department of Health, 2012) of care, compassion, competence, communication, commitment also includes courage. Courage is often needed in challenging others and the status quo. These 6Cs need to be embedded in organisations across health and social care and then there will be better outcomes, better experiences for patients, clients and employees, and a better use of resources. This involves a focus on a positive organisational culture, listening to staff, the right research and education in place and the right staff in the right places at the right times.

The COVID-19 pandemic has had a tremendous impact across the world in terms of wellbeing and psychological health. People who are especially vulnerable and thrive on social interaction for example those with mental health issues, individuals with learning disabilities, children, young people, those with long term conditions and socially isolated older people were especially struggling during times of lockdown. Some services to support these individuals changed to virtual meetings and support, but engaging in this way was not possible for many extremely elderly older people. Other services struggled to adapt to online ways of communication or phone contact, or they simply were not possible. Pandemic associated social isolation had a negative impact on child development generally and development of children and young people's social and communication skills. Postnatal depression, depression generally, self-harming and suicidal thoughts and behaviour were prevalent. In addition, health care practitioners put their lives at risk by exposing themselves to people with COVID, and they worked extreme hours under extreme pressures in the hospital environment. In community settings practitioners in South Carolina in America reported that they struggled with not being in the office, having difficult virtual conversations and not being able to see clients. They had difficulty in connecting with others and found it difficult not being in the office during reflective supervision. In the UK health visitors were the second highest group, after midwives, to report feeling unwell due to work stress (Baldwin, 2022). The Emotional Wellbeing at Work (EWW) programme was implemented by the Institute of Health Visiting in 2020 as result. https://ihv.org.uk/training-and-events/training-programme/courses/emotional-wellbeing-at-work-programme (Accessed 26/08/2023).

This programme focused on enhancing emotional wellbeing through EWW Champions and cascading a programme to health visitors. The programme had excellent feedback and focused on:

- Mindfulness and self-compassion
- Relationships at work and finding support
- Giving, gratitude and tolerating emotions
- Racial and cultural identity and inclusivity
- Growth mindsets and goal setting
- Group and team approaches in relation to trauma, challenges and professional status issues (Baldwin, 2022).

Another example of listening to staff during COVID-19 was in Northumbria Health care NHS Foundation Trust. Northumbria Health care NHS Foundation Trust, (2021) a provider of hospital, community and social care in north-east England, uses real time staff experience data to drive improvement and innovation. In the 2019 NHS Staff Survey, the trust scored highest nationally for health and wellbeing, morale, and equality, diversity and inclusion. As the pandemic started, the trust adapted its staff engagement platform to develop Corona Voice – a short web-based survey that enabled staff to raise issues, voice concerns and share their experiences in real time. Each week, staff were asked to rate their motivation for work on a scale of 1–10, alongside a varying set of 3–4 additional questions. Dedicated data analysts and researchers at Open Lab at Newcastle University supported measurement and evaluation of the data within the patient and staff experience teams. The trust used this data to inform an evolving action plan focused on meeting the changing physical, social and emotional wellbeing needs of staff during the peak of the pandemic and beyond.

As leaders we need to stay engaged with patients so that we know what their needs are, and whether these are being met. We also need to be focused leaders and know what to defer, delegate and ditch (Oshikanlu, 2016). This is not easy to work out sometimes, and we might not have anyone to delegate to. However, the principle is important; we do not always need to do everything, and there are key priorities that can emerge at any time.

Waddington (2016) talks about the compassion gap and how compassion is often missing in relation to how we treat our colleagues. Acting compassionately can be difficult at times.

> Foster (2009) says that to energise for excellence in care, we need to ensure that the staffing is right; then we can deliver quality care, the impact of which can be measured. The result will be an enhanced patient or client experience, which in turn will mean a far better nursing experience. However, it is essential that this positive culture is led from the top and from the interface with the patients and clients we care for. Leadership needs to take place at all levels to ensure that problems are identified and solved as quickly as possible. More than that, the focus has to be on the quality of the care experience, and how we convey the importance of this to all members of our teams.
>
> (Chambers and Ryder, 2012 p156).

Dewar (2012) advocates creative ways of helping individuals and teams to think about the meaning of compassionate care. These could involve the use of photographs and images, poetry and role enactment to develop the thinking of those involved in care. Pearson (2006) talks about the invisibility and lack of recognition and value placed on small acts of compassion. These are perceived as "simple not clever, basic not exquisite, peripheral and not central" (Pearson, 2006, p22). This devalues and minimises the importance of these small acts which should be central to everyday practice. Making small changes and appreciating the importance of emotional contagion and social learning is crucial (Stephenson, 2016).

Covey's circle of concern and circle of influence in his book, (*The 7 Habits of Effective People* 1989) highlights interesting strategies for us to take. Proactive people focus on what they can do, and what they can influence, whereas reactive people focus their energy on things outside their control and often feel victimised and full of blame. Devoting your time to things that you cannot influence depletes your energy and is a waste of time and make you hypercritical and overly negative. Positive energy enlarges our circle of influence, whereas negative energy reduces our circle of influence.

"We all have a leadership role in creating a culture where approaches that lack compassion are not tolerated, and where developmental opportunities exist to enhance compassionate care" (Chambers and Ryder, 2009, p195). However, it is also important to acknowledge that "great change and challenging times need great leadership and great leaders" (Chambers and Ryder, 2012, p159). It is also worth bearing in mind the Serenity prayer "God grant me the serenity to accept the things that I cannot change, the courage to change the things I can, and the wisdom to know the difference" (Niebuhr). http://en.wikipedia.org/wiki/Serenity_Prayer. Not all change is possible at every given time but we need to look for opportunities to make changes when these are possible, this is another sign of a great leader.

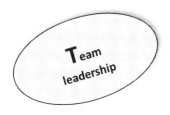

Team leadership has been a theme throughout the book and each chapter has finished with points about individual, team and organisational leadership. However, there are some additional thoughts about leadership. As team leaders we need to be:

- Compassionate
- Resilient
- Able to manage our stress
- Positive
- Ready to take the lead on compassion
- Emotionally intelligent and self-aware
- Problem solving
- Mindful
- Able to predict and de-escalate conflict
- Challenge issues when we need to in a positive and constructive way.

We also need to be able to focus on excellence and compassionate approaches and have the following competencies:

- Have an understanding about what a culture of excellence and compassion feels like.
- Focus on how we could take a lead in creating a culture of excellence.
- Understand how this benefits the organisation in terms of maximising resources and encouraging a positive staff morale.
- Challenge assumptions and create an environment of team learning.
- Focus on strategies for patients, staff and our own wellbeing which we can take forward and know how we can do this.
- Think about what our feelings are about our work environment at the moment.
- Know how we would rate our ability to be compassionate.

In the previous book (Chambers and Ryder, 2019) I identified six elements in relation to positive and compassionate care (see Fig 6.1). These are challenging in a stressful and resource limited care environment. However, we need to increase connectiveness to ensure that we take a lead on creating and sustaining a positive and compassionate care environment. These are:

- Excellence – the focus needs to be on achieving this.
- Exceptional and extraordinary – striving for this at all times.
- Enhanced wellbeing and positivity – focusing on these for staff.
- Expected – high standards need to be perceived as the norm.
- Encouraged – new initiatives and excellent care supported.
- Enabled – ways to facilitate initiatives need to be explored.
- Exalted – celebrating what is working well.

This leadership approach should be seen as a team approach to compassionate care and ensuring that the culture is positive and compassionate. This builds a team intelligence or an emotionally intelligent team approach. This involves team members being constructively challenged on their approaches to care, patients or colleagues which makes team members feel psychologically safe because all team members are being seen as accountable for their actions. There is then a positive approach through a no blame culture and non-judgemental approaches and attitudes. There is also an emphasis on understanding the motivation, drivers and

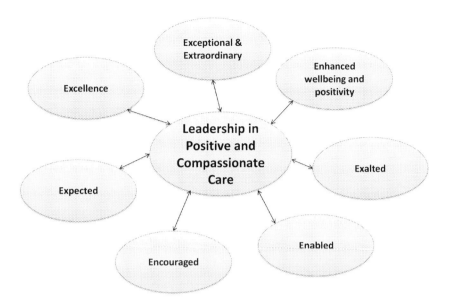

Figure 6.1 Leadership in positive and compassionate care

values of other members of the team, building a team understanding which also enhances psychological safety within the team and a team identity and team spirit. It is essential to predict and identify stressors to team members and solve issues before they get to be a crisis affecting patient care or team dynamics. This is much less time consuming and damaging to all. This also means that constructive conversations take place so that resources are used to best effect, the team is higher performing and staff turnover is lower and team morale, motivation and team spirit are higher.

Having applied all the different elements of the RESPECT model (Chambers and Ryder, 2009) it can be seen that this could be an effective way of managing our roles through respect:

- Respecting that our roles are stressful
- Respecting ourselves, our colleagues, our patients, our role, our profession and our organisation
- Using the RESPECT toolkit focuses on compassionate and positive practice.

To conclude the importance of our individual, team and organisational leadership will be discussed in relation to compassionate care, stress management, resilience and positivity.

RECOMMENDATIONS FOR LEADERSHIP AS INDIVIDUAL PRACTITIONERS, LEADERS AND ORGANISATIONS

So, to sum up, compassion is noticing that others are struggling and wanting to make a difference to alleviate this. This involves empathy and sensing and understanding that distress, but this also involves taking action to help. This is true compassion and people will never forget your actions because it is not about what you did, but how you make people feel as a result of your actions. This deepens our relationships with people in our home and professional lives, with our patients and our colleagues.

Compassion, empathy and communication are often seen as being "soft skills" but there is a wealth of evidence to prove that using these enhances health in the patients we care for, thereby saving valuable money as well as distress. For us though, as health care practitioners, being compassionate and kind is also associated with less burnout, and this enhances our health and wellbeing too. Trzeciak et al (2023) say that being kind and giving "is linked with a longer life, and can buffer the effects of stressful events and mortality risk. Specifically, kindness can reduce risk factors for cardiovascular disease, including counteracting high blood pressure. Kindness and compassion may also help us to maintain vitality and cognitive function as we age. Focusing on selfless acts has even been shown to have pain relieving effects. Numerous studies show that selfless giving to others is associated with happiness, wellbeing, resilience and resistance to burnout, fewer depression symptoms, and better relationships" (Trzeciak et al, 2023, p3). So being compassionate is crucial to us personally, but we need to genuinely care about ourselves and others to bring about these benefits to ourselves and others.

As leaders we need to focus on relational approaches and developing and sustaining a compassionate culture in our work environment and this will encourage others to be more compassionate, and reduce work stress and reduce team absence, sickness and turnover. Again, we need to genuinely care for the people we work with, as well as our patients, and those we love and enjoy spending time with.

Trzeciak et al (2023) say that in order to do this we need to:

- Start small – just 20–40 seconds of being more compassionate and appearing to have time for others lowers anxiety and stress.
- Be thankful and focus on being grateful and look for opportunities to be compassionate. There can be on average nine unique opportunities to demonstrate compassion every day.
- Be purposeful – ask what you can do to help, rather than asking whether someone needs help. What would lighten their load, help them to feel better and thrive more? So, focus not on whether they need help but how you can help them.
- Look for common ground – particularly with those who are more unlike us. It is easier to be compassionate to those who are most similar to us, so we need to expand our compassion towards those who are less easy to evoke our empathy.
- Celebrate compassion – in your organisation or workplace and show that you have noticed small acts of kindness. This encourages greater compassion and virtuous circles to develop, and it reassures us that kindness is more common than we realise.
- Elevate – we feel worse when we witness negativity, rudeness and unkindness and much better when we see compassion, kindness and heroism. So, we need to be aware of how we act has a real impact on others, for good or bad.
- Know your power – if compassion was our superpower what would this look like. We can cause immense change and be that tipping point if we chose to.

So being compassionate is part of the art of nursing and the art of leadership, but it is based on strong scientific evidence.

Halligan says that "the real compassion test is how we behave when we are stressed, rushed, hassled and no one is watching" (Halligan, 2014). "However, if your compassion does not include yourself, it is incomplete" (Kornfield, 1996).

"If you want others to be happy, practice compassion. If you want to be happy, practice compassion" (Dalai Lama XIV). www.positivepschology.com/compassion-meditation (Accessed 26/08/23).

In order to do this, as was highlighted in Chapter 4, we need to think about how we can:

> Do all the good that you can
> In all the ways that you can
> In all the places you can
> At all the times that you can
> To all the people you can
> As long as ever you can.
>
> Attributed to John Wesley but author unknown cited in
> Skovholt and Trooter-Mathjison (2016, p 136)

Focusing on leadership in compassionate care, stress management, resilience and positivity as individual practitioners and leaders

In the first book (Chambers and Ryder, 2009) the key components of compassionate care were highlighted, which are:

- Empathy and sensitivity
- Dignity and respect
- Listening and responding
- Diversity and cultural competence
- Choice and priorities
- Empowerment and advocacy.

The first book finished by highlighting the main challenges for compassionate care. Namely inadequate resourcing, the culture of the care environment and individual nurse attitude.

These challenges were taken forward in the second book which focused on the importance of everyone at every level of the team and organisation taking a lead to enhance care and take a lead on the changes needed (Chambers and Ryder, 2012). Cultural, attitudinal and resourcing challenges were identified, all of which needed positive principles and actions to create leadership and excellence in compassionate care (Figure 2.5 in Chapter 2 of this book). Positive principles and actions in relation to these leadership areas involve focusing on relational and transformational leadership. Transactional leadership is a much more top-down approach and Goodrich (2009 and cited in Chambers and Ryder 2012 p 22) differentiates between high and low levels of transactional leadership where things are either efficient but impersonal or unpleasant and inefficient. With relational or transformational leadership everything works when relational levels are high, whereas things are warm but chaotic if levels are low. Therefore, the most compassionate and effective leadership is where there are high levels of both transactional and relational leadership. Personal and professional leadership attributes were also identified (Chambers and Ryder 2012, p157 and replicated in Figure 2.6 in chapter 2 of this book) in relation to leading excellence in compassionate care; these attributes are personal, quality, leadership, team leading and educational attributes and all are needed to take a lead in developing and sustaining compassionate environments.

Book 3 (Chambers and Ryder, 2019), like this book, focused on the importance of a compassionate care environment and the importance of us having stress management, resilience, wellbeing and positivity strategies in place. Cultural competence is key to a compassionate care environment and as Campinha-Bacote (2002) says this is a process not an event, and her model highlights the importance of cultural awareness, cultural knowledge, cultural skill, cultural encounters and cultural desire. Papadopoulos says that culturally competent leadership (2018 p 65, also in Chapter 5 of this book) "takes time, education, good role models, a clinical environment that promotes and nurtures compassion and lots of practice" (Papadopoulos, 2018, p65). This involves cultural awareness, cultural knowledge, cultural competence, cultural sensitivity, cultural values and cultural principles. If these are not in place patients, their loved ones and staff from different cultural backgrounds will not feel understood or valued. Compassion focused leadership involves developing a sustainable culture of care (Chambers and Ryder 2019, p 58) and compassion-focused leadership involves practice development, individual development, communication development, team development, staff development, evidence-based practice and compassion development. So, culturally competent and compassionate leadership at team and organisational level are key to developing appropriate stress management strategies at that level. Resilient, positive and wellbeing orientated strategies need to be accessible to all members of the team.

It might be helpful to paint a visual picture in relation to stress management and resilience strategies. Using Bunyan's Pilgrim's Progress analogy (1678) we need to move from the **land of stress-based practice and leadership** to the **land of compassion and resilience based practice and leadership**. In the land of stress there is the **swamp of stress** which can be characterised by unhelpful, ineffective and blaming leadership and management. In this land there is too little staff support, and poor communication between patients and staff, and between colleagues. There is too little time with too few staff and resources and too many patient needs. This leads to physical, psychological, organisational and behavioural stress. The river takes us towards compassionate and resilient based practice and leadership. However, **rocks in the river** could be dangerous standards of care, depersonalisation and distancing and stress symptoms such as long term physical and emotional in health can lead to the **waterfall of ill health**

The raft of stress helps us out of the swamp and this involves knowing what stress is, what our stressors are, and recognising signs of stress and understanding the costs that these bring. We need to avoid negative coping strategies and create a balance of physical, social, emotional and intellectual health. The **bridge of resilience** involves understanding resilience and positive change management. The tools that can be helpful are:

- Mindfulness
- Reflection
- Appreciative inquiry
- Restorative supervision
- Reflection alone and with others
- Compassionate resilience
- Positivity
- Flexible autonomous empathy
- Team resilience
- Self-care and compassion
- Focusing on health and wellbeing.

In the **Land of compassion and resilience-based practice and leadership** we have **happy**:

Patients – through holistic patient-centred care where patients are involved in decision making and there are high levels of communication and practice.

Practitioners – who self-aware, engaged, emotionally intelligent and feel valued.

Leaders – who are humble, inspiring, courageous, passionate, enthusiastic and valuing.

Culture – which focuses on values-based employment, education and a positive culture and climate.

Individual stress can lead to burnout and increased stress in ourselves, our friends and family, the patients in our care and the teams where we work. There are so many benefits or working in a well-functioning team but there are a lot of challenges of working within poorly functioning teams, or teams where bullying attitudes prevail or we do not feel valued or appreciated.

From an individual perspective we need to remember that we decided on a career in health care in order to care, so not being able to do so exhausts us and leads to compassion fatigue, not vice versa (as discussed in Chapter 3). Remember we cannot be burnt out unless we were on fire to start with. So, we were engaged and motivated before, so what is compromising that now? We need to practice self-compassion in order to be able to be compassionate towards others. We need to think about what stress management strategies will work best for us. We also need to develop strategies to develop resilience and positivity because these go hand in hand. We need to be drains not radiators and increase virtuous circles and upward trends and emotions rather than vicious circles which do the opposite. Without this positivity there is no bounce back because the mind returns to the negative if we do not make a real effort to focus on the positives. Once we are feeling more positive we can focus on our wellbeing strategies.

Focusing on leadership in compassionate care, stress management, resilience and positivity as organisations

As health care practitioners we need to take an individual approach and take a lead at team, educational and organisational level wherever possible.

INDIVIDUAL COMPASSIONATE LEADERSHIP

- Deal with emotions in a healthy manner.
- Respond to the emotions of patients.
- Stay true to our feelings and values wherever possible.
- Use problem solving rather than avoidance and seek social and psychological support.
- Create a distance from work when at home.
- Use strategies to deal with insomnia, stress, low self-esteem and use humour appropriately.
- The RESPECT model is a toolkit to help us to maintain your compassionate and positive practice (Chambers and Ryder, 2019).

TEAM AND COMPASSIONATE LEADERSHIP

- Work engagement and work enthusiasm approaches.
- Team spirit and encouragement.
- Enthusiastic approaches.
- Communication, support and team meetings.
- Improved relationships with supervisors and support.
- More appreciation and feeling valued with positive feedback.
- Choice of days off / control over work to help with work overload and control.
- Monitor staffing levels and work/home demands plus working hours, as much as possible.

- Team leadership which supports empowering leadership leading to best care and healthy engaged staff.
- High level MDT collaboration, liaison and decision making.
- Debriefing opportunities, especially in end-of-life care, high dependency and following distressing situations when secondary distress could become a factor.
- Psychological support and create positive leadership.
- Supportive culture focusing on staff emotional wellbeing.
- Time for relaxation, fun and humour as a team.
- Avoidance of professional exhaustion and burnout and compassion fatigue and depersonalisation, or a lack of stimulation and boreout (Kompanje (2018) through a supportive culture, compassion, stress management and resilience training strategies.
- Identification and treatment and CPB on resilience.
- Deal with work pressures, work distress, discrimination, harassment and dehumanising attitudes at work where possible and encourage healthy and happy teams and workplaces.
- Encourage conflict anticipation, prediction, identification, de-escalation strategies.
- Adapt our roles as possible through job crafting and employ staff with a good person role fit with the values that are needed in the role.
- Focus on transformational leadership approaches and take a lead on compassionate care and encourage a positive environment in practice.
- *Create a compassionate culture by being compassionate towards patients, colleagues, managers and ourselves and taking a lead on this.*

EDUCATIONAL COMPASSIONATE LEADERSHIP

- Prepare and support students and new members of the team adequately through a focus on:

  - Conflict management and resolution
  - Stress management workshops and resources
  - Training in resilience and self-care
  - Death awareness and coping with death competence
  - Maximise compassion satisfaction and minimise compassion fatigue & burnout
  - Emotional intelligence and emotional resilience
  - Vicarious trauma and secondary stress from distressing patient situations
  - Promote work engagement, compassion satisfaction, exquisite empathy, meaning centred approaches, self-awareness, self-care and vicarious post-traumatic growth.

ORGANISATIONAL COMPASSIONATE LEADERSHIP

- Reflection and Schwartz rounds
- Mentorship and supervision opportunities
- Recruitment and selection giving realistic information concerning the new role and ensuring appropriate values plus a good person/job match
- Appropriate staffing/workload when possible
- Increased awareness and strategies concerning workplace bullying and stress from challenging patients and relatives
- Realistic, person-centred targets
- Ensuring adequate equipment, for example, PPE etc

- Taking turns in high pressure roles
- Redeployment to less intense areas if possible
- Shift patterns that allow sufficient rest between shifts
- Organisational culture which reflects shared values and the 6 Cs
- Provide specialist support for staff who are suffering from long COVID-19
- Provide high level mental health support for depression, anxiety etc.

I hope that you have found this book helpful as a guide to helping you to develop your own strategies. All four books have followed the theme of the centrality of compassionate care, and the importance of leadership at all levels in making this happen. The last two books (Chambers and Ryder 2019 and this book) have focused on the necessity of self-care and stress management, and the importance of resilience, positivity and wellbeing strategies. I hope that you are as inspired by the student case studies as I am and many of these have taken place through the COVID-19 pandemic, which is particularly impressive. I know that you have gone to extreme measures to carry out your role through the pandemic, and since. Thank you for all that you have done. I hope that you can feel as positive as you can about what you have done to help and care for others through this terrible time. Celebrating this within nursing is important, as is getting the help that is needed for those who have been severely damaged by the experience.

I hope that you have found the aide mémoires, exercises, questions and information in this book helpful to you in developing your own strategies to manage your stress and focus on your wellbeing. Try to stay as well, positive and happy as you can, and try to encourage this as much as possible in others, in your teams and organisations.

REFERENCES

Abel J, Clarke L. (2020) *The Compassion Project: A Case for Hope and Human Kindness from the Town that Beat Loneliness.* London: Octopus Publishing Group Ltd.

Agnew T. (2022) Reflective Practice 1: Aims, Principles and Role in Revalidation. *Nursing Times*, 118(5): 18–20.

Aked J, Marks N, Cordon C, Thompson S. (2008) *Five Ways to Wellbeing.* https://neweconomics.org/2008/10/five-ways-to-wellbeing (Accessed 13/9/23).

Alban-Metcalfe J, Alimo-Metcalfe B. (2018) Engaging Leadership: A Better Approach to Leading a Team? *Nursing Times*, 114(6): 21–24.

Alimo-Metcalfe B, Alban-Metcalfe J. (2006) More (Good) Leaders for the Public Sector. *International Journal of Public Sector Management*, 19(4): 293–315.

Atkins P, Parker S. (2012) Understanding Individual Compassion in Organizations: The Role of Appraisals and Psychological Flexibility. *The Academy of Management Review*, 37(4): 524–46.

Baines E. (2023) Survey Reveals Nurses Fear Another Mid Staffs is Likely. *Nursing Times*, 119(5): 8–9.

Baldwin, S. (2022) Supporting Nursing, Midwifery and Allied Health Professional Teams Through Restorative Clinical Supervision, *British Journal of Nursing*, 31(20): 1058–62.

Ball J, Ejebu O-Z, Saville C. (2022) What Keeps Nurses in Nursing? A Scoping Review into Nurse Retention. *Nursing Times* [online], 118(11). https://www.nursingtimes.net/roles/nurse-managers/what-keeps-nurses-in-nursing-a-scoping-review-into-nurse-retention-10-10-2022/.

Ballatt J, Campling P. (2011) *Intelligent Kindness: Reforming the Culture of Health care.* London: Royal College of Psychiatrists.

Bauer-Wu S, Fontaine D. (2015). Prioritizing Clinician Wellbeing: The University of Virginia's Compassionate Care Initiative. *Global Advances in Health and Medicine*, 4(5): 16–22.

Boo S. (2022) *Kindness a Pocket Guide: How it Empowers Health and Success and Why we Need to Prioritise it Now.* London: Kindness Advantage publishing.

Boynton B. (2022) Improving Communication Requires Tough Soft Skill Development, *MedPageTodayProfessional*.https://www.kevinmd.com/2022/08/improving-communication-requires-tough-soft-skill-development.html.

Bunyan J. (1678) *The Pilgrim's Progress from This World to That Which Is to Come*. https://www.gutenberg.org/files/131/131-h/131-h.htm (Accessed 15/9/23).

Campinha-Bacote J. (2002) The Process of Cultural Competence in the Delivery of Health care Services: A Model of Care. *Journal of Transcultural Nursing*, 13(3): 181–84.

Campling P. (2013/14) Intelligent Kindness: Reforming the Culture of Health care in the Wake of the Francis Report. *Journal of Holistic Health care*, 10(3): 5–9.

Chambers C, Ryder E. (2009). *Compassion and Caring in Nursing*. Oxford: Radcliffe Publishing.

Chambers C, Ryder E. (2012) *Excellence in Compassionate Nursing Care*. London: Radcliffe Publishing.

Chambers C, Ryder E. (2019) *Supporting Compassionate Health care Practice*. Abingdon: Routledge.

Clegg S, Hardy C, Lawrence T, Nord W (eds). (2006) *The SAGE Handbook of Organization Studies* (2006). London: SAGE Publications Ltd.

Clouston, T. (2015) *Challenging Stress, Burnout and Rust-Out: Finding Balance in Busy Lives*, London: Jessica Kingsley Publishers.

Covey S. (1989) *The 7 Habits of Highly Effective People*. New York: Simon Schuster.

Creighton L, Smart A. (2022) Professionalism in Nursing 2: Working as Part of a Team. *Nursing Times*, 118(5): 27–30.

Csikszentmihalyi M. (2002) *Flow: The Classic Work on How to Achieve Happiness*. London: Rider.

Daloz L. (1986) *Effective Teaching and Mentoring*. San Francisco: Jossey-Bass.

Davidson J. *Connor-Davidson Resilience Scale (CDRISC) Manual* 19/8/2018. www.cd-risc.com (Accessed 27/7/23).

de Zulueta P. (2013) Compassion in 21st Century Medicine: Is it Sustainable? *Clinical Ethics*, 8(4): 119–28.

Demerouti, E. (2008) The Oldenburg Burnout Inventory: A Good Alternative to Measure Burnout and Engagement. *Handbook of Stress and Burnout in Health Care*. Hauppauge, NY: Nova Science Publishers.

Department of Health (2012) *Compassion in Practice – Nursing, Midwifery and Care Staff: Our Vision and Strategy*. London: Department of Health.

Deutser B. (2018) *Leading Clarity: The Breakthrough Strategy to Unleash People, Profit, and Performance*, Hoboken, New Jersey: John Wiley & Sons.

Dewar B. (2012) Using Creative Methods in Practice Development to Understand and Develop Compassionate Care. *International Practice Development Journal*, 2(1) https://www.fons.org/Resources/Documents/Journal/Vol2No1/IPDJ_0201_02.pdf.

Diener E, Oishi S, Tay L. (eds) (2018) *Handbook of Well-being*. Salt Lake City, UT: DEF publishers.

Driscoll J, Stacey G, Harrison-Dening K, Boyd C, Shaw T. (2019) Enhancing the Quality of Clinical Supervision in Nursing Practice. *Nursing Standard*, 34(5): 43–50.

Eaton M. (2010) Why Change Programs Fail, *Human Resource Management International Digest*, 18(2): 37–42.

Egan J. (2019) *Thrive: Accentuating the Positive in the Emergency Department*. https://openrepository.aut.ac.nz/items/38f11ec2-214d-4b43-a1b5-9627b929621f (Accessed 27/7/23).

Fleming N. (2006) *VARK Visual, Aural/Auditory, Read/Write, Kinesthetic*. New Zealand: Bonwell Green Mountain Falls.

Foster D. (2009) Developing an Effective Framework to Deliver Nursing Quality. *Second Annual Nursing Times Nursing Quality Conference Delivering High Quality Nursing Care:* Nov 18, London.

Francis R. (2013) *The Francis Report (Report of the Mid-Staffordshire NHS Foundation Trust public inquiry) and the Government's Response*. https://researchbriefings.files.parliament.uk/documents/SN06690/SN06690.pdf (Accessed 27/7/23).

Fredrickson B. (2009) *Positivity: Groundbreaking Research Reveals How to Embrace the Hidden Strength of Positive Emotions, Overcome Negativity, and Thrive*. Oxford: Oneworld Publications.

Frost P, Dutton J, Maitlis S, Lilius J, Kanov J, Warline M. (2006) *Seeing Organizations Differently: Three Lenses on Compassion*. In: Clegg S, Hardy C, Lawrence T, Nord W. (eds) (2006) *The SAGE Handbook of Organization Studies*. London: SAGE Publications Ltd.

Geis E. (2022) Work, Relax and Play: A Wellbeing Programme for Student Nurses. *Nursing Times*, 118(7). https://www.nursingtimes.net/roles/nurse-educators/work-relax-and-play-a-wellbeing-programme-for-student-nurses-06-06-2022/.

George M. (2017a) The Effect of Introducing New Public Management Practices on Compassion Within the NHS. *Nursing Times*, 113(7): 30–34.

George M. (2017b) How Traditional Management Approaches Damage Staff Wellbeing. *Nursing Times*, 117(7): 35–38.

Gibbons S, Newberry M. (2023) Exploring Self-compassion as a Means of Emotion Regulation in Teaching. *Teacher Development*, 27(1): 19–35.

Gilbert P, Choden. (2013) *Mindful Compassion*. London: Robinson.

Gilbert P. (2010) *The Compassionate Mind*. London, Constable.

Gladwell M. (2000) *The Tipping Point*. Boston: Little, Brown and Company.

Goetz J, Keltner D, Simon-Thomas E. (2010) Compassion: An Evolutionary Analysis and Empirical Review. *Psychological Bulletin*, 136(3): 351–74.

Goodrich J, Cornwell J. (2008) *Seeing the Person in the Patient*. London: The King's Fund.

Goodrich J. Transactional and Relational Aspects of Care. In: Goodrich J. Understanding the Patient Experience of Care. *Second Annual Nursing Times Nursing Quality Conference Delivering High Quality Nursing Care*. 2009 Nov 18; London.

Greenwood G. (2022) How Imposter Syndrome Can Help Shape Professional Identity. *Nursing Times [online]*, 118(11). https://www.nursingtimes.net/roles/nurse-educators/how-imposter-syndrome-can-help-shape-professional-identity-10-10-2022/.

Griffiths K. (2022) Using Restorative Supervision to Help Nurses During the COVID-19 pandemic. *Nursing Times [online]*, 118(3). https://www.nursingtimes.net/roles/newly-qualified-nurses/using-restorative-supervision-to-help-nurses-during-the-covid-19-pandemic-14-02-2022/.

Halligan A. (2014) The NHS Needs Compassionate Leadership. *Journal of Holistic Health care*, 11(1): 4.

Health Connections Mendip. https://healthconnectionsmendip.org/our-model/videos/.

Health Education England. (2023) The Role of Reflection in Developing Resilience. https://london.hee.nhs.uk/reflective-writing-role-reflection-developing-resilience (Accessed 27/7/23).

Higgins A, McBennett P. (2007) The Petals of Recovery in a Mental Health Context. *British Journal of Nursing*, 16(14): 852–56.

Honey P, Mumford A. (1986) *The Manual of Learning Styles*. Maidenhead, Berks: Peter Honey Associates.

Hougaard R, Carter J, Hobson N. (2020) Compassionate Leadership is Necessary – But Not Sufficient. *Harvard Business Review*. https://hbr.org/2020/12/compassionate-leadership-is-necessary-but-not-sufficient (Accessed 28/7/23).

Kline N. (2002) *Time to Think: Listening to Ignite the Human Mind*. London, Cassell and Co.

Kompanje E. (2018) Burnout, Boreout and Compassion Fatigue on the ICU: It is Not About Work Stress, But About Lack of Existential Significance and Professional Performance. *Intensive Care Medicine*, 44(5): 690–91.

Kornfield J. (1996) *Buddha's Little Instruction Book*. London: Rider

Leffert N, Benson P, Scales P, Sharma A, Dyanne R, Blyth D. (1998) *Developmental Assets: Measurement and Prediction of Risk Behaviors Among Adolescents*. In: Peterson C, Seligman M. (2004) *Character Strengths and Virtues: A Handbook and Classification*. Oxford University Press: American Psychological Association.

Lilius J, Kanov J, Dutton J, Worling M, Maitlis S. (2011) *Compassion Revealed: What we Know About Compassion at Work (and Where we Need to Know More)*. Online: http://www.academia.edu/26719043/compassion_revealed_what_we_know_about_compassion_at_work_and_where_we_need_to_know_more_?email_work_card==title (Accessed 27/7/23)

Maben J, Peccei R, Adams M, Robert G, Murrells T. (2012) "Poppets and Parcels": The Links Between Staff Experience of Work and Acutely Ill Older Peoples' Experience of Hospital Care. *International Journal of Older People Nursing*, 7(2): 83–94.

Maben J, Bridges J. (2020) COVID-19: Supporting Nurses' Psychological and Mental Health. *Journal of Clinical Nursing*, 29(15–16): 2742–50.

McCauley C, Fick-Cooper L. (2020) *Direction Alignment, Commitment: Achieving Better Results through Leadership.* Greensboro NC: Center for Creative Leadership CCL Press.

Michaelson J, Mahony S, Schifferes J. (2012*) Measuring Wellbeing: A Guide for Practitioners.* London: New Economics Foundation.

Miles, B. (2023) A Review of the Potential Impact of Professional Nurse Advocates in Reducing Stress and Burnout in Dstrict Nursing. *British Journal of Community Nursing* 28(3). https://www.britishjournalofcommunitynursing.com/content/professional/a-review-of-the-potential-impact-of-professional-nurse-advocates-in-reducing-stress-and-burnout-in-district-nursing/.

Miller W, Rollnick S. (2002) *Motivational Interviewing: Preparing People for Change* (2nd ed). New York: Guildford Press.

Miller W, Rollnick S. (2012) *Motivational Interviewing* (3rd ed.). New York: Guildford Press.

Murray S, Magill J, Pinfold M. (2012) Transforming Culture in the Critical Care Environment – The Building Block of the Journey. *International Practice Development Journal.* https://www.fons.org/Resources/Documents/Journal/Vol2No1/IPDJ_0201_05.pdf (Accessed 27/7/23).

NHS England (2017) *A-EQUIP: A New Model of Midwifery Supervision.* https://www.england.nhs.uk/publication/a-equip-a-model-of-clinical-midwifery-supervision/ (Accessed 27/7/23).

NHS Providers (2020) *The NHS Staff Survey 2019.* https://nhsproviders.org/media/689188/nhs-staff-survey-results-2019-nhs-providers-otdb.pdf (Accessed 27/7/23).

Northumbria Health care NHS Trust (2021), *Northumbria Trust to Enable Health care Innovation.* https://www.northumbria.nhs.uk/media-centre/news-and-blogs/news-stories/northumbria-trust-enable-healthcare-innovation (Accessed 27/7/23).

Nursing & Midwifery Council (2018) *The Code.* London: NMC.

Nyatanga B. (2013) Bringing Compassion Back Into Caring: An Equation of Reciprocation. *British Journal of Community Nursing*, 18(6): 299.

Oshikanlu R. (2016) Defer, Delegate or Ditch. *Journal of Health Visiting*, 4(4). https://www.magonlinelibrary.com/doi/abs/10.12968/johv.2016.4.4.178.

Papadopoulos I. (2018) *Culturally Competent Compassion: A Guide for Health care Students and Practitioners.* Abingdon, Oxon: Routledge.

Pearson, A. (2006) Powerful Caring. *Nursing Standard*, 20(48): 20–22.

Peterson C, Seligman M. (2004) *Character Strengths and Virtues: A Handbook and Classification.* Oxford University Press: American Psychological Association.

Picard A. (2016) Remembering Kate Granger, a Champion of Human Connection. *The Globe and Mail.* www.theglobeandmail.com/opinion/a-champion-of-human-connection-in-doctor-patient-care/article31107734 (Accessed 26/8/22).

Radcliffe M. (2014) Noticing Good is as Important as Noticing Bad, Just Not as Popular. *Nursing Times*, 110(12): 9.

Radcliffe M. (2020) Great Practice Makes Me Feel Better About the World. *Nursing Times*, 116(2): 15.

Radcliffe M. (2022a) The Best Nurses Always Feel as Though They Don't Know Enough. *Nursing Times*, 118(3): 15.

Radcliffe M. (2022b) Too Often, Issues Affecting Nurse Wellbeing are Met With a Shrug. *Nursing Times*, 118(8): 17.

Ross S, Jabbal J, Chouhan K, Maguire D, Randhawa M, Dahir S. (2020) *Workforce Health Inequalities and Inclusion in NHS Providers.* London: The Kings Fund.

Russell S, Daly R, Dodds P, Madden G, Maidens G, Parry-Hughes M, Whiteman S, Scales C, Weeks L. (2022) Using Online Practice Action Learning Sets for Clinical Supervision. *Nursing Times*, 118(5): 21–26.

Saarikoski M, Isoaho H, Warne T, Leino-Kilpi H. (2008) The Nurse Teacher in Clinical Practice: Developing the New Sub-dimension to the Clinical Learning Environment and Supervision (CLES) Scale. *International Journal of Nursing Studi*es, 45(8): 1233–37.

Saarikoski M, Strandell Laine C. (2018) *The CLES-Scale. An Evaluation Tool for Health care Education.* New York: Springer International Publishing.

Schein E, Schein P. (2018) *Humble Leadership: The Power of Relationships, Openness and Trust.* Oakland, California: Berrett-Koehler Publishers Inc.

Schwartz K. (2012) A Patient's Story. *The Boston Globe Magazine*. Available at: https://www. bostonglobe.com/magazine/1995/07/16/patient-story/q8ihHg8LfyinPA25Tg5JRN/story. html (Accessed 28/7/23).

Seligman, M. (2002). *Authentic Happiness: Using the New Positive Psychology to Realize Your Potential for Lasting Fulfilment*. New York: Free Press.

Seligman M. (2011) *Flourish: A Visionary New Understanding of Happiness and Well-being*. Boston: Nicholas Brealey Publishing.

Seligman M. (2016) *The Pursuit of Happiness* www.pursuit-of-happiness.org (Accessed 28/7/23).

Shaller D. (2007) *Patient-Centered Care: What Does It Take?* The Commonwealth Fund: Shaller Consulting. In: Goodrich J, Cornwell J. (2008) *Seeing the Person in the Patient*. London: The King's Fund.

Shaw J. (2022) *Intelligent Kindness in UK Student Nurse Practice Placements? A Mixed Methods Study*. PhD thesis unpublished. Leeds Beckett University.

Shuttleworth, A. (2015) Make a Change – Even Small Things Can Have a Huge Effect. *Nursing Times*, 111(11). https://www.nursingtimes.net/opinion/comment-make-a-change-even-small-things-can-have-a-huge-effect-09-03-2015/.

Skovholt T, Trotter-Mathison M. (2016) *The Resilient Practitioner: Burnout and Compassion Fatigue Prevention and Self-care Strategies for the Helping Professions*. London: Routledge.

Smith B, Dalen J, Wiggins K, Tooley E, Christopher P, Bernard J. (2008). The Brief Resilience Scale: Assessing the Ability to Bounce Back. *International Journal of Behavioral Medicine*, 15(3): 194–200.

Smith S, James A, Brogan A, Adamson E, Gentleman M. (2016) Reflections About Experiences of Compassionate Care from Award Winning Undergraduate Nurses – What, So what… Now What? *Journal of Compassionate Health Care*, 3(6): 1–11.

Solihull Approach (2015) *Welcome to the Solihull approach*. www.solihullapproachparenting. com (Accessed 26/7/23).

Squires A, Astle A, Barratt J, Belle L, Charlton S, Greaves C, Haines S, Worrell J. (2022) How Staff Burnout and Change Were Escalated by the COVID-19 Pandemic, *Nursing Times*, 118(11): 18–21.

Stainer L, Humphries B, Uren C, Watson A, Johns C. (2022) Practice Supervisors' and Assessors' Experiences in the COVID-19 Pandemic. *Nursing Times*, 118(8): 52–54.

Stephenson J (2016) Nursing Expert Calls for More Ward-based 'Social Learning'. *Nursing Times*, 112(26): 6.

Style C. (2011) *Brilliant Positive Psychology*. Harlow: Pearson Education Limited.

Su R, Tay L, Biener E. (2014) The Development and Validation of the Comprehensive Inventory of Thriving (CIT) and the Brief Inventory of Thriving (BIT). *Applied Psychology Health Well-Being*, 6(3): 251–79.

The Dalai Lama, *"If you want others to be happy, practice compassion. If you want to be happy, practice compassion"*. Found in https://positivepsychology.com/compassion-meditation/ (Accessed 27/7/23).

The Kings Fund. (2011) *The Future of Leadership and Management in the NHS: No More Heroes*. London: The Kings Fund.

Trzekiak S, Mazzarelli A. (2019) *Compassionomics: The Revolutionary Scientific Evidence That Caring Makes a Difference*. Pensacola: Studer Group.

Trzekiak S, Mazzarelli A, Seppälä E. (2023) Leading with Compassion has Research-Backed Benefits. *Harvard Business Review*. https://hbr.org/2023/02/leading-with-compassion-has-research-backed-benefits (Accessed 13/09/2023).

Waddington, K. (2016) The Compassion Gap in UK Universities. *International Practice Development Journal*, 6(1): 10. https://www.fons.org/library/journal/volume6-issue1/article10.

Wallbank S. (2016) *The Restorative Resilience Model of Supervision. A Reader Exploring Resilience to Workplace Stress in Health and Social Care Professionals*. Hove: Pavilion Publishing and Media Ltd.

Warr P, Nielsen K. (2018) *Wellbeing and Work Performance*. In: Diener E, Oishi S, Tay L. (eds) *Handbook of Well-being*. Salt Lake City, UT: DEF Publishers.

Weaver L. (2016) Is Compassion the Missing Ingredient in Optimal Health? https://www.drlibby.com/health-wellbeing/is-compassion-the-missing-ingredient-in-optimal-health/ (Accessed 28/7/23).

Webb L. (2012) *How to Be Happy*. West Sussex: Capstone Publishing Ltd.

West M, Dawson J, Admasachew L. (2011) *NHS Staff Management and Health Service Quality: Results from the NHS Staff Survey and Related Data*. https://www.gov.uk/government/publications/nhs-staff-management-and-health-service-quality (Accessed 27/7/23).

West M, Dawson J, Admasachew L, Topakas A. (2011) *NHS Staff Management and Health Service Quality*. London: Department of Health and Social Care

West M, Armit K, Loewenthal L, Eckert R, West T, Lee A. (2015) *Leadership and Leadership Development in Health care*. London: The King's Fund.

West M, Markiewicz L.(2016) *Effective Team Working in Health Care*. In: *The Oxford Handbook of Health Care Management*. Ferlie E, Montgomery K, Pedersen A. Oxford: Oxford University Press

West M, Chowla R. (2017) *Compassionate Leadership for Compassionate Health care*. In: Gilbert P. (2017) *Compassion: Concepts, Research and Applications*. London: Routledge.

West M, Dyrbye L, Shanafelt T. (2018) Physician Burnout: Contributors, Consequences and Solutions. *Journal of Internal Medicine*, 283(6): 516–29.

West M, Bailey S. (2019) *Five Myths of Compassionate Leadership*. https://www.kingsfund.org.uk/blog/2019/05/five-myths-compassionate-leadership (Accessed 28/7/23)

West M, Coia D. (2019) *Caring for Doctors, Caring for Patients*. London: General Medical Council.

West M, Bailey S, Williams E. (2020) *The Courage of Compassion: Supporting Nurses and Midwives to Deliver High-quality Care*. London: The Kings Fund. https://www.kingsfund.org.uk/sites/default/files/2020-09/The%20courage%20of%20compassion%20full%20report_0.pdf (Accessed 28/7/23).

West M. (2021) *Compassionate Leadership: Sustaining Wisdom, Humanity and Presence in Health and Social Care*. London: The Swirling Leaf Press

West T, Daker P, Dawson J, Lyubovnikova J, Buttergeig S, West M. (2021) The Relationship Between Leader Support, Staff Influence Over Decision Making, Work Pressure and Patient Satisfaction: A Cross Sectional Analysis of NHS datasets in England. *BMJ Open*, 12(2). https://bmjopen.bmj.com/content/12/2/e052778.

West M, Dawson J. (2022) *Employee Engagement and NHS Performance*. London: The King's Fund.

Wheeler P. (2023) Leadership Lessons From the Cockpit. *Coaching Toward Happiness: Applying Positive Psychology in Your Coaching, Work and Life*. (Email accessed 31/08/23).

Xanthopoulou D, Bakker A, Ilies R. (2012) Everyday Working Life: Explaining Within-person Fluctuations in Employee Well-being. *Human Relations*, 65(9): 1051–69.

Youngson R. (2012) *Time to Care*. New Zealand: Rebelheart Publishers.

Youngson R. (2016) *From HERO to HEALER: Awakening the Inner Activist*. Scotts Valley, California: CreateSpace Independent Publishing Platform.

Index

and mindfulness 242; and PTSD 108–9; and resilience 137, 184–5; and self-care 165, 168; signals of 111–13, **112**; stages of 110; and stress 88, 107–8; and work engagement 216–19
burnout tests 111, 116–18
burns sufferers 98
busyaholics 12–13

caffeine 93, 111, 170
cardiac arrest 281–2
care *see* quality of care
care environments: compassionate 11; culture of 49–50; and resourcing 34, 41, 43
care experience xviii, 5, 44, 301
CARE framework (Connect, Adapt, Routinize, Exercise) 163
CARE heuristic (Compassion, Awareness Resilient Responding and Empowerment) 185
care homes, compassionate leadership in 290–1
careaholics 12–13
caring: about and for 10; indicators of 25–6
caring burnout 63
caring conversations 27, 31, 284
caring cultures 54, 277, 287, 294
caring environments 28, 32, 47
Case, Molly 56–8
case studies xix, 2
catastrophising 147, 237, 240, 244, 248
celebration 14, 23, 27–8, 33
challenge: lack of 99, 105; in RESPECT model xix, 2, 34, 295–6, 299
challenging behaviour 69–70
change: ambivalence to 46; assessing 97; initiating and promoting 50, 297; personal commitment to 297
change as a challenge 122, 137, 175, 178
change management 47, 212, 248, 306
change talk 46–7
character, education of 144
character strengths and virtues 145, 229, 244, 262, 298
charismatic leadership 28, 275
chronic burnout 107
circle of concern 301
circle of influence 181, 301
CLECC (Creating Learning Environments for Compassionate Care) 166–7
CLERM (Clinical Learning Environment Relationship Model) 286
CLES (Clinical Learning Environment Supervision Scale) 286
clinical supervision 51, 70; and

compassionate culture 32, 63, 73; and COVID-19 163; group 181, 278–9; and kindness 70; resilience-based 245, 278–9; and workplace culture 165
coaching leadership 267
coercive leadership 267
cognitive behavioural therapy (CBT) 109, 138, 146–7, 150, 265
cognitive empathy 245
collaboration xviii, 154, 163, 205, 266, 274
collaborative approaches 99, 103
collaborative leadership 72
collaborative MDT working 124–5, 179, 183, 185–6, 308
collaborative problem solving 157, 293
collaborative relationships 179
collaborative team working 206
collaborative working 33
collective leadership 28, 180, 275–6, 291, 294
Colwell, Maria 187
comfort zones: optimum 241; for students 282; working outside 84, 87–8, 100, 134
commanding leadership 267
commiseration 215
commitment 69, 175, 205, 275–6; in 6Cs 247, 273, 299; sense of 137; *see also* organisational commitment
common ground 159, 206, 213, 304
communication: adaptation of 20–1; breaking down barriers to 135–6; different levels of 216; effective 48, 180, 272; unacceptable 172; unambiguous 25
communication skills 60, 201; advanced 40, 69; and assertiveness 222; and challenging behaviour 69–70; and conflict management 157; and conflict resolution 155; and emotional intelligence 245; and patient advocacy 55–6; for students 284; and team leadership 272
communication strategies: and compassion fatigue 100; and conflict resolution 155; in COVID-19 79, 85; positive 60; and teamwork 278
community connections 96, 234, 261
community nursing 40–1
compassion: and brain imaging 222; challenges of 11, 39, 214; components and attributes of 25; culturally competent 214; essential features of xvii, 8; experiences of 276; focus on 2; as great medicine *19*; impact on organisations 41–5; importance of 17–21; lenses of 298–9; as motivation 143; in nursing practice 58; to ourselves (*see* self-compassion); personal review **8–10**;

respect 55, 64; culture of 113, 183; dignity and xvii, 8, 305; for feelings 211; lack of 111; mutual 259, 278, 286; for patients 171, 207, 265; as soft skill 266; treating everyone with 213–14; as value 247
RESPECT toolkit xix, 2, *34–5*, 255, 295–303, 307
respectfulness 34, 50, 56, 160, 179, 218, 246
responsibility: for colleagues 68; collective 275; and conflict management 156, 158–9; duty of 141; taking 14, 49, 139, 211, 275
restlessness 63, 92, 116, 146
restorative supervision 278–9, 281
ripple effect 237, 261–2
Robson, Steve 68
role ambiguity and conflict 100, 108, 110, 123, 183
role modelling xvii–xviii, 32–3, 35, 278; for compassion 6, 53–4, 72; moral 145; for student nurses 81
Roosevelt, Eleanor 238
RULE approach 46, 257
rushaholics 13
rust-out 88

sadness 81, 86, 179, 182; assessment of 229–31
salutogenesis 69, 137
satiation 107
SBAR (Situation, Background, Assessment & Recommendations) approach 261, 278
Schwartz, Ken 164
Schwartz Centre rounds 50, 164, 179; and compassionate leadership 279; and practitioner wellbeing 166; and resilience training 106; and trauma 248
secondary distress 308
secondary traumatic stress (STS) 109–10, 242
secondary victims 15, 62
self-acceptance 241
self-actualisation 212
self-awareness 15, 59, 112, 133, 138, 195; and clinical supervision 278; and conflict resolution 155–6, 158; and educational leadership 286; and emotional intelligence 202–3, 205, 207–8, 212; and intelligences 214; and mentoring 274; and mindfulness 242; and resilience 173; and self-care 165, 169; as soft skill 266
self-care 100, 113, 161–71, 245, 309; and compassionate leadership 270, 279–81; and resilience 138, 173; strategies *124–5*,

185; understanding need for 133
self-compassion 2, 14–15, 35, 164–5, 273; and appreciative inquiry 30; and educational leadership 285; and EI 211; and mindfulness 241–2; and professional boundaries 52; and resilience 138; and RESPECT model 35; and self-care 164–5, 167–8; strategies for **244**
self-concept 232
self-confidence 286
self-control 266
self-criticism 166, 168, 241
self-determination 235
self-development, time for 165
self-doubt 285
self-efficacy 19, 46, 72; and engagement 64; and locus of control 175; and resilience 137, 185; and salutogenesis 69; and self-care 171; training around 108; and work engagement 220
self-esteem 69, 85, 87, 115, 185, 262; and conflict 153; enhancing 197–9, 201; and happiness 234; higher 167; low 108, 111; and self-care 124; and stress 93; and wellbeing 235; and work engagement 218, 220
self-forgiveness 15
self-harm 84
self-image 108
self-judgement 169, 242
self-kindness 167, 169
self-knowledge 158, 169, 212
self-leadership 214
selflessness 246, 304
self-management 59, 195, 202, 205, 245
self-perception 208
self-protection 138
self-regulation 182, 205, 245, 262
self-reliance 136
self-sabotage 14, 179
self-soothing 109, 240–1, 281
self-talk 166
self-value 286
sense of belonging 137, 181, 229, 259, 286
sense of coherence 137, 140, 178, 239
sense of humour 259; as coping strategy 173; maintaining 171; poor 64; and salutogenesis 69; and self-care 270
sense of purpose 69, 137, 140, 179, 234, 239, 262–3, 272
sensitivity 6; empathy and xvii, 8, 51, 303, 305; lack of 70; over- 111; to patients 51, 133, 201; and stress 58–9; to suffering 50, 276; *see also* cultural sensitivity
serenity prayer 175, 301
servant leadership 271, 287

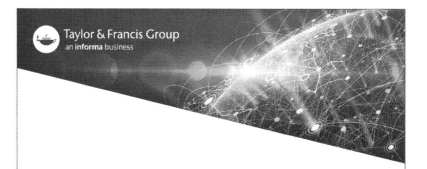

Printed in the United States
by Baker & Taylor Publisher Services